Textbook of
Pharmacognosy and Phytochemistry

Textbook of
Pharmacognosy and Phytochemistry

Sapna Malviya MPharm, PhD
Associate Professor and Head
Department of Pharmaceutical Sciences
Modern Institute of Pharmaceutical Sciences, Indore, MP

Swati Rawat MPharm, PhD
Professor
Department of Pharmaceutical Sciences, and
Principal, SND College of Pharmacy, Yeola, Nashik, Mh

Neelesh Malviya MPharm, PhD
Associate Professor
Department of Pharmacognosy
Smriti College of Pharmaceutical Education, Indore, MP

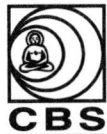

CBS Publishers & Distributors Pvt Ltd

New Delhi • Bengaluru • Chennai • Kochi • Kolkata • Mumbai
Bhopal • Bhubaneswar • Hyderabad • Jharkhand • Nagpur • Patna • Pune
Uttarakhand • Dhaka (Bangladesh)

Disclaimer

Science and technology are constantly changing fields. New research and experience broaden the scope of information and knowledge. The authors have tried their best in giving information available to them while preparing the material of this book. Although, all efforts have been made to ensure optimum accuracy of the material, yet it is quite possible some errors might have been left uncorrected. The publisher, printer and the authors will not be held responsible for any inadvertent errors or inaccuracies.

Textbook of
Pharmacognosy and Phytochemistry

ISBN: 978-81-239-2395-6

Copyright © Authors and Publisher

First Edition: 2015
Reprint: 2019, 2020

All rights reserved. No part of this book may be reproduced or transmitted in any form or by any means, electronic or mechanical, including photocopying, recording, or any information storage and retrieval system without permission, in writing, from the authors and the publisher.

Published by Satish Kumar Jain and produced by Varun Jain for
CBS Publishers & Distributors Pvt Ltd
4819/XI Prahlad Street, 24 Ansari Road, Daryaganj, New Delhi 110 002, India.
Ph: 23289259, 23266861, 23266867   Website: www.cbspd.com
Fax: 011-23243014   e-mail: delhi@cbspd.com; cbspubs@airtelmail.in.
Corporate Office: 204 FIE, Industrial Area, Patparganj, Delhi 110 092
Ph: 4934 4934   Fax: 4934 4935   e-mail: publishing@cbspd.com; publicity@cbspd.com

Branches

- **Bengaluru:** Seema House 2975, 17th Cross, K.R. Road, Banasankari 2nd Stage, Bengaluru 560 070, Karnataka
  Ph: +91-80-26771678/79   Fax: +91-80-26771680   e-mail: bangalore@cbspd.com
- **Chennai:** 7, Subbaraya Street, Shenoy Nagar, Chennai 600 030, Tamil Nadu
  Ph: +91-44-26680620, 26681266   Fax: +91-44-42032115   e-mail: chennai@cbspd.com
- **Kochi:** 42/1325, 1326, Power House Road, Opposite KSEB Power House, Ernakulam 682 018, Kochi, Kerala
  Ph: +91-484-4059061-65   Fax: +91-484-4059065   e-mail: kochi@cbspd.com
- **Kolkata:** 6/B, Ground Floor, Rameswar Shaw Road, Kolkata-700 014, West Bengal
  Ph: +91-33-22891126, 22891127, 22891128   e-mail: kolkata@cbspd.com
- **Mumbai:** 83-C, Dr E Moses Road, Worli, Mumbai-400018, Maharashtra
  Ph: +91-22-24902340/41   Fax: +91-22-24902342   e-mail: mumbai@cbspd.com

Representatives

• Bhopal	0-8319310552	• Bhubaneswar	0-9911037372	• Hyderabad	0-9885175004	• Jharkhand	0-9811541605
• Nagpur	0-9421945513	• Patna	0-9334159340	• Pune	0-9623451994	• Uttarakhand	0-9716462459
• Dhaka (Bangladesh)	01912-003485						

Printed at Mudrak, Noida, UP, India

Preface

It is indeed our pleasure to present to you this book *Textbook of Pharmacognosy and Phytochemistry*. Pharmacognosy has steadily metamorphosed into a dynamic, wide planked and multidimensional study, embracing in its fold biology, chemistry, biochemistry, pharmacology and other collateral disciplines. Pharmacognosy embraces a number of scientific and other disciplines providing a unified and comprehensive treatment of medicinal plants.

The aim of this book is to acquaint pharmacy students with primary and updated knowledge of pharmacognosy, to take them through the maze of medicinal plant features and help them learn pharmacognosy as efficiently as possible.

The theme of the book is to introduce medicinal plant biotechnology, medicinal and aromatic plant substances, phytopharmaceuticals and marker constituents, drugs from marine sources, drugs from mineral origin, enzymes and protein substances, aromatherapy, flavoring agents, sweeteners and bitter plant substances, plant anatomy, cosmeceuticals, poisonous teratogenic and hallucinogenic plants, Ayurvedic pharmacy and standardization of Ayurvedic formulations, biomedicinal value of important herbs, plant tissue culture, studies of different families and chromatography profiling of important herbs.

We convey our deep sense of gratitude to all those who have assisted us throughout by providing contributions to the text, carrying out literature searches and helping us with the organization of the manuscript, as without their dedicated help, this edition would not have been possible. We are immensely thankful to Shweta Gandhi, Swati Yadav, Anamika Singh, Rizwana Khan and Neha Agarwal for their decisive and energetic support during the write-up stage.

We thank CBS Publishers & Distributors, New Delhi, for their usual helpful assistance and understanding; and Prof. Anil Kharia, Principal, Modern Institute of Pharmaceutical Sciences, Indore, for his constant encouragement. There is a final debt that we can never repay which we owe to God for the strength and guidance bestowed upon us right from the beginning.

We shall gratefully accept the criticism and welcome remarkable suggestions from the readers, faculty and the students to improve the quality of book in its future editions.

Sapna Malviya
Swati Rawat
Neelesh Malviya

Contents

Preface   v

1. **Introduction**   1–26
   History and Scope of Pharmacognosy 1
   Indian and Alternative System of Medicine 6
   Sources of Crude Drugs 15
   Drug Discovery from Natural Substances 19

2. **Medicinal Plant Biotechnology**   27–60
   Biosynthetic pathway of phytoconstituents 27
   Radioactive Tracer Technique 53

3. **Medicinal and Aromatic Plant Substances**   61–78
   Cultivation of Medicinal Plants 61
   Fastors Affecting Cultivation 62
   Methods of Pest Control 68
   Endogenous Factors 69
   Requirement of Packaging Materials 76

4. **Phytopharmaceuticals and Marker Constituents**   79–90
   Characteristics of Good Marker 79
   Phytopharmaceuticals with their Marker Constituent 80

5. **Drugs Derived from Natural Sources**   91–205
   5.1 Carbohydrates 91
   5.2 Glycosides 104
   5.3 Terpenoids, Volatile Oils and Resins 135
   5.4 Alkaloids 158
   5.5 Tannins 185
   5.6 Lipids, Fats and Waxes 193

6. **Drugs from Marine Sources**   206–212
   Marine Drugs 206
   Marine Toxins 210
   Algal Toxin 210

7. **Drugs from Mineral Origin**   213–217
   Shilajit 213
   Asbestos 214
   Kaolin 215
   Bentonite 215
   Kieselguhr 216

8. **Enzymes and Protein Substances**   218–224
   Enzymes 218
   Protein 222

9. Aromatherapy 225–232
- Eucalyptus 229
- Geranium 229
- Jasmine 230
- Rose 230
- Sandalwood 231
- Peppermint 232

10. Flavoring Agents, Sweeteners and Bitter Plant Substances 233–242
- Flavouring Agents 233
- Sweetning Agents 239
- Plant Bitters 240

11. Plant Anatomy 243–259
- Tissus and Tissue Systems 243
- Anatomy of Monocot and Dicot Stems 253
- Anatomy of Dicot and Monocot Leaves 255
- Anatomy of Monocot and Dicot Roots 257

12. Cosmeceuticals 260–268
- Structure of the Skin 261
- Origin of Botanical Extracts 264
- Characterization of Casmetic Care Products 264

13. Poisonous Teratogenic and Hallucinogenic Plants 269–278
- Poisonous Plants 269

14. Ayurvedic Pharmacy and Standardization of Ayurvedic Formulation 279–288
- History of Ayurveda 279
- Quality Control and Standards 283

15. Plant Tissue Culture 289–305
- History of Plant Tissue Culture 289
- Equipment and Apparatus 291
- Sterilization of Glasswares and Equipment 293
- Types of Plant Tissue Culture 298
- Applications of PTC (Plant Tissue Culture) 305

16. Study of Different Families 306–313
- Floral Formula and Floral Diagram 306
- Families with their Description 306

17. Quality Control and Standardization of Herbal Drugs and Formulation 314–327
- Plant Identification 314
- Parameters for Quality Control of Herbal Drugs 321

18. Morphological, Microscopic and Analytical Profile of Important Herbs 328–343

19. Chromatography 344–353
- Types of Chromatography with their Description 345

20. Herbal Drug Interactions 354–357

21. Phytonutrients: The Natural Drugs of Future 358–364
- Nutraceuticals 358

Bibliography 365
Index 369

Introduction

HISTORY AND SCOPE OF PHARMACOGNOSY

Definition

Pharmacognosy is the study of medicines derived from natural sources. The *American Society of Pharmacognosy* defines pharmacognosy as "the study of the physical, chemical, biochemical and biological properties of drugs, drug substances or potential drugs or drug substances of natural origin as well as the search for new drugs from natural sources. The term pharmacognosy was introduced by Seydler in 1815, has been derived from the two Greek words: i) *pharmakon*, which means a **drug** and ii) *gnosis*, which means **to acquire knowledge of.** It deals with:

1. Properties, sources, identification and nature of raw materials.
2. Study of medicinal plants and their crude products known as herbal drugs.
3. History, cultivation, collection, distribution, preparation, commerce of herbal clings used in treatment of various disorders including allergens, immunizing products, flavoring agents, insecticides, rodenticides, and herbicides.

Historical Development (Table 1.1)

Pharmacognosy is regarded as the mother of all sciences due to its origin in the health-related activities of the human race. The primitive man sought to alleviate his sufferings of illness and injuries by using plants and crude drugs. After sometimes, communities emerged who acquired expertise in cultivation, collection, selection, testing and using medicinal plants for treating diseases. Later these people became to be known as 'Medicine Men', who monopolized the knowledge of drugs and hide that knowledge in some mysterious incantations. They transferred this secret knowledge only to their trusted predecessors of the successive generations. Initially, the transfer of the acquired knowledge from generation to generation used to be done verbally by the use of signs and symbols. As civilization progressed, transfer and recording of the knowledge were done in writing.

The apothecary (pharmacist-physician), used to do all the works of collection, processing, preparation and dispensing of the medicaments (the works of the pharmacist) and also diagnosing the disease and prescribing the drug (the works of the physician). Thus, at this point, pharmacy and medicine started developing along two separate paths:

a. One group specialized in diagnosing the disease and prescribing the drug and became known as the physicians or doctors.
b. The other group specialized in collecting, processing, preparing and dispensing the drug and became known as the apothecaries or pharmacists.

In this way, pharmacognosy progressed gradually and formed the basis and beginning of both pharmacy and medicine.

Table 1.1: Historical development of pharmacognosy

Contributors	Milestone
Sumerian clay slab	The ancient evidence (approximately 5000 years old) of natural plants for medical *preparation* has been found on a Sumerian clay slab in Nagpur. It comprised 12 recipes for preparation referring to over 250 plants and some alkaloids, such as poppy and henbane.
Shen Nung (2838–2698 BC)	The emperor taught China to cultivate hemp as a fiber and later on for food and oil and wrote Chinese book on roots and grasses "Pen Ts'ao which consists of dried parts 365 drugs, such as the great yellow gentian, ginseng, jimson weed, cinnamon bark, and ephedra.
Babylonians (about 3000 BC)	Illustrated medical treatment of plants with their properties.
Pen Ts'ao Kang Mu (3000–2730 BC)	He has written Chinese Pharmacopoeia including recipes and therapeutic uses of many Chinese traditional medicines.
Egyptian contributors (1550 BC)	*Ebers Papurus* is the most important medical papyri of ancient Egypt known as **Papyrus Ebers** which is collection of 800 prescriptions referring to 700 plant species. It provides good knowledge of human anatomy and medicinal uses of hundreds of plants which made them capable of embalming dead bodies for making mummies, e.g. henbane, mandrake, opium, pomegranate, caster oil, aloe, onion, fig, willow and coriander.
Charaka (300 BC)	Charaka wrote famous Ayurvedic treatise *Charaka Samhita*. It includes a rational approach to the causation and cure of disease with introduction of objective methods of clinical examination.
Sushruta (600 BC)	*Sushruta Samhita* contains 184 chapters and description of 1120 illnesses, 700 medicinal plants, a detailed study on anatomy, 64 preparations from mineral sources and 57 preparations based on animal sources.
Hippocrates (460–377 BC)	He is regarded as the **Father of medicine** for his contribution to human anatomy, physiology and development of medicinal plants. He classified medicinal plants on the basis of physiological action. His literature consists of 300 medicinal plants, like garlic against intestine parasites, opium, henbane, and deadly nightshade were used as narcotics, oak and pomegranate as astringents.
Aristotle (384–322 BC)	He described medicinal importance of about 500 plants with their description and uses.
Theophrastus (371–287 BC)	He is known as **father of botany,** founded botanical science with his books "*De Causis Plantarium*"—Plant Etiology and "*De Historia Plantarium*"—Plant History. He classified more than 500 medicinal plants, like cinnamon, mint, pomegranate and cardamom.
Aulus Cornelius Celsus (25 BC–50 AD)	In his work "*De medicina*", he quoted approximately 250 medicinal plants, such as aloe, henbane, flax, poppy, pepper, cinnamon, cardamom.

(Contd.)

Table 1.1: Historical development of pharmacognosy (*Contd.*)

Contributors	Milestone
Dioscorides (1st Century AD)	The Greek physician also known as **"The father of Pharmacognosy,"** published five volumes of a book, entitled '*De Materia Madica*' in 78 AD, which offers plenty of data on collection, storage and uses of 944 drugs, 600 are of plant origin, with descriptions of the outward appearance, locality, mode of collection, making of the medicinal preparations, and their therapeutic effect.
Pliny the Elder (23–79 AD)	He wrote about approximately 1000 medicinal plants in his book "Historia naturalis".
Galen (130–200 AD)	The most distinguished Greek pharmacist cum physician, described methods of preparing pharmaceutical formulations containing plant and animal drugs. He compiled the first list of drugs with similar or identical action (parallel drugs), which are interchangeable and introduced several new plant drugs in therapy that Dioscorides had not described, for instance, *Uvae ursi folium*, used as an uroantiseptic and a mild diuretic.
Charles the Great (742–814 AD)	He quoted 100 plants such as sage, sea onion, iris, mint, common centaury, poppy, marsh mallow.
Paracelsus (1493–1541)	He was a Swiss physician and firm believer of astrologically, supported *Signatura doctrinae* that is continuously emphasizing belief in observations. According to this belief, God designated his own sign on the healing substances, which indicated their application for certain diseases. For example, *Hypericum perforatum* L. would be beneficial for treatment of wounds and stings as plant leaves appears as if they had been stung. On the basis of his idea that the body was a chemical system which had to be balanced not only internally, but which also had to be in harmony with its environment, he introduced new chemical substances into medicine, like use of the metal mercury for the treatment of syphilis.
Linnaeus (1707–1788)	He was a Swedish botanist considered as **father of modern botany**. He was first naturalist to classify plants and intiated two Latin names the identifying genus, with an initial capital letter, and species to classify all plants with an initial small letter. For the naming, a polynomial system was employed where the first word denoted the genus while the remaining polynomial phrase explained other features of the plant, e.g. the willow clusius was named *Salix pumila angustifolia antera*.
Wilhelm Adam Sertürner (1783–1841)	The German pharmacist isolated alkaloids with many potent physiologically active compounds including quinine, atropine, cocaine, and tubocurarine.
Schleiden (1804–1881)	He not only contributed to the knowledge of the structure of plants, but was the first to recognize that drugs of different origin might be determined by their cellular differences.
ARBs	They introduced numerous new plants in pharmacotherapy, like aloe, deadly nightshade, henbane, coffee, ginger, strychnos, saffron, curcuma, pepper and cinnamon.

Scope

The object of pharmacognosy is the study of drugs and the plants yielding them. The main object is not only to determine the identity of the drug and its origin, but the study of its constituents and the factors influencing their

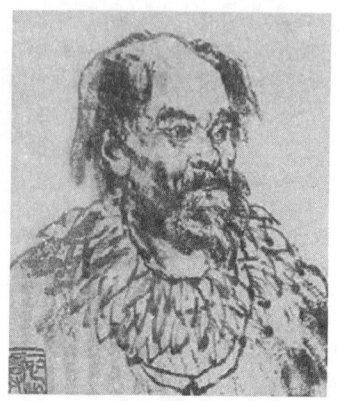
Shen Nung (2838–2698 BC)

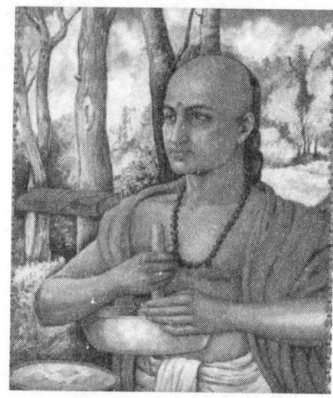
Saint Charaka (300 BC)

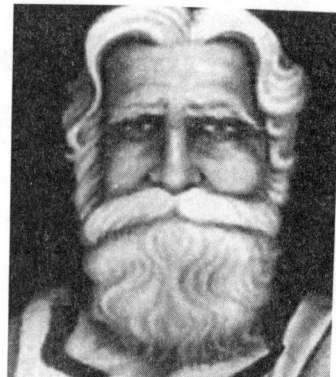
Saint Sushruta (600 BC)

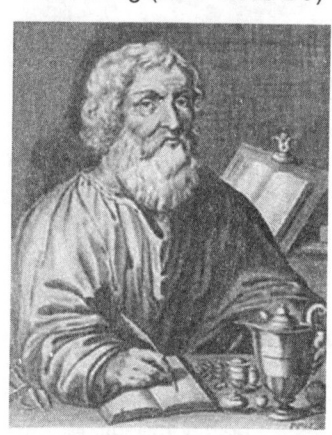
Hippocrates (460–377 BC)

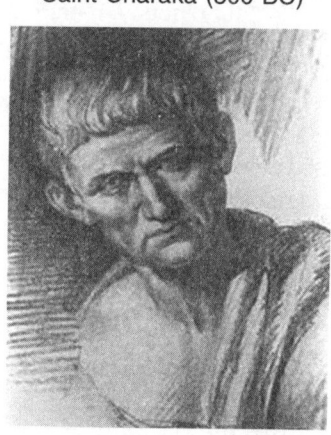
Aristotle (384–322 BC)

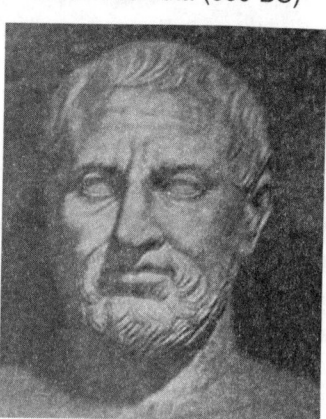
Theophrastus (371–287 BC)

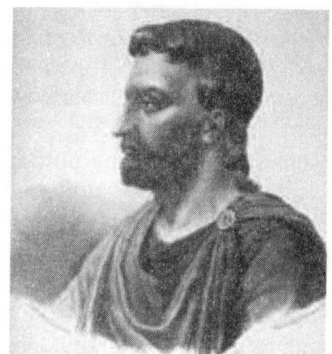
Aulus Cornelius Celsus (25 BC–50 AD)

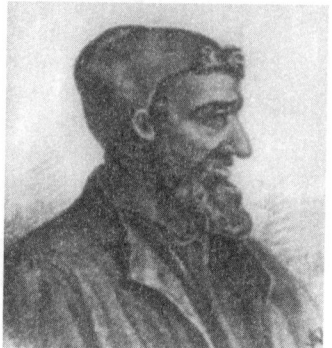
Galen (130–200 AD)

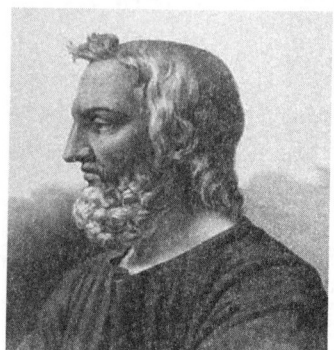
Pedanius Dioscorides (40–90 AD)

variation in the living plant as well as after collection.

Pharmacognosy gives a sound knowledge of the vegetable drugs under botany and animal drugs under zoology. It also includes plant taxonomy, plant breeding, plant pathology, and plant genetics and by this knowledge one can improve the cultivation methods for both medicinal and aromatic plants. Phytochemistry (plant chemistry) has significant improvement which includes a variety of substances that are accumulated by plants and synthesized by plants. Methods of collection, curing, drying, and assaying affect the price of drugs and, as far as economics is concerned, pharmacognosy is intimately associated with phases of pharmacy administration dealing with prescription pricing. The relationship of pharmacognosy between operative pharmacy and dispensing pharmacy is obvious when one considers the number of plant and animal products handled by the pharmacist in todays time. Because of his knowledge of drug constituents and their physical and chemical properties, the pharmacist is able to predict incompatibilities in actual compounding. In dispensing non-compounded prescription specialties, he is conversant with a vast store of information permitting him to confer intelligently with his fellow colleagues in the medical, dental, and nursing professions. In the pursuit of pharmacognosy, we examine drugs which for the most part consist of broken fragments, and from these pieces, frequently microscopic in size, the plants from which they are derived must be determined. Again, particles which resemble each other or are obtained from very closely related species must be separated. Parts of other plants growing with them in the soil must be distinguished and standards established showing how much of this extraneous material is permissible, and these standards must be so framed that drugs collected at widely separated points will be of uniform quality and efficiency. The ultimate aim of the science of pharmacognosy is to obtain knowledge of the chemical nature and the properties of all commercial products, from their origin in nature to the final changes produced by the manufacturer. The pharmacognosy is the vital link between:

- **A vital contribution to the advancement of natural and physical science:** Advanced technologies of cultivation, purification, identification (characterization) of pharmaceuticals from nature help in the improvement of collection, processing, and storage of pharmaceuticals. Pharmacognosy also gives knowledge of chemotaxonomy, and biogenic pathways for the formation of acute ingredients.

- **A vital link between pharmacology and medicinal chemistry:** Pharmacognosy is an important link between pharmaceuticals and basic science, as well as ayurvedic and allopathic systems of medicine. So pharmacognosy is a science of active principles of crude drugs and which can help in dispensing, formulating, and manufacturing of dosage forms. In other words, the complete knowledge of pharmacognosy will help in the recent trend that is in industries.

Problems of Pharmacognosy

- The problems of pharmacognosy take us at once into the field where the origin of the drugs can be studied at first hand. A second phase of the subject is the study of pure morphology dealing with the development of certain structures as the stipes in cubeb, or the origin of tissues in seeds, and scars or markings in roots and rhizomes. The difference in constituents of different parts of the same plant, as the oils in the leaves and bark of cinnamon or difference in the

proportion of alkaloids in the different kinds of cinchona, offers a most fertile opportunity for the application of physiological studies.
- Furthermore, when we approach the subject of the cultivation of medicinal plants we are confronted with the problems of hybridization and mutation. In the historical study of drugs, such phases are considered as the origin of their introduction into medicine, the dissemination of information concerning their uses among other nations, the official recognition by some, of the more important pharmacopoeias, and finally the facts regarding their real usefulness as supplied by modern pharmacological investigations and clinical experience. The study of synonyms is one of the most important departments of pharmacognosy. While there have been some attempts to treat the synonyms of drug names and their derivation, nothing has been written which is adequate to the needs of this subject.
- It is one of the most difficult phases of pharmacognosy, and requires that researchers be acquainted not only with the principles of scientific nomenclature, but that he shall be familiar with the several languages and the historical development of pharmacognosy. Finally, there is a phase of pharmacognostical work, which is the division that relates to the study of drugs from the time they are shipped by the collector until they reach the retail pharmacist or even the consumer.
- This subject cannot be ignored because it involves the study of the packing of drugs, the conditions of storage, and the changes in the quality of drugs in passing from hand to hand. While few drugs remain more or less unaltered, or may be improved on storing for a limited time, a large number of the valuable drugs require that they be kept under special conditions, for a very limited period of time.
- As indicating the importance of the subject, various pharmacopoeias are giving explicit directions regarding the manner in which certain drugs shall be kept and how long will be the retention of their active constituents. This study requires an intimate acquaintance of the pharmacognosist with the collector, the appraiser's stores, the wholesale warehouse, and the retail drug store. It should also be stated that in practice we have a scientific and a practical pharmacognosy.

INDIAN AND ALTERNATIVE SYSTEM OF MEDICINE

Systems of Medicine: Conventional, Alternative and Traditional

Traditional medicine (TM) is the sum total of knowledge, skills and practices based on the theories, beliefs and experiences indigenous to different cultures that are used to maintain health, as well as to prevent, diagnose, improve or treat physical and mental illnesses. Traditional medicine covers a wide variety of therapies and practices that has been adopted by other populations which vary from country to country and region to region and is often termed as "alternative or complementary medicine". This system is appropriate for people of the culture in which they originate, and can be applied as complementary and alternative mean for treating illness not responding to conventional therapies. It includes mind/body interventions, biologically based interventions, body-based manipulation therapies and energy/metaphysical therapies.

According to WHO, traditional medicine has been used for thousands of years. As these practices are adopted by new populations, they faced challenge, such as:
- International diversity
- National policy and regulation

- Safety, effectiveness and quality
- Knowledge and sustainability
- Patient safety and use

The Indian medical tradition prevails at two levels: (1) the classical system, which includes Ayurveda, Siddha, and Unani traditions and is characterized by institutionally trained doctors and also well-developed theories to support its practices; and (2) the folk system, termed *Lok Parampara*, which an oral tradition is passed on from father to son or mother to daughter. The folk tradition is rich, vibrant, and diverse and includes:

- Knowledge and belief regarding foods—*Pathyam* and *Apathyam* (i.e. foods to be preferred or avoided)
- Knowledge of diagnostic procedures and preventive measures
- Knowledge of *Rutucharya* or adaptation of food and regimen to suit the seasons
- Yoga and physical practices for disease prevention.

Traditional Chinese Medicine

Traditional Chinese medicine (TCM), originated in ancient China, is the quintessence of the Chinese culture heritage, and has a long history of 5000 years. TCM is a comprehensive, holistic oriental healing art that includes acupuncture, herbal medicine, massage, diet and exercise therapy. The principles of TCM are centered on the theory of harmony between two opposite forces, Yin and Yang, which is the crux of health, whereas disease results from disharmony between these forces. TCM is to view how human body works, what causes illness, and how to treat illness that attempts to bring the body, mind and spirit into harmony. The underlying concept of TCM is that the human body is regarded as an organic whole, and there exists an organic connection between all tissues and structures, and other parts have distinct functions but are all interdependent. In this view, health and disease relate to balance of the functions.

The Theoretical Framework of TCM (Fig. 1.1)

1. **Eight principles:** The chief principles which are used to analyze symptoms and categorize conditions include cold/heat, interior/exterior, excess/deficiency and Yin/Yang.

2. **Five elements:** The five elements include fire, earth, metal, water, and wood which explain how the body works; these elements correspond to particular organs and tissues in the body. Fire is essential in sparking and maintaining physiological processes, whereas water is nourishing, moistening and cooling. For health to be maintained, a balance is needed between water and fire, that is, between Yin and Yang.

3. **Yin–yang theory:** Health is maintained by achieving and then maintaining the balance between these opposing forces. Imbalance results from a blockage of vital energy that flows throughout the body and causes disease. Each individual phenomenon possesses both a yin and a yang aspect. Yin and yang are natural complements in the sense that they depend upon and counterbalance each other. There is fine balance between the two opposing but interrelated and inseparable forces of nature.

The following principles may be observed in the application of the theory of yin and yang to medicine:

- Yin and yang are divisible
- Yin and yang are interdependent
- Yin and yang counterbalance each other
- Mutual convertibility of yin and yang

Table 1.2 shows comparison of yin and yang.

Table 1.2: Comparison of yin and yang

Yin	Yang
Earth	Sky
Night	Day
Winter	Summer
Cold	Heat
Dark	Light
Dorsal	Ventral
Interiority	Exteriority
Decrease	Increase
Woman	Man

Treatment of TCM

TCM emphasizes individualized treatment. The traditionally used four methods to evaluate condition: (i) observing (especially the tongue), (ii) hearing/smelling, (iii) asking/interviewing, and (iv) touching/palpating (especially the pulse). The most commonly used are Chinese herbal medicine and acupuncture by stimulating specific points on the body, most often by inserting thin metal needles through the skin, practitioners seek to remove blockages in the flow of qi.

Ayurveda

Ayurveda, the traditional system of medicine which is one of the world's oldest medical systems has been practiced for well over 6000 years. The word Ayurveda is derived from two words in Sanskrit *Ayus*, meaning "life" from birth to death, and *veda*, meaning "knowledge" or science. Ayurveda indicates the science by which life in its totality is understood. It is a way of life that describes the diet, medicine and behavior that are beneficial or harmful for life. The World Health Organization (WHO) estimated that about 80% of the population in developing countries rely almost exclusively on traditional

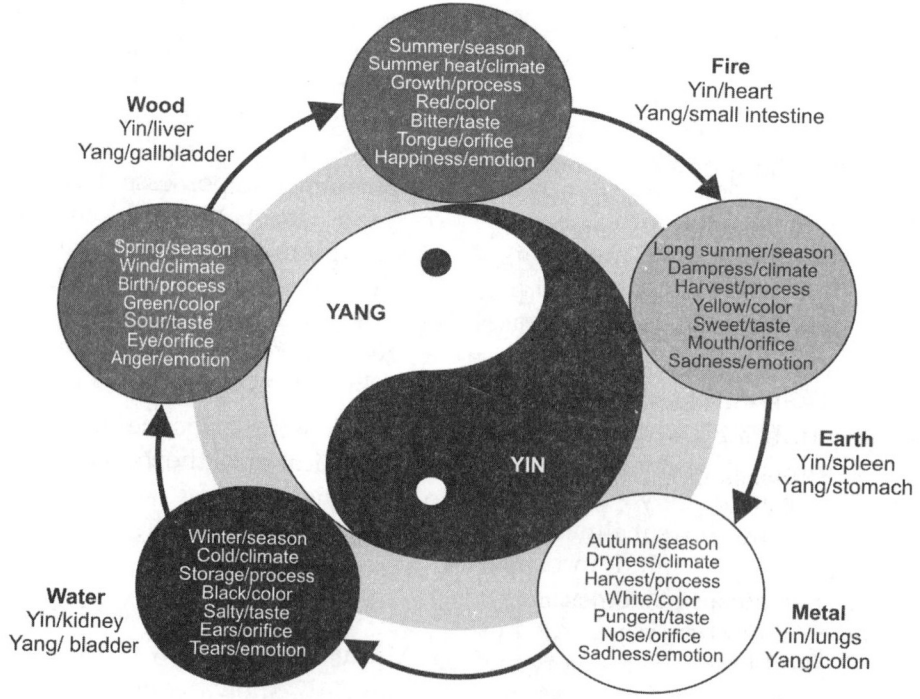

Fig. 1.1: Theoretical concepts of TCM

Table 1.3: Contribution in field of Ayurveda

Charaka	Sushruta	Ashtanga Hridaya
Charaka Samhita, prime work on the basic concepts of Ayurveda, is the oldest of the three and was probably first compiled around 1500 BC. It is a systematic work divided into eight Sthanas or sections, which are further divided into 120 chapters.	Sushruta explains about sophisticated descriptions of diseases and surgical instruments. It represents Dhanwantri School of surgeons.	The important authority in Ayurveda flourished about the seventh century AD is Vagbhatta of Sindh, His treatise called Ashtanga Hridaya. It is a combination of surgery and medicine.

medicine for their primary health care needs. Ayurveda covers most of the community care in India. It is preventive as well as a curative system of medicine.

The material scattered in the Vedas was collected, subjected to rigid tests of efficacy and systematically arranged in books written in the post-vedic period, such compilations of knowledge were called Samhitas. Three authentic works of Ayurveda are Charaka Samhita, Sushruta Samhita and Ashtanga Hridaya Samhita, great trio called the Brihatrayi has enjoyed much popularity and respect for the last two thousand years (Table 1.3).

The Ayurveda, mother of all healing, represents a model of health and disease and to integrate and balance the body, mind, and spirit. This is believed to help people to live their lives in harmony with nature, nature here being both without, and within, one's relationship with the outside world as well as with one's own body. It examines the individual's relationship with food and herbs, the weather and the seasons, fellow human beings and, ultimately, with itself (Table 1.4).

Ayurvedic medicine has several key foundations that pertain to health and disease. The approach to health care is based on their applications (Fig. 1.2). Panchamahabhutas, represents five fundamental categories of matter. State of balance of Dosha represents health while imbalance to the disease. Tridoshas, like *Vata* **is dry, cold, light, mobile, clear, rough, subtle;** *Pitta* **is slightly oily, hot, intense, light, fluid, free flowing, foul smelling and** *Kapha* **is oily, cold, heavy, stable, viscid, smooth, soft.** Dosha and Dhatus have relation with each other in health and disease. Sustenance of Mala in appropriate limits, sustain the life. Agni is considered as biological fire. It performs digestion of food, tissue metabolism and molecular metabolism.

Siddha System of Medicine

The word *Siddha* comes from the word *Siddhi*, meaning an object to be attained or perfection of heavenly bliss that is achievement. The Siddha system of medicine is based on remedies derived from the vegetable kingdom.

Principle: The fundamental principle on which Siddha is guided is that "nature is man" and "man is nature" and thus both are essentially one. According to Siddha system, the human body, food and the drugs are the replica of the universe, irrespective of their origin. Moreover, they believe that the

Table 1.4: Eight limbs of Ashtanga Ayurveda

Kaya chikitsa	Medical therapeutics
Shalakya Tantra	Diseases of eye, ear, nose and throat
Shalya Tantra	Surgery
Surgery	
Kaumarabhritya	Pediatrics, obstetrics and gynecology
Agada Tantra	Toxicology
Bhutavidya	Psychology and psychiatry
Rasayana	Rejuvenation

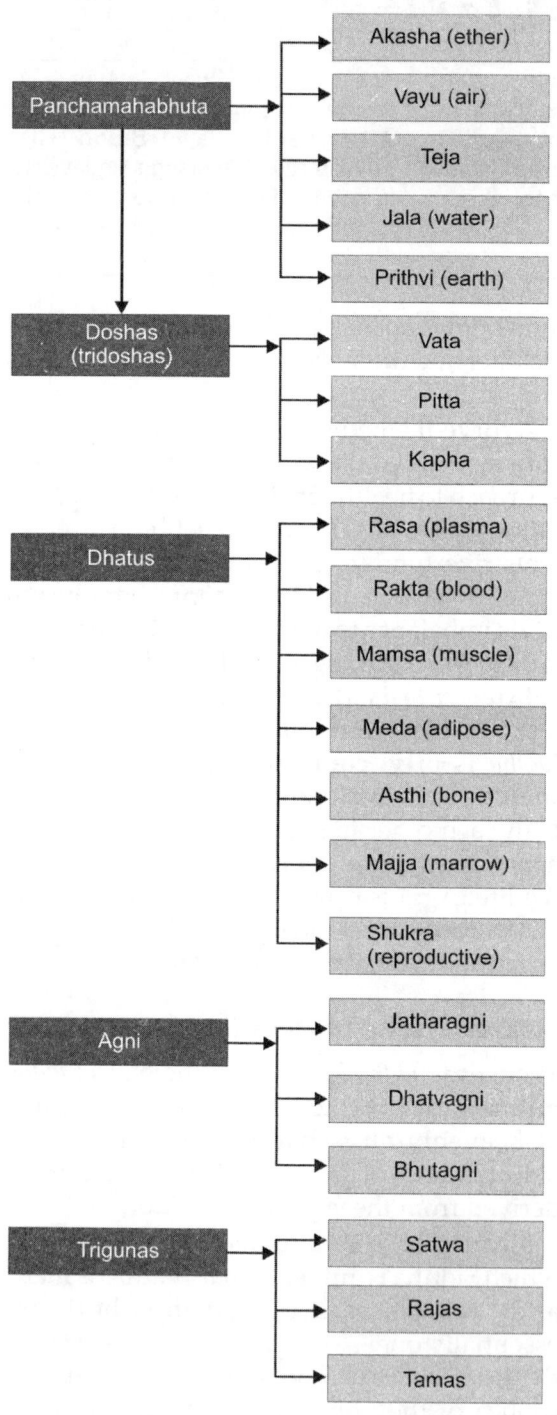

Fig. 1.2: Approach of Ayurveda

universe holds two main entities, namely matter and energy—Siva (male) and Shakti (female). The two are inseparable and co-exist as matter cannot subsist without the energy in it and vice versa.

They are also the primordial elements, Bhutas known as *Munn* (solid), *Neer* (fluid), *Thee* (radiance), *Vayu* (gas), and *Akasam* (ether).

Eight methods of diagnosis in Siddha system of medicine are:

1. Pulse diagnosis.
2. Examination of the tongue
3. Examination of the complexion
4. Examination of the speech
5. Examination of the eyes
6. Examination of the palpitation
7. Examination of the urine
8. Examination of the stool

All the traditional forms whether Ayurveda, Siddha, or Unani advocate that without these three humors, the individual cannot be normal and any imbalance that occurs in these three factors results in disease or death. If all three factors work properly and without any change, the body will be healthy and disease free. Imbalance due to astral or cosmic influence, poison or poisonous substances, or psychological or other factors causes these three factors and disease.

Unani System of Medicine

Unani system of medicine recognizes the influence of surroundings and ecological conditions on the state of health of human beings. It was compiled centuries back by Hippocrates, the great scholar. A balanced relationship between the six essential factors keeps the humors and the temperament on the right track. The non-essential factors, like habit, habitat, cosmic and terrestrial influences, social factors, profession, etc. influence only those who come across them. Unani system aims at restoring the equilibrium of various elements and faculties of the human body.

Principles and Philosophies

The proper functioning of human body depends on six factors as given in Table 1.5.

Table 1.5: Factors of Unani system of medicine

Umoor-e tabaiya viz. arkan/anasir	Elements
Mizaj	Temperament
Akhlat	Humors
Aaza	Organs
Arwah	Vital forces
Quwa	Faculties
Afaal	Functions

The humoral theory presupposes the presence of four humors, viz **Dam** (blood), **Balgham** (phlegm), **Safra** (yellow bile) and **Sauda** (black bile) in the body (Fig. 1.3). The temperaments of persons are expressed as sanguine, phlegmatic, choleric and melancholic according to the preponderance of humors—blood, phlegm, yellow bile and black bile, respectively. The humors themselves are assigned temperaments: blood is hot and moist, phlegm cold and moist, yellow bile hot and dry and black bile cold and dry.

The six factors of health help in determining the state of a person. The primary six factors are examined in relation with health and disease. They are:
- The air of one's environment
- Food and beverages
- Movement and rest
- Sleep and wakefulness
- Eating and evacuation
- Emotion

Diagnosis

Unani systems of medicine take into account the complete personality of the person during diagnosis. This is because every individual possesses specific basic structure, psychic

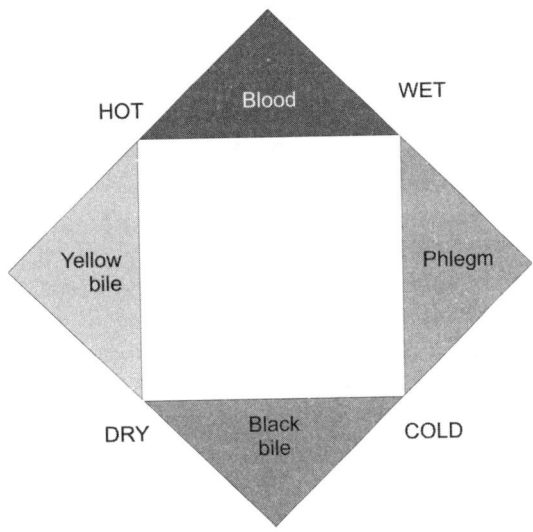

Fig. 1.3: Four humors in Unani system of medicine

makeup, self-defense mechanism, reactions to environmental factors, likes and dislikes. Thus, Unani healing mechanism is customized for each patient individually. Basically, the Unani diagnostic involves examination of the pulse, urine and stool.

Homeopathy (Table 1.6)

The term Homeopathy was coined by Hanhemann in 1807, which is derived from the Greek word *"homeo"*, meaning like or similar and *"pathos"*, meaning disease or suffering. It is a natural system of healing which employs extremely small doses of wholesome organs, tissues, metabolic factors, recombinant materials, plants, animals and minerals to stimulate the body's immune system. Thus, it is an established system of medicine based on the principle of treating like with like. Homeopathy presents contemporary wisdom as it uses medicine solutions that are diluted to a point beyond that which is measurable by normal scientific means.

Diagnosis

Homeopathy involves a careful observation of the patient and the symptoms of the disease exhibited by him. This includes detailed examination of patient's history including all the aspects of his life, such as physical, mental and emotional. It also includes various incidents in his life, which might have led to the problem. This information is then translated into a complex blueprint of mental and physical symptoms, comprising of the likes, dislikes, innate predispositions and even the body type of the person.

Naprapathy

Naprapathy is a branch of alternative medicine, a manipulative therapy that focuses on the evaluation and treatment of neuromusculoskeletal conditions. Naprapathy emphasizes health restoration and maintenance as well as disease prevention, also referred to as naprapathy and considered a universal healing system. Naprapathy was developed in the late 1800s by Dr. Oakley Smith.

There are six fundamental principles of naprapathy, which will appear similar to other systems of health care:

1. The healing power of nature
2. Identification and treatment of the cause of the disease
3. First do no harm
4. The doctor as teacher

Table 1.6: The principles of homeopathy

Principles	Description
Law of simila	It is based on the principle Like Cures Like. The substances that produce the same symptoms of a disease can be used to cure that disease.
Law of simplex	A *complex* remedy is made from a number of substances combined in a single dose. The sequential matching of substance to symptoms that is made possible with a simplex remedy enables a truly safe and maximally therapeutic effect.
Law of minimum	The smallest quantities of dose produce the least possible excitation of the vital force and yet sufficient to affect the necessary change in it. The minimum dose action is thus, appropriate as a gentle remedial effect and has led to the discovery of a more practical process called potentization.
Doctrine of drug proving	Drug proving is a systematic investigation of pathogenic (disease-producing) power of medicine on healthy human being of different ages, both sexes and of various constitutions.
Theory of chronic disease	The chronic diseases are caused by chronic miasms. The miasms are psora, syphilis and sycosis. Psora is the real fundamental cause and producer of innumerable forms of disease. It is the mother of all diseases and at least 7/8th of all the chronic maladies spring from it while the remaining eighth spring from syphilis and sycosis. Cure is only possible by proper anti-miasmatic treatment.
Theory of vital force	The material organism without the vital force is capable of no sensation, no function, no self-preservation; it derives all sensations, and performs all functions of life solely by means of the immaterial being (the vital force) which animates the material organism in health and disease.
Doctrine of drug dynamization	The principle of dilution in homeopathy is related with the process known as "dynamization" or "potentization", where a remedy is diluted in alcohol or water. It is then shaken vigorously against an elastic body, the process of which is known as succussion.

5. Treatment of the whole person
6. Prevention

Naturopathy

Naturopathy believes that all the diseases occur due to the accumulation of morbid matter into the body. When opportunity is given for its removal, it provides cure and relief. Also, it considers that the human body is self-sufficient as it possesses inherent self-constructing and self-healing powers. Naturopathic medicine is an eclectic practice of healthcare united by core underlying principles. Naturopathy is based on the recognition that the body possesses not only a natural ability to resist disease but inherent mechanisms of recovery and self-regulation'. The application of this concept gives rise to the use of natural methods to assist the healing process: the use of food, sunshine, water, rest and relaxation. It treats the disease with the help of stimulation, as well as increases and supports the person's inherent healing capacity. The therapies used in naturopathy are chosen in accordance with the natural healing process of the nature. All the naturopathic medicines include the six principles of healing.

- Do no harm (Primum No Nocere)
- Healing power of nature (Vis Mediatrix Naturae)
- Identify and treat the cause (Tolle Causam)
- Heal the whole person (Tolle Totum)
- Physician as teacher (Docere)
- Prevention is the best cure (Prevention)

Flower Essences

Bach Flowers/Australian Bush Flower Essences

These 38 remedies became the Bach Flower Remedies. Although each remedy addresses a specific emotional state: Fear, uncertainty, insufficient interest in present circumstances, loneliness, oversensitivity to influences and ideas, despondency and despair, and overcare for the welfare of others.

Probably the best known of the Bach Flower Essences, Rescue Remedy is made up of five individual remedies:

- Cherry plum—for the fear of losing control
- Clematis—to bring a person back into the present
- Rock rose—the emergency remedy when there is extreme fear or terror
- Star of Bethlehem—for great distress and shock
- Impatiens—for impatience and stress

Rescue Remedy is a good general remedy indicated for any emergency, shock or stress. An accident or injury, receiving bad news, nervousness and anxiety are all instances where Rescue Remedy can be used. It can be taken every few minutes, if necessary until the person feels calmer. Rescue Remedy is also incorporated into a cream, which is especially beneficial for children.

Aromatherapy

Aromatherapy is categorized as a form of complementary and alternative medicine (CAM). Aromatherapy has roots that can be traced back at least 5,000 years to ancient China, India, Persia, and Egypt. The word aromatherapy is used to describe the use of essential oils for aromatic inhalation, compresses, and topical application through massage. Aromatherapy is an intervention that uses essential oils which are the concentrated aromatic part of the plant extracted from plants inhaled through the nose to produce relaxation, pain reduction, and alleviation of conditions, such as bronchitis. Essential oils stimulate the nerves and the olfactory system. The oils are picked up by the nerve endings and passed on until they eventually reach the pituitary gland. This, in turn, affects the adrenals, thereby reducing stress.

Aromatherapy basics oils are extracted from flowers, twigs, leaves, bark, or from a fruit's rind of plants. For example, sandalwood oils are from the wood, rose oils from the flowers, and some basil oils from the leaves. The most common method is steam distillation. The other methods include hydrodiffusion, mechanical expression or pressing, enfleurage (using fixed oil or fats to absorb aromatic volatile oils), and solvent extraction.

Aromatherapy seems to produce some positive benefit as supportive treatment; however, evidence is limited at this time. Based on current literature, the following conclusions can be made as described in Table 1.7.

Yoga and Meditation

The word 'yoga' means union, joining or to link together as one whole. Yoga is the art and science of resolving the inherent opposition in all things to create a union of body, mind and soul. Meditation is an integral component, and the essence of yoga. The eight (*asta*) limbs (*angas*) of Astanga yoga are as described in Table 1.8.

Yoga, the sister science to Ayurveda, has a highly evolved and integrated system for connecting the mind and body. Various techniques for breathing (Pranayama) integrate the connections among autonomic body functions, which can be brought under conscious control. Asanas (the yogic postures) do not merely tone and strengthen muscles, but are aimed at strengthening and toning internal organs and their interrelated systems as well. Slow intense concentration introduces the feel of each muscle group as it moves, and awareness is stimulated.

Meditation is part of yoga and other healing disciplines, but it is also thought of as being a separate activity. Often, meditation and prayer are misclassified together. The difference is that meditation is personal and internal, whereas prayer is aimed at an external or internal

Table 1.8: Eight limbs of yoga

Yama	Our attitudes to our environment
Niyama	Our attitudes towards ourselves
Asana	Physical exercises
Pranayama	Breath control
Pratayahara	Meditative sense control
Dharana	Meditative concentration
Dhyana	Meditative contemplation
Samadhi	Meditative absorption

Table 1.7: Aromatherapy and its health benefits

Inhalation by lavender	Antispasmodic, antidepressant, anti-inflammatory
	Sedative
	Antiviral and antibacterial
Inhalation by rosemary	Enhance alertness and pain reliever
	Enhance memory and stimulates circulation
Inhalation by rose	Antibacterial, antidepressant, antiseptic, antispasmodic, astringent, diuretic, sedative
Massage by neroli	Relieve anxiety in cardiac surgery
Tea tree oil	Antifungal and antibacterial
Massage by chamomile	Anti-inflammatory, antiallergenic, relaxant and antidepressant
Inhalation by peppermint	Digestive, antiseptic, decongestant and stimulant
Inhalation by eucalyptus	Decongestant, antiviral, antibacterial and stimulant
Inhalation by geranium	Antiseptic, antifungal, anti-inflammatory and diuretic
Massage by bergamot	Antidepressant and anti-inflammatory

sense of God or spirituality. A good way of considering meditation is as "mind hygiene" keeping the paths and the channels of the mind open, and allowing the waste to be expelled. In Ayurveda, the mind is considered an organ of no greater importance than the bowels or bladder. The mind, however, processes mental and emotional energies in the forms of images and communications.

SOURCES OF CRUDE DRUGS

The term crude drug generally applies the harvested and usually dried plant or animal sources of pharmaceutically or medicinally useful products before they have undergone extensive processing or modification. However, the term is also applied to include pharmaceutical products from mineral kingdom in original form and not necessarily only of organic origin, such as kaolin, bentonite, etc. Crude drugs can thus be defined as to the natural products that have not been advanced in value or improved in condition by any process or treatment beyond that which is essential for their proper packing and prevention from deterioration. Crude drug is recognized in the official pharmacopoeia, intended for use in the diagnosis, cure, mitigation, treatment or prevention of disease in man or other animals and intended to affect the structure or any function of the body of man or other animals.

Classification of Crude Drugs (Table 1.10)

Drugs may be arranged in different ways to suit the aim and convenience of students. The particular sequence and arrangement to follow the study of the individual drugs is referred to a system of classification of drugs. A method of classification should be precise, simple, easy to use and free from ambiguities and unnecessary confusions. Crude drugs have wide distributions, so each classification has its advantages and disadvantages. Vegetable drugs are usually classified for study in one or other of the following ways (Fig. 1.4).

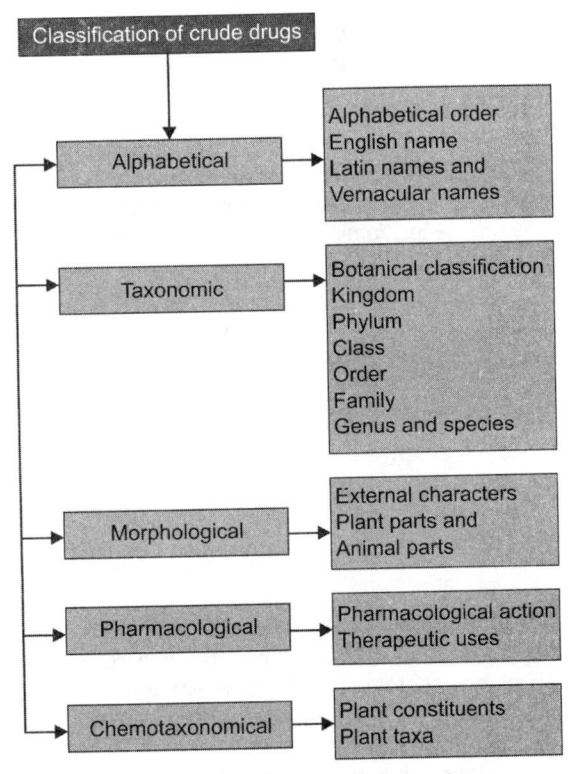

Fig. 1.4: Classification of crude drugs

S.no	Parts	Examples of crude drugs
	Table 1.9: Crude drugs with their examples	
1.	Entire plants or animals	Mentha viridis, Lobelia inflate, Cochineal
2.	Entire organs of plants or animals	Cassia acutifolia, Eugenia caryophyllata, Foeniculum vulgare, Linum usitatissimum, Glycyrrhiza glabra and thyroid gland
3.	Minerals	Chalk, kaolin and talc
4.	Substances derived from plants or animals (unorganized)	Papaver somniferum, Astragalus gummifer and musk

Table 1.10: Elaborate classification of crude drugs with their benefits and drawbacks

Classification of crude drug	Benefits and drawbacks
Alphabetical classification The simplest way of classification and crude drugs are arranged in alphabetical order of their Common names (English) and Latin names or vernacular names (local language names). This system of classification is accepted in pharmacopoeias like Indian pharmacopoeia, British pharmacopoeia, British Herbal pharmacopoeia and dictionaries and reference books.	**Benefits** Easy system location, tracing and addition of drug entries. No repetition of entries. Devoid of confusion. **Drawbacks** There is no relationship between previous and successive drug entries. **Examples:** *Curcuma zedoaria, Cassia acutifolia, Rauwolfia vomitoria, Styrax benzoin, Cinchona calisaya.*
Taxonomical classification Botanical classification and is based on principles of natural relationship and evolutionary developments. They are classified on basis of Kingdom, phylum, order, family genus and species.	**Benefits** Helpful in studying evolutionary changes. **Drawbacks** It cannot give detailed information about systematic pharmacognostic parameters like chemical constituents and biological activity. It's insufficient to correlate evolutionary and systematic pharmacognostic parameters. **Thallophyta** • Kingdom: Bacteria • Phylum: Actinobacteria • Class: Actinobacteria • Order: Bifidobacteriales • Family: Bifidobacteriaceae • Genus: *Bifidobacterium*
Morphological classification It is based on classification in which drugs are arranged according to the external characters of the plant parts or animal parts. The drugs are grouped as organized and unorganized. **Organized drugs** are obtained from the direct cellular tissues of plants and part, e.g. leaves, flower, woods, barks, rhizomes, entire plants etc. **Unorganized drugs** are those which don't contain any cellular plant tissues prepared from plants by physical processes such as incision, drying or extraction with a solvent, e.g. resins, volatile oil, fixed oils and fats, gums and waxes	**Benefits** Convenient for practical study It is more helpful to determine and observe adulteration of drugs. **Drawbacks** It does not explain about chemical constituents and therapeutic actions of drugs. **Examples:** Refer to Table 1.11 **Examples:** Refer to Table 1.12

(Contd.)

Table 1.10: Elaborate classification of crude drugs with their benefits and drawbacks (*Contd.*)

Classification of crude drug	Benefits and drawbacks
Pharmacological classification The pharmacological action or therapeutic use is termed as pharmacological or therapeutic classification of drug. Drugs like digitalis, squill and strophanthus having cardiotonic action are grouped together irrespective of their parts used or phylogenetic relationship or the nature of phytoconstituents they contain. Table 1.13 gives an outline of pharmacological classification of drugs.	**Benefits** It is more relevant and mostly followed method. For suggesting substitutes of drugs. Drugs with different pharmacological action on the body get classified separately in more than one group that causes confusion. **Examples:** Refer to Table 1.13
Chemical classification (Table 1.14) The crude drugs are divided according to the chemical nature of their most important constituent. It depends upon the grouping of drugs with identical constituents.	**Benefits** It is a popular approach for phytochemical studies. **Drawbacks** In cases of drugs possess a number of chemical constituents belonging to different groups of compounds, confusion can arises **Examples:** Refer to Table 1.14
Chemotaxonomy classification This classification attempts to review plant constituents according to plant taxa. It is based on the existence of relationship between constituents in various plants.	**Benefits** It is the latest classification and gives more opportunity for interpretating correlation between chemical constituents, their biosynthesis and their possible action.

Table 1.11: List of organized drugs with examples

S.no	Organized drugs	Examples
1	Leaves	Digitalis, senna, tulsi, mint
2	Flowering parts	Clove, saffron, chamomile
3	Fruits	Coriander, fennel, amla, bael, cardamom.
4	Seeds	Kaladana, nutmeg, nux vomica, ispaghula
5	Woods	Sandalwood, quassia
6	Barks	Cinchona, cinnamon, cassia, cascara.
7	Roots and rhizomes	Ginger, garlic, rauwolfia, podophyllum, rhubarb, shatavari
8	Plants and herbs	Vinca, grgot, kalmegh, datura
9	Hair and fibres	Jute, silk, cotton, flax.

Table 1.12: List of unorganized drugs with examples

S.no	Unorganized drugs	Examples
1	Resins	Guggul, tolu balsam, asafoetida, benzoin
2	Waxes	Spermaceti, carnauba wax, yellow beeswax
3	Gums	Indian gum, guar gum, tragacenth, acacia
4	Volatile oil	Peppermint, lemon, clove, rosemary, eucalyptus.
5	Fixed oils and fats	Cod-liver, cotton seed, almond, kokum butter

(*Contd.*)

Table 1.12: List of unorganized drugs with examples *(Contd.)*

S.no	Unorganized drugs	Examples
6	Dried juice	Aloe, kino
7	Dried latex	Papain, opium
8	Dried extracts	Pale catechu, black catechu, pectin, agar
9	Animal products	Honey, cod-liver oil, gelatin, bees wax, lactose.
10	Fossil organism and minerals	Kaolin, kiesslguhr, bentonite, talc.

Table 1.13: Pharmacological classification of crude drugs

Activity	Crude drugs
Analgesic and narcotic	Morphine, codeine
Anti-inflammatory	Colchicum, turmeric
Carminatives	Fennel, coriander, clove
CNS stimulant	Strychnine, brucine, caffeine
Mydriatics	Atropine, homatropine
Antiamoebic	Ipecac root, kurchi bark
Myotics	Physostigmine, pilocarpine
Hypertensive	Ephedrine
Hypotensive	Reserpine, veratrine
Vermifuge	Pelletierine
Local anesthetic	Cocaine
Antimalarial	Quinine
Antiemetic	Emetine
Muscle relaxant	Curare
Antispasmodic	Papaverine
Uterine stimulant	Ergometrine
Antigout	Colchicines
Antiasthmatic	Ephedra, lobelia
Purgatives	Senna, thubarb
Expectorant	Tulsi, balsam of tolu

Table 1.14: Chemical classification of crude drugs

Carbohydrates

Carbohydrates are compounds containing the elements carbon, hydrogen, and oxygen. They are either aldehyde or ketonic alcohols in which hydrogen and oxygen are present in the same ratio as in water.

Examples

Acacia arabica, Astragalus gummifer, Cyamopsis tetragonolobus and *Plantago ovata*

Glycosides

Glycosides are non-reducing substances that, on hydrolysis brought about by reagents or enzymes, yield one or more reducing sugars among the products of hydrolysis. The non-sugar part of the molecule is called the aglycone or genin; the sugar component is called the glycone.

Examples

Anthraquinone glycosides: *Cassia acutifolia, Aloe perryi, Rheum emodi.*
Saponins glycosides: *Glycyrrhiza glabra, Terminalia arjuna*
Cyanophore glycosides: *Prunus serotina*
Isothiocyanate glycosides: *Brassica alba*

(Contd.)

Table 1.14: Chemical classification of crude drugs (Contd.)

	Cardiac glycosides: *Strophanthus Kombe*, *Digitalis purpurea*
	Bitter glycosides: *Picraena excelsa*, *Swertia chirata*
Tannins Tannins are complex organic, non-nitrogenous derivatives of polyhydroxy benzoic acids.	**Examples** *Emblica officinalis*, *Terminalia arjuna*, *Uncaria gambier*, *Acacia catechu* and *Terminilia chebula*
Volatile oils Volatile oils are odorous principles found in various parts of the plant. They are called volatile oils because they are volatile in steam and at higher temperatures evaporate.	**Examples** *Foeniculum vulgare*, *Peucedanum graveolens*, *Carum Carvi*
Lipids The term *lipid* refers to fixed oils, fats, and waxes. They are esters of long-chain fatty acids and alcohols and closely related derivatives. They are stored in seeds, spores, and vegetative perennial organs, such as bulbs.	**Examples** **Fixed oils**: *Ricinus communis*, *Oleum olivae*, *Prunus amygdalus* and *Hyoprion brevirostris* **Fats**: *Theobroma cacao* **Waxes**: *Apis mellifera*, *Prunus amygdalus*
Resins and resin combinations The term *resins are* brittle secretions or exudations of plant tissues, either produced normally or as the result of pathogenic conditions. Resins, as a class, are hard, transparent or translucent brittle substances. They are generally heavier than water (sp. gr. 0.9–1.25).	**Examples** *Podophyllum hexandrum*, *Cannabis sativa*, *Ipomoea purga*, *Capsicum annuum*, *Curcuma longa*, *Ferula foetida*, and *Zingiber officinalis*.
Alkaloids The term *alkaloid* can be defined as a plant base. Alkaloids mean "alkali-like," referring to the basic nature of these plant constituents. They are essentially basic nitrogenous compounds of vegetable origin, possessing some marked physiological action.	**Examples** **Pyridine and piperidine**: *Lobelia inflata*, *Nicotiana tabacum* **Tropane**: *Theobroma cacao*, *Atropa belladonna*, *Datura metel* and *Hyoscymus niger* **Quinoline**: *Cinchona calisaya* **Isoquinoline**: *Papaver somniferum*, *Cephaelis ipecacuanha* **Indole**: *Claviceps purpurea*, *Rauwolfia serpentina* **Purine**: Tea, coffee **Protein**: Gelatin, ficin, papain **Vitamins**: Yeast **Triterpenes**: Rasna, colocynth

DRUG DISCOVERY FROM NATURAL SUBSTANCES (Fig. 1.5)

A multifaceted approach of drug discovery from medicinal plants involves combining botanical, biological, phytochemical, and molecular techniques. New and important leads against various pharmacological targets including cancer, HIV/AIDS, Alzheimer's, malaria, and pain continues to be provided by medicinal plant drug discovery. Something

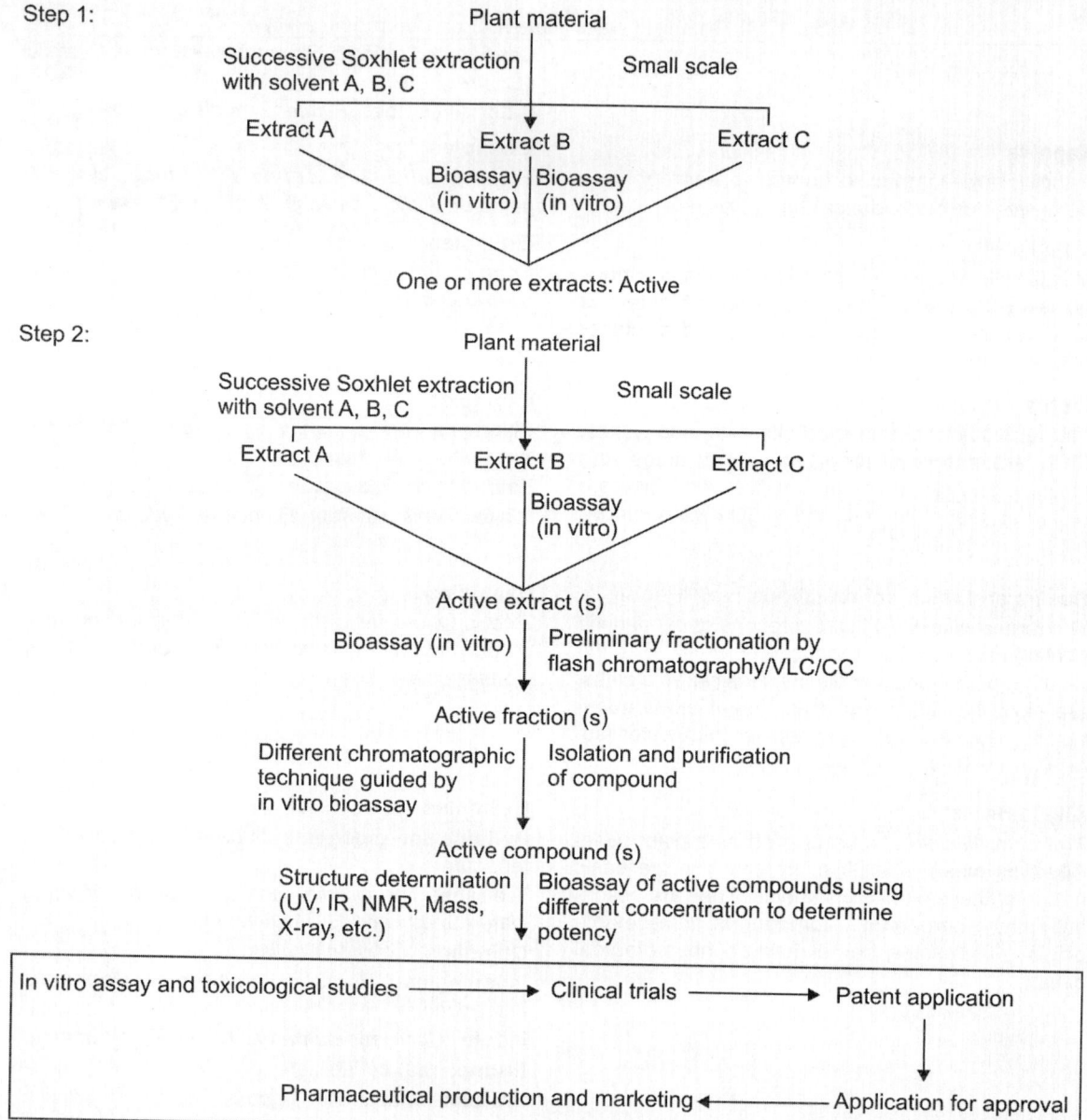

Fig. 1.5: A generic protocol for the drug discovery from natural products using a bioassay-guided approach

that is present in or produced by nature and not artificial or man-made is an adjective referring to *natural*. The term *natural products* refers to herbs, herbal concoctions, dietary supplements, traditional medicine, or alternative medicine. A remarkable resurgence of interest in natural product research over the areas of separation science, spectroscopic techniques, and microplate-based ultra sensitive in vitro assays. The preisolation analysis of crude extracts or fractions from different natural sources, isolation and

Table 1.15: Difference between modern medicine and traditional remedies

	Modern medicine	Traditional remedy
Mechanism	Specific molecular target	Holistic function
Objective	Treatment of diseases and/or symptoms	Restoring homeostasis
Action	Fast	Gradual
Indication	Acute and chronic diseases	Chronic diseases
Patient	Considered as a group	Individualized therapy

online detection of natural products, chemotaxonomic studies, chemical finger printing, quality control of herbal products, dereplication of natural products, and metabolomic studies have made possible by various available hyphenated techniques, e.g. GC-MS, LC-PDA, LC-MS, LC-FTIR, LC-and NMR, LC-NMR-MS, CE-MS. Plants are the structural anchors of the ecosystem in which these organisms live. The rapid loss of plant life has far-reaching consequences, and their loss will adversely affect future drug discovery.

Strategies for research in the area of natural products have evolved significantly over the last few decades. These can be broadly divided into two categories (Table 1.15):

1. Older strategies

a. Chemistry of compounds from natural sources was focused, not activity.
b. Isolation and identification of compounds from natural sources followed by in vivo biological activity testing.
c. Selection of organisms primarily based on folkloric reputations, or traditional uses, ethno pharmacological information.
d. Chemotaxonomic investigation.

2. Modern strategies

a. In vitro bioassay-guided isolation and identification of active "lead" compounds from natural sources.
b. Production of natural products libraries and active compounds in cell or tissue culture, genetic manipulation, natural combinatorial chemistry.
c. More focused on bioactivity and introduction of the concepts of dereplication, chemical finger printing, and metabolomics.
d. Selection of organisms based on ethnopharmacological information, folkloric reputations, or traditional uses, and also those randomly selected.

Background of Natural Products as Therapeutic Agents

For centuries, people have been using herbs for healing; in fact, medicinal application of natural products can be traced back for at least 5000 years, while Western medicine has a relatively short history of a few hundred years. Today, there are more than 85,000 plant species that have been documented for medical use globally. The World Health Organization (WHO) estimates that almost 75% of the world's population have therapeutic experience with herbal remedies.

Natural products are generally either of prebiotic origin or originate from microbes, plants, or animal sources. Natural products are chemicals which include such classes of compounds as terpenoids, polyketides, amino acids, peptides, proteins, carbohydrates, lipids, nucleic acid bases, RNA, DNA. Botanical drugs, as defined by the FDA, contain ingredients from fresh or dried plants, plant parts, isolated or combined chemical components of plant origin, algae, macroscopic fungi, or combinations thereof. They can be used in the diagnosis, cure, mitigation, treatment or prevention of diseases in humans. They may be available as a solution, powder, tablet, capsule, topical or injectable, etc. This drug class often has unique features, such as complex mixtures and a **lack of distinct bioactive components**. The isolation of morphine from opium in the early 19th century opened a new evidence-based drug discovery. During 1983–1994, about 40% of the new drugs approved in North America were derived from natural compounds, and approximately 70% of the new chemical entities (NCEs) reported between 1981 and mid-2006 resulted from studies on natural product. A recent survey involves modernization and globalization, shows that a majority of clinical researches on botanical drugs in the 21st century are focusing on the efficacy and safety.

Natural Product Research and Development: An Update

The current data on natural product research and development is:
- According to WHO approximately 80% of the world's population rely primarily on traditional medicines.
- Over 100 chemical substances that are considered to be important drugs, have been derived from 100 different plants.
- Approximately 75% of these substances were discovered as a direct result of the isolation of active substances from plants used in traditional medicine.
- 39% of the 520 new drugs approved during the period 1983–1994 were either natural products or derivatives of natural products.
- Approximately 250 discrete chemical structure prototypes have been used up to 1995.

Natural products today are most likely going to continue to exist and grow to become even more valuable as sources of new drug leads. The interest in natural products as a platform for drug discovery has waxed and waned in popularity with various pharmaceutical companies. The overwhelming concern today in the pharmaceutical industry is to:

- Improve the ability to find new drugs and to accelerate the speed with which new drugs are discovered and developed. This will only be successfully accomplished, if the procedures for drug target elucidation and lead compound identification and optimization are optimized.
- The costs of drug discovery and drug development continue to increase at astronomical rates, yet despite these expenditures, there is a decrease in the number of new medicines introduced into the world market.
- The degree of chemical diversity found in natural products is broader than that from any other source, and the degree of novelty of molecular structure found in natural products is greater than that determined from any other source.

Screening for Natural Product Activity

A screen is an assay or biological assay that provides a tool to test the presence and level of a target activity in a specific sample. Screens can be designed in such a fashion as to monitor only a single biological activity. Bioassays in a screening program should be rapid, simple to conduct, relevant, capable of being automated, cost. The classical approach is to design a screen or screening program that will permit the use of the assay or assays to provide guidance to successive steps in purification. An advantage of this is that the effectiveness and efficiency of purification can also be simultaneously evaluated at the same time as biological activity is being enhanced. Ultimately, after sufficient purification, a chemical structure can be determined for the active moiety.

Some objectives should be kept in mind when preparing natural product extracts for their ultimate introduction into the screening process.

- Every attempt should be made to stop ongoing biological processes.
- Steps should be taken to provide chemical stability of the compounds in the extract.
- Efforts need to be made to minimize losses of material.
- Sample preparation costs need to be minimized.

Natural products have been subjected to bioassay-directed isolation, a crude natural product mixture is subjected to fractionation and the individual fractions then bioassayed for specific biological activity. This process continues repetitively with comparison of individual fraction assay data to a bioassay database. Modern separation/chemical characterization approaches can eliminate much of this problem by identification of the compounds before they are subjected to bioassay. Indeed the coupling of such techniques to biological screens can improve the quality of the assay result and shorten research and development time frames. These new tandem approaches are termed fractionation-driven bioassays.

- The first step is the chromatographic separation of compounds from the complex source mixture.
- In the second step, the physico-chemical properties or chemical reactivities of the separated compounds are analyzed.

The former is referred to as the **fractionation-driven bioassay**. A crude natural product mixture is subjected to fractionation and the individual fractions then subjected to NMR spectroscopy or MS/MS. The structures of the compounds in the individual fractions are identified; and, if the structures are known, their biological activity profiles are evaluated from an existing database. If they are unknown, then the compounds are subjected to bioassay.

In latter, known as isolate and assay approach, a crude natural product mixture is subjected to automated fractionation and purification. The individual fractions are then subjected to bioassay. Desirable biological activity serves as the trigger to subject the sample to NMR or MS/MS and ascertain the structure(s). If the material is a previously known compound, it may well be discarded, depending on its biological activity or toxicological profile. If the material is a novel compound, the structure can be optimized.

Extraction of Natural Products

Extraction is carried out for following reasons:
1. The generation and supply of larger amounts of an already known compound so that more extensive biological testing, such as pharmacology and toxicology, can be performed on the material.
2. The purification of a small amount of material for initial biological and chemical characterization to be performed.
3. To purify sufficient material in order to conduct complete structural studies and further biological activity characterization.

Isolation and Purification of Natural Products

Natural products are typically secondary metabolites and are smaller in size, chemically more diverse in structure, and present in smaller concentrations than the more homogeneous proteins, carbohydrates, lipids, nucleic acids. An important concept of purification is that the relationship between purity of compound achieved during natural product extraction and the amount of effort expended to achieve such a level of purity is almost exponential in nature. Natural products are isolated and purified for one of two reasons:

1. To ascertain what the natural product is, and
2. To carry out sufficient experimental work necessary to biologically characterize or profile the compound.

Before initiating an isolation and purification, there are a number of basic steps to be analysed.

Identify the type of chemical constituent: (1) An unknown compound associated with a particular biological activity, (2) a previously known compound present in a specific organism, (3) a group of compounds within an organism that are all structurally related to each other, (4) all of the metabolites produced by one natural product source that are not produced by another closely related source, or (5) all of the molecules of a particular organism.

Type of purity: A natural product compound is to be used for biological testing, it is important to know not only the degree of purity of the material but also the nature of the impurities.

In a purification scheme no step delivers the desired material in 100% yield. Each extraction step results in the loss of material, and when working to attain very high levels of purity, losses can be extreme.

Type of fractionation: All separation processes involve the division of a mixture into a number of discrete fractions. This process is called fractionation. Such fractions can be physically separated, such as the two phases of a **liquid–liquid extraction** or they may not be physically separated, such as the continuous eluate from a chromatography column. The eluate from a chromatography column can then be artificially divided into fractions via the use of a fraction collector. The method of fractionation depends on the sample and the goals of the separation.

Nature of the compound: It depends on its acid/base properties (pKa, pKb), molecular charge, stability, and solubility (hydrophilicity/lipophilicity).

Desired activity localized: Plant, tree, moss, bacteria, vertebrate, invertebrate, insect, terrestrial, or marine-based components or parts in which the desired activity or compound is present in greater concentration as opposed to other parts in which the compound is present in lesser amounts.

A variety of different techniques can be used for the isolation and purification of natural product compounds. These techniques include solid-phase extraction, high performance liquid chromatography (HPLC), gradient high-performance liquid chromatography, bioautography; thin-layer chromatography (TLC), countercurrent chromatography, droplet countercurrent chromatography, vacuum column chromatography, desalting, liquid–liquid chromatography, paper chromatography, ion exchange chromatography, size exclusion chromatography, affinity chromatography, acid–base switching technology, centrifugal partition chromatography, liquid–solid chromatography, microwave-assisted extraction, pressurized solvent extraction, large scale solvent extraction, and super critical fluid extraction.

Structure Identification of Natural Products

The chemical structures of natural product compounds are tremendously diverse and can be very elegant in their nature. Modern technology has made structure identification simpler and faster by techniques as MS, MS/MS, IR, Fourier transform infrared spectroscopy (FTIR), NMR, Fourier transform nuclear magnetic resonance (FTNMR) spectroscopy, and others (Table 1.16). Structure determination pertinent to the area of natural products has come from the field of computer-assisted structure elucidation (CASE). Advancements in chromatography, spectrometry, and spectroscopy together with breakthroughs in the coupling of these technologies are important steps in the production of a fully automated and integrated natural products structure determination instrument, which will provide significant advantage to the early, rapid, and facile identification of new natural-product based drug opportunities.

Table 1.16: Natural product testing with its purity

Testing	Purity
Pharmacological or pharmacokinetic testing	99%
Chemical characterization via NMR, IR and MS/MS spectroscopy	95 to 99%
X-ray crystallographic studies	99.9%
Analysis of the ultraviolet spectrum	50%

Synthesis of Natural Products

Natural product compound has been screened for biological activity, isolated, purified, its structure identified, and the pharmacological profile refined, the journey is not over. The molecule may turn out to be too complex in nature and too expensive to be synthesized. Any given natural product compound may possess unacceptable physicochemical, pharmacodynamic, pharmacokinetic, or bioavailability properties or demonstrate excessive toxicity and will therefore require optimization of its chemical structure. **Optimization** involves a dissection of the lead molecule and the synthetic addition, removal, replacement, or modification of substituent groups so as to enhance the utility and efficacy of the molecule. The synthesis of a complicated molecule is a very difficult task since every group and atom must be placed in a proper position and with the correct stereochemistry.

Development of Natural Products

Regulatory Guidelines and Nonclinical Development

The classical model of drug development is composed of three phases: discovery, development, and marketing.

Discovery is the first of these phases and is composed of two essential components, drug discovery and drug design.

Development is the second of these phases and is composed of two large components, preclinical studies and clinical studies. The development phase, although lengthy, expensive, and time consuming is meant to ensure the safety and efficacy of compounds and to decrease the hazard and risk of exposure for humans.

Preclinical studies begin some of the more rigorous testings that a potential candidate must successfully endure and survive. The major objectives of any preclinical development program should be:

1. Development of a good manufacturing practices (GMP)
2. The creation of a usable and tolerable preclinical formulation(s) and efficacious clinical formulation(s).
3. Complete pharmacologic and pharmacokinetic profiling of the test article.
4. Performance of proper toxicology studies to support an investigational new drug (IND) application, and
5. Construction of a complete and detailed informational platform to permit the recommendation of an initial human dose in phase I studies.

Nonclinical or preclinical studies are the same thing and are composed of studies on drug processes, pharmacology, and toxicology.

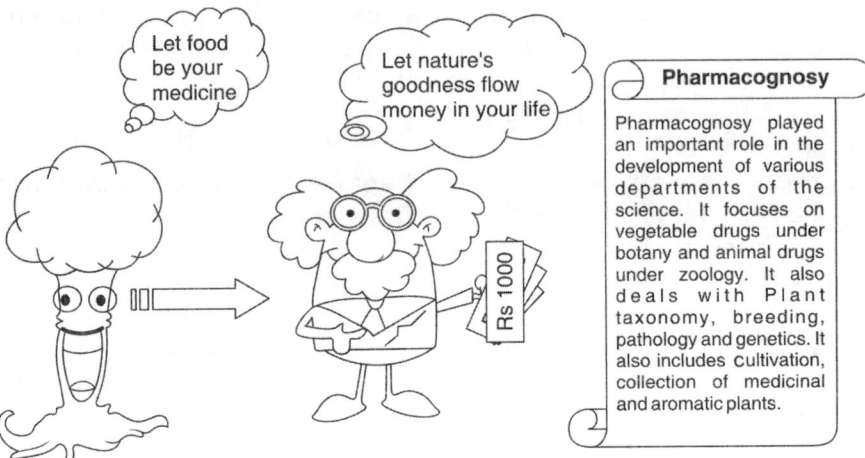

Scope of pharmacognosy

Toxicology studies have a profound quality assurance component, which facilitate validation of the data by a regulatory agency. These studies typically include mutagenicity, genotoxicity, and cytotoxicity studies; acute studies; subchronic studies; chronic studies; reproductive and developmental toxicity studies; carcinogenicity studies; immunotoxicity assessments.

- **Phase I** studies represent the first exposure of a drug to humans. These studies examine the effects of single and multiple increasing doses in small numbers of normal and/or patient volunteers, tolerance level, basic pharmacokinetic studies, the routes of metabolism, excretion, and elimination and assess the amounts of active and inactive or toxic metabolites. Typically only a small number of volunteers are involved.
- **Phase II** studies represent that a drug candidate is tested in humans for efficacy. In phase II studies, optimization of dose of drug is done by different dose-range finding to maximize its efficacy, and to minimize any compound-associated intolerance. These studies typically involve up to several hundred patients.
- The last clinical studies that need to be performed before submitting a complete information package for regulatory approval is **phase III studies**. These studies will verify efficacy and safety and detect adverse reactions and contraindications. These are very large studies composed of hundreds to thousands of volunteer patients, depending upon the therapeutic indication.
- **Phase IV** studies are postmarketing surveillance studies, which are conducted after a drug has been approved for sale. These studies typically involve adverse reaction reporting, surveys and general sampling, and testing evaluations.

2

Medicinal Plant Biotechnology

BIOSYNTHETIC PATHWAY OF PHYTOCONSTITUENTS

All organisms need to transform and inter-convert a vast number of organic compounds to enable them to live, grow, and reproduce. They need to provide themselves with energy in the form of ATP, and supply of building blocks to construct their own tissues.

The important molecules of life are carbohydrates, proteins, fats, and nucleic acids (Table 2.1).

Table 2.1: Molecules of life with their composition

Molecules of life	Composition
Carbohydrates	Sugar units
Proteins	Amino acids
Fats	Polymeric materials
Nucleic acids	Nucleotides

A metabolic pathway is a series of chemical reactions occurring within a cell, catalyzed by enzymes, resulting in either the formation of a metabolic product to be used or stored by the cell, or the initiation of another metabolic pathway. Mainly metabolic pathways are concerned with modifying and synthesizing molecules like carbohydrates, proteins, fats and nucleic acids from basic compounds. These processes demonstrate the fundamental unity of all living matters, and are collectively described as **primary metabolism** (Table 2.2) with the compounds involved in the pathways being termed **primary metabolites**. Primary metabolic pathways, which synthesize, degrade, and generally interconvert compounds commonly encountered in all organisms. They are needed for general growth and physiological development of plant which is widely distributed in nature and is also utilized as food by man. Typically, primary metabolites are found across all species within broad phylogenetic groupings, and are produced using the same pathway (or nearly the same pathway) in all these species (Fig. 2.1).

Table 2.2: List of primary metabolism

Primary metabolism is the routine chemical process that plant need to carry out to survive and reproduce
1. Photosynthesis
2. Glycolysis
3. Citric acid cycle
4. Amino acid synthesis
5. Transamination
6. Protein and enzyme synthesis
7. Coenzyme synthesis
8. Number Absorption
9. Reproduction and cells
10. Duplication of genetic materials

The secondary metabolites, such as alkaloids, glycosides, flavonoids, volatile oils, etc. (Table 2.3), are biosynthetically derived from primary metabolites. Secondary metabolites, by contrast, are often species-specific (or found in only a small set of species in a narrow phylogenetic group), and without these compounds the organism suffers from

Table 2.3: List of important secondary metabolites

Plant drug	Secondary metabolite	Activity
Cinnamomum zeylanicum	Quinine alkaloids	Antimalarial
Catharanthus roseus	Vincristin and vinblastin	Anticancer
Taxus species	Taxol	Anticancer
Papaver somniferum	Morphine	Analgesic
Digitalis purpurea	Digitalis glycosides	Cardiotonics

Table 2.4: List of major metabolic pathways

Cellular respiration	Glycolysis
	Anaerobic respiration
	Kreb's cycle/citric acid cycle
	Oxidative phosphorylation
Creation of energetic compounds from non-living matter	Photosynthesis (plants, algae, cyanobacteria)
	Chemosynthesis (some bacteria)
Other pathways occurring in living organisms	Fatty acid oxidation (β-oxidation)
	Gluconeogenesis
	HMG-CoA reductase pathway (isoprene prenylation)
	Pentose phosphate pathway (hexose monophosphate)
	Porphyrin synthesis (or heme synthesis) pathway
	Urea cycle

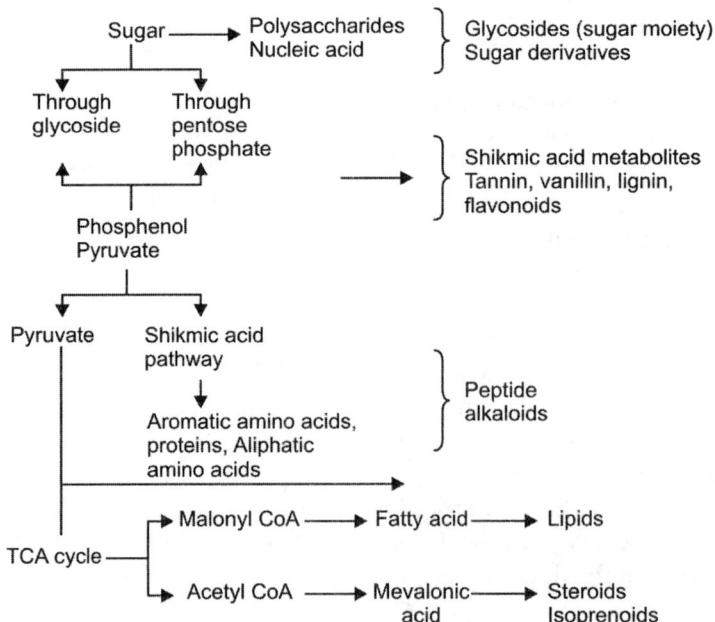

Fig. 2.1: Primary and secondary metabolites derived from carbon metabolism in plants

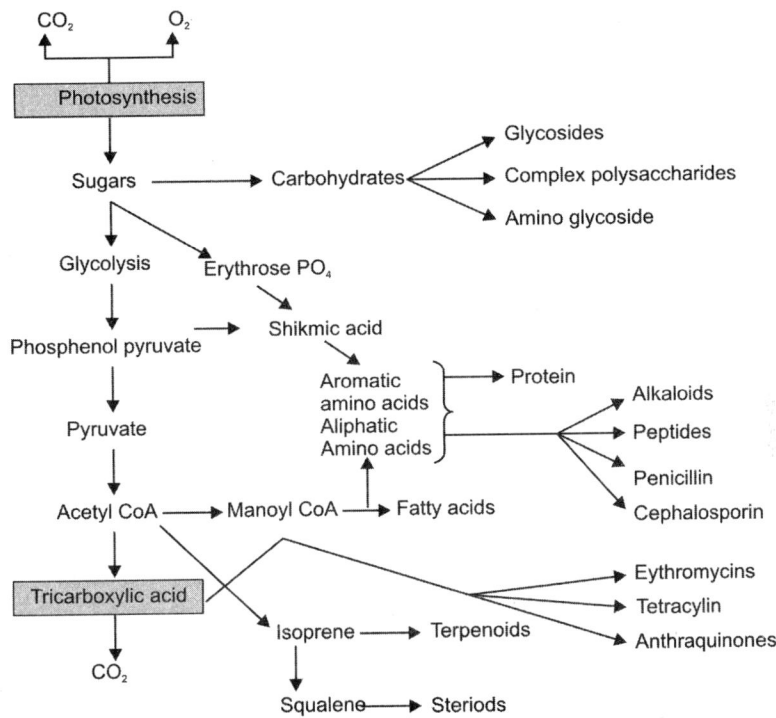

Fig. 2.2: Inter-relationships of biosynthetic pathways leading to secondary constituents in plants

only a mild impairment, lowered survivability/fecundity, esthetic differences, or else no change in phenotype at all. They are produced for easily appreciated reasons, e.g. as toxic materials providing defence against predators, as volatile attractants towards the same or other species, or as coloring agents to attract or warn other species, but it is logical to assume that all do play some vital role for the well-being of the producer (Fig. 2.2).

Important features of secondary metabolites:

- They are unnecessarily restricted to a taxonomic group.
- They provide most of the pharmacologically active natural products. Though secondary metabolites present in lesser quantities, but they are main constituents responsible for medicinal utility hence are expensive to produce.
- They produce due to any environmental stresses or any abnormal condition, and serve as defensive, protective or offensive chemicals against microorganisms, insects and higher herbivorous predators.
- They also act as waste or secretory products of plant metabolism and are of pharmaceutical importance.

Biosynthesis of Aromatic Compounds

Shikimic acid pathway: The shikmic acid pathway is a key intermediate from carbohydrate for the biosynthesis of C_6–C_3 units (phenyl propane derivative). The shikimic acid pathway converts simple carbohydrate precursors derived from glycolysis and the pentose phosphate pathway to the aromatic amino acids. The shikimic acid pathway is present in plants, fungi, and bacteria but is not found in animals (Fig. 2.3).

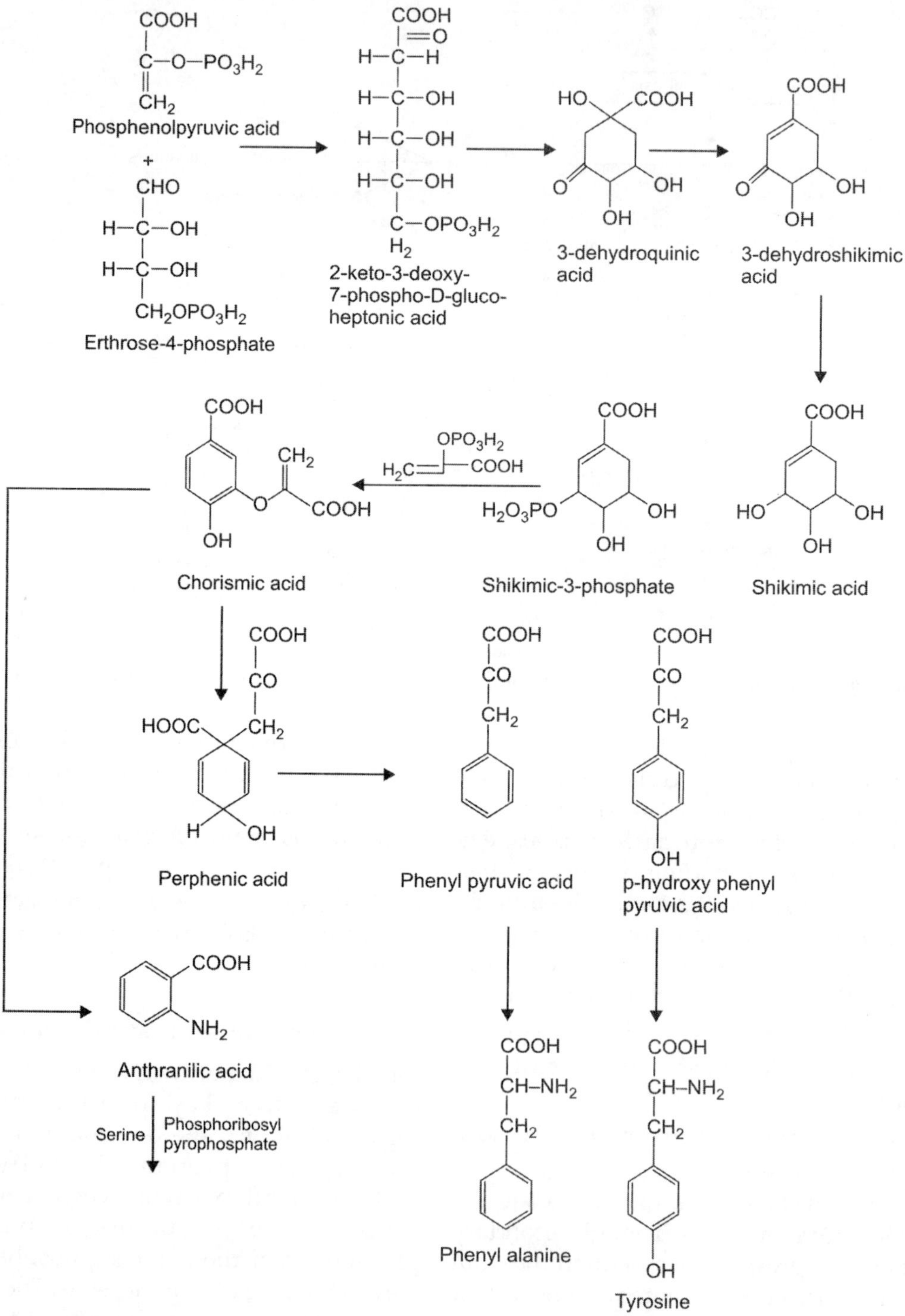

Fig. 2.3: Shikimic acid pathway

Amino acids: Amino acids occur in plants both in the form of free state and as the basic units of proteins and other metabolites. They arise at various levels of glycolytic and TCA systems (Table 2.5 and Fig. 2.4).

Basic Metabolic Pathways

Glycolysis (EMI: Embden-Meyerhof pathway): Glycolysis represents an anabolic pathway common in both aerobic and anaerobic organisms. **Glycolysis** is the metabolic pathway that converts glucose, $C_6H_{12}O_6$, into pyruvate. The free energy released in this process is used to form the high energy compounds, ATP (adenosine triphosphate) and NADH (reduced nicotinamide adenine dinucleotide) (Fig. 2.5).

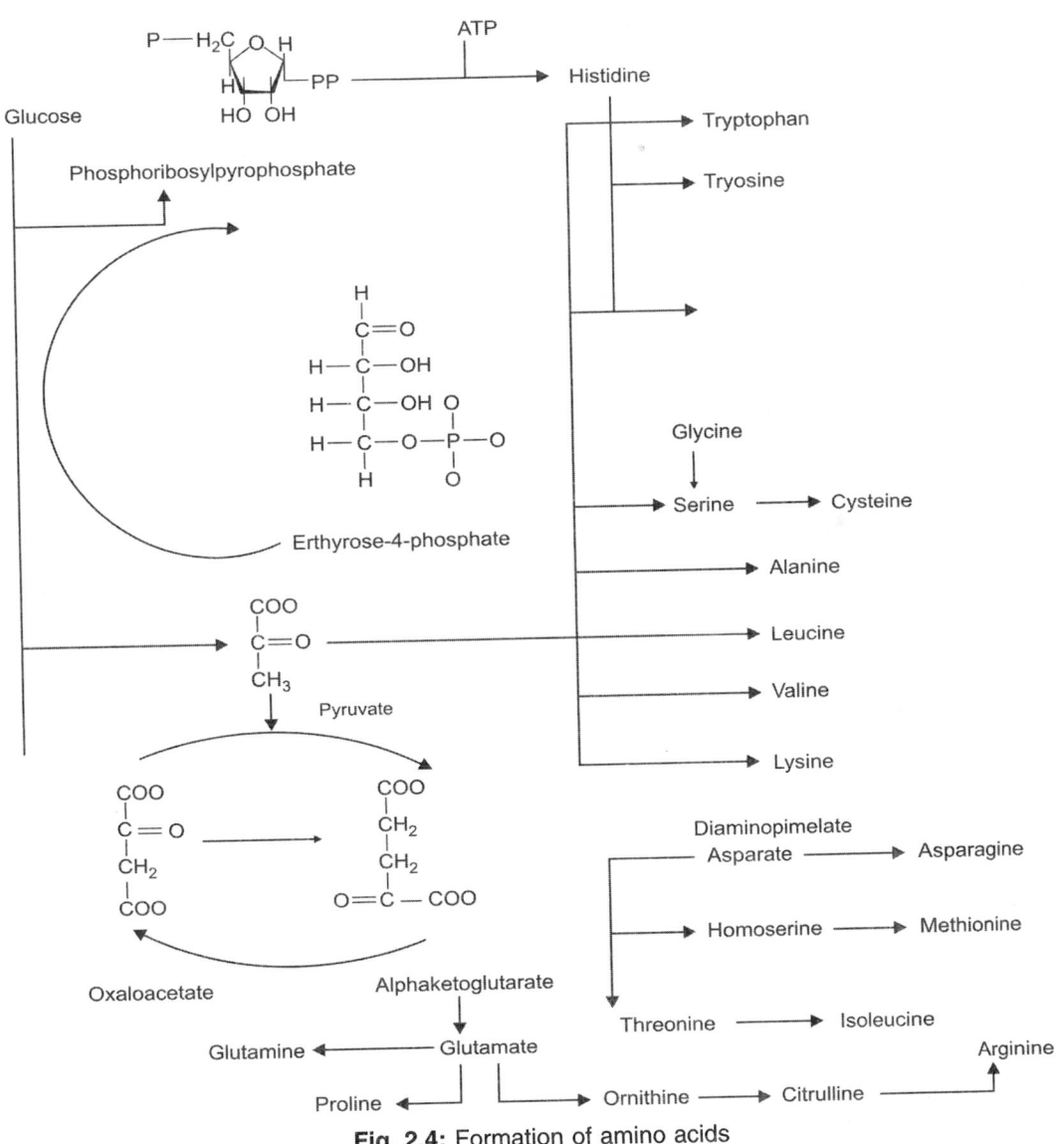

Fig. 2.4: Formation of amino acids

Table. 2.5: Amino acids and their precursors

Amino acids	Precursors
Glutamate family	α-ketoglutarate
Aspartate family	Oxaloacetate
Alanine-valine-leucine group	Pyruvate
Serine-glycine group	3-phosphoglycerate
Aromatic amino acids	Phosphoenolpyruvate
	Erythrose-4-phosphate

Biosynthesis of Glycosides

The term 'glycoside' is a very general one which embraces all the many and varied combinations of sugars and aglycones. The metabolic process of glycoside formation essentially consists of two parts. The first part of biosynthesis is the reactions by means of which various type of aglycones are formed, whereas the other part of biosynthesis process takes into account metabolic pathway involving coupling of aglycone with sugar moiety. The synthesis of glycosides in plant cells involves interaction of nucleotide glycoside, such as UDP-glucose with alcoholic or phenolic group of a second compound aglycone. The principal pathway of glycoside formation involves the transfer of uridylyl group from uridine triphosphate (UTP) to sugar-1-phosphate and the enzymes catalyzing this reaction are known as uridylyltransferases. The subsequent reaction controlled by enzymatic system glycosyltransferases involves transfer of sugar from uridine diphosphate to aglycone moiety resulting in formation of glycoside.

1. UTP + sugar-1-phosphate $\xleftarrow{\text{Uridylyl-transferases}}$ UDP-sugar + PP_1

2. UTP + sugar + aglycone $\xleftarrow{\text{Glycosyl-transferases}}$ Glycoside UDP

Biosynthesis of Alkaloids

Alkaloid derived from ornithine: Ornithine is incorporated into both pyrrolidine specifically and asymmetrically into pyrrolidine ring of tropane nucleus, the α-carbon of ornithine becoming the C_1 of tropine nucleus.

Alkaloids derived from lysine: In biogenesis of the anabasine, lupinine, and isopelletierine precursor are lysine.

Alkaloids derived from phenylalanine, tyrosine and related amino acids: These amino acids and their decarboxylation products serve as the precursor for ephedrine, colchicines and opium alkaloids.

MORPHINE

(5α,6α)-17-methyl-7,8-didehydro-4,5-epoxymorphinan-3,6-diol

Chemistry

- Its molecular composition is $C_{17}H_{19}NO_3$ and levorotatory in nature.
- Chemically, it has phenanthrene type of nucleus and due to presence of phenolic hydroxyl group, it is soluble in alkali hydroxides except ammonium hydroxide.
- Morphine on acetylation or benzoylation gives diacetyl morphine or dibenzoyl derivatives,

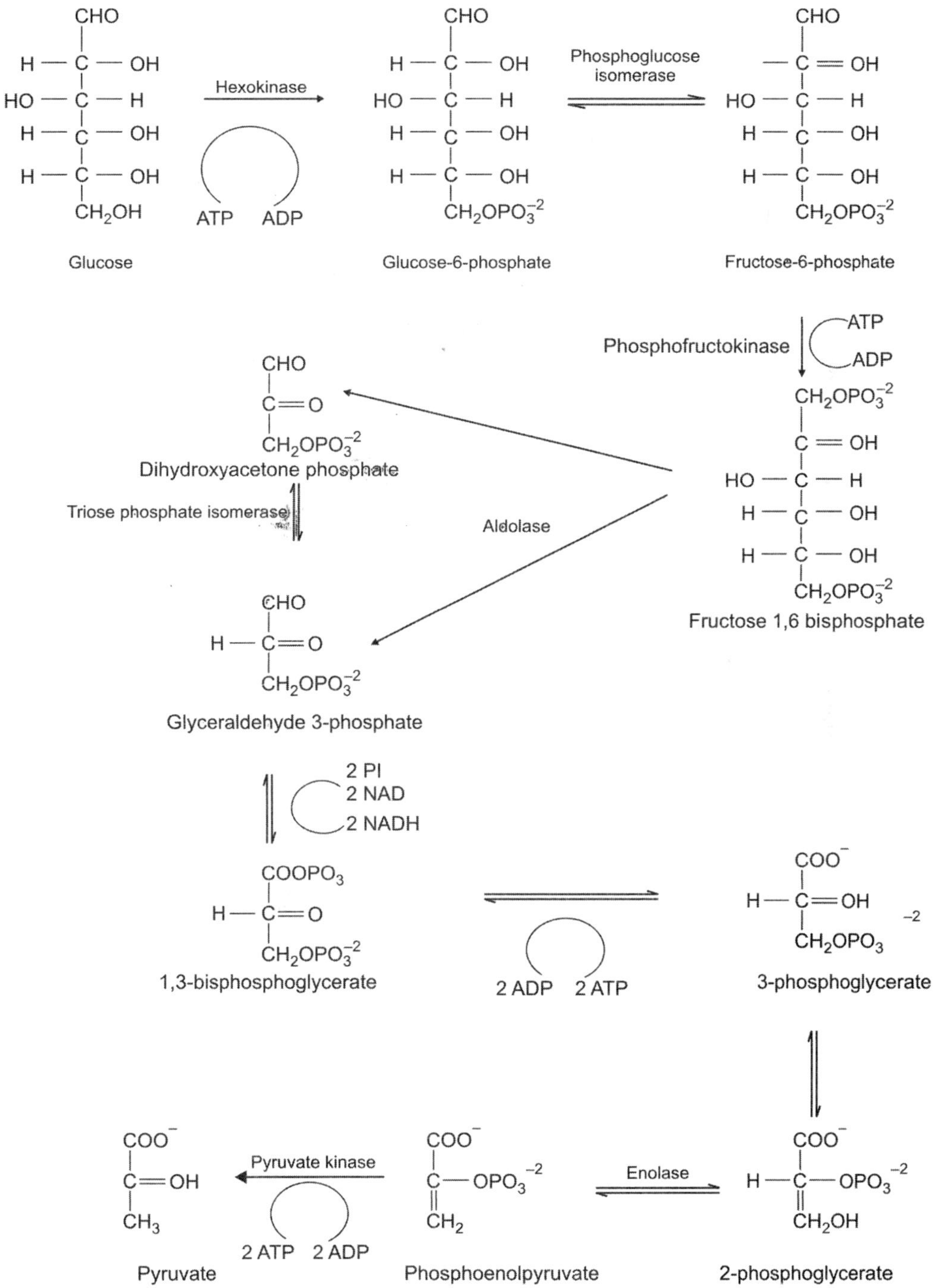

Fig. 2.5: Glycolysis (EMI: Embden-Meyerhof pathway)

Pharmacognosy and Phytochemistry

A biosynthetic pathway scheme is shown, beginning from Phosphoenol pyruvic acid and Erythrose-4-phosphate, proceeding through the shikimate pathway to form aromatic amino acids and benzylisoquinoline alkaloids.

Key intermediates and steps depicted:

- Phosphoenol pyruvic acid + Erythrose-4-phosphate → 2-keto, 3-Deoxy, 7-phospho D-Glucohepturic acid
- Cyclisation → 3-Dehydro quinic acid
- → 3-Dehydro shikmic acid (NADH, NAD)
- Reduction (NADH, NAD) → Shikmic acid
- Phosphorylation (ATP → ADP) → 3-Phospho shikmic acid
- Condensation → Chorismic acid (Unstable)
- → Prephinic acid (−H_2O, −CO_2)
- → Phenyl pyruvic acid → Phenylalanine
- → p-hydroxy phenyl pyruvic acid → Tyrosine
- → 3,4 dihydroxy phenyl pyruvic acid ⇌ 3,4 dihydroxy phenyl alanine → 3,4 dihydroxy phenyl ethylamine
- Condensation → Norlaudanosoline carboxylic acid
- −CO_2, H^+ → 1, 2 dehydro norlaudainosoline
- Reduction → Papaverine (MeO groups)
- → Norlaudnosoline
- → Key intermediate in the formation of benzyl-isoquinoline phenanthrene type alkaloid

(Contd.)

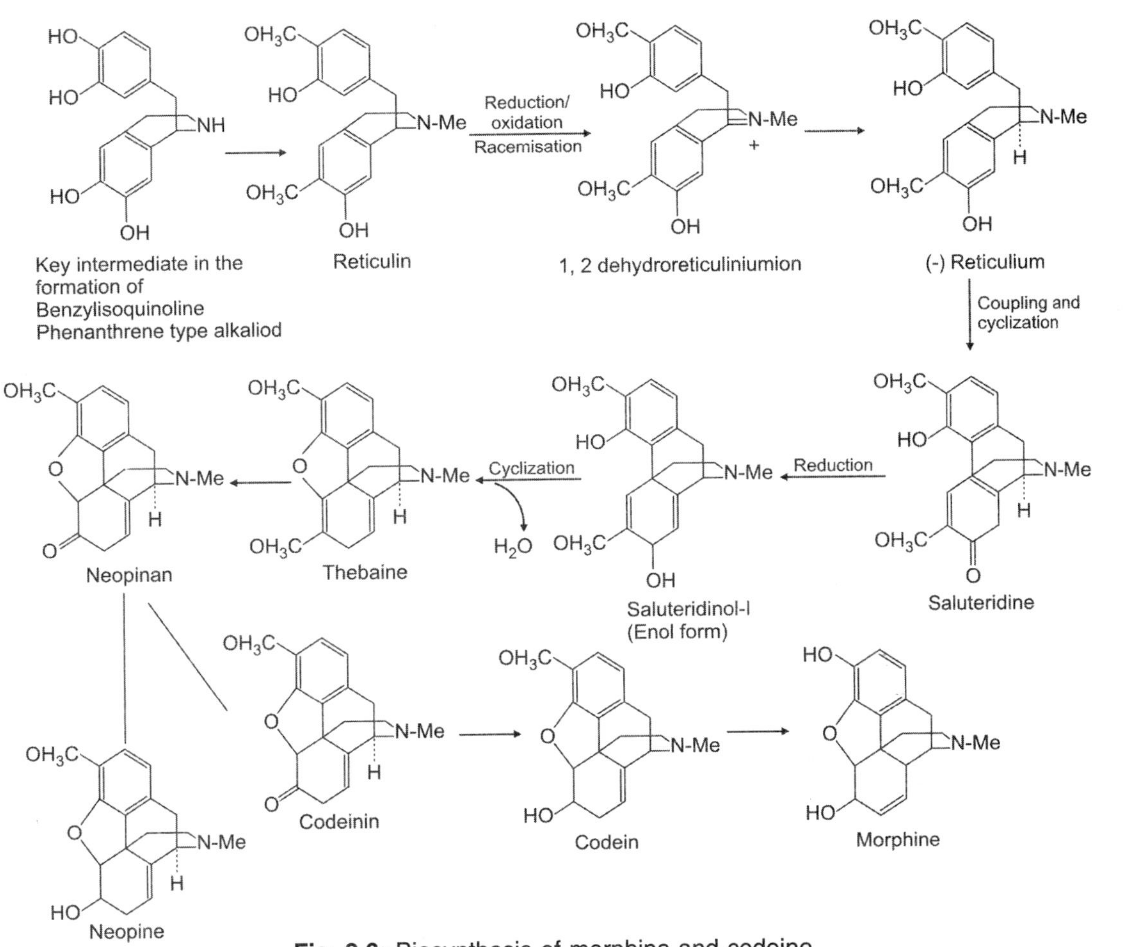

Fig. 2.6: Biosynthesis of morphine and codeine

which indicates presence of two hydroxyl groups. On treatment with halogen acids, morphine forms monohalogen product indicating that an alcoholic hydroxyl group.

- Due to the presence of phenolic hydroxyl group, morphine is soluble in alkali hydroxides except ammonium hydroxides (Fig. 2.6).

Biological Source

Morphine is obtained from dried latex by incision from the unripe capsules of *Papaver somniferum* belonging to family Papaveraceae.

Pharmacological Activity

Morphine possesses powerful analgesic and narcotic activity, and exerts depressant action on central nervous system (CNS). Morphine exerts stimulating effect on the spinal cord and vomiting center. Morphine reduces intestinal motility and used in treatment of diarrhea (See Fig. 2.6).

EPHEDRINE

(1R,2S)-2-(methylamino)-1-phenylpropan-1-ol

Chemistry

1. Ephedrine is amino alkaloids ($C_{10}H_{15}NO$), is biosynthesized through phenyl alanine.
2. Ephedrine exhibits optical isomerism and has two chiral centers, giving rise to four stereoisomers (1R, 2S and 1S, 2R) ephedrine, while pseudoephedrine (1R, 2R and 1S, 2S).

3. The dextrorotatory (+)- or d-enantiomer is (1S, 2R)-ephedrine, whereas the levorotatory (")- or l- form is (1R, 2S)-ephedrine.
4. Ephedrine is a sympathomimetic amine.
5. The principal mechanism is indirect stimulation of the adrenergic receptor system, and increasing the activity of noradrenaline at the postsynaptic α- and β-receptors.

Biological Source
It is obtained from dried aerial parts of *Ephedra gerardiana*, *Ephedra sinica*, *Ephedra nebrodensis* belonging to family Ephedraceae.

Pharmacological Activity
1. Ephedrine and pseudoephedrine act as a bronchodilator, but pseudoephedrine has considerably less effect.
2. Ephedrine promotes weight loss.
3. Ephedrine also decreases gastric emptying.
4. Ephedrine is CNS stimulant.
5. Ephedrine increases the force of myocardial contraction and relaxes bronchial smooth muscles as well as uterine smooth muscles (Fig. 2.7).

ERGOMETRINE
(8β)-N-[(2S)-1-hydroxy-2-propanyl]-6-methyl-9,10-didehydroergoline-8-carboxamide

Biological Source: A fungal sclerotium of *claviceps purpurea* in ovary of rye plant belonging to family clavicipitatceae.

Chemistry
Ergometrine has molecular formula $C_{19}H_{23}N_3O_2$. It is synthesized by esterification of D-lysergic acid using 2-aminopropanol in dimethylformamide and direct treatment of the reaction mixture with phosgene.

Pharmacology
- It has a medical use in obstetrics to facilitate delivery of the placenta and to prevent bleeding after childbirth by causing smooth muscle tissue in the blood vessel walls to narrow, thereby reducing blood flow.
- It can induce spasm of the coronary arteries. It is used to diagnose angina.
- Ergometrine increases peristaltic activity and potentiates the action of neostigmine on the gut.
- It produces direct vasoconstrictor effect to reduce the bleeding.
- It has no adrenergic blocking activity (Fig. 2.8).

ATROPINE
(3-endo)-8-methyl-8-azabicyclo oct-3-yl tropate

Chemistry
Atropine is a racemic mixture of *d*-hyoscyamine and *l*-hyoscyamine, with physiological effects due to *l*-hyoscyamine. The molecular formula is $C_{17}H_{23}NO_3$

Biological Source
Atropine is a naturally occurring tropane alkaloid extracted from deadly nightshade (*Atropa belladonna*), Jimson weed (*Datura stramonium*) and mandrake (*Mandragora officinarum*) of the family Solanaceae.

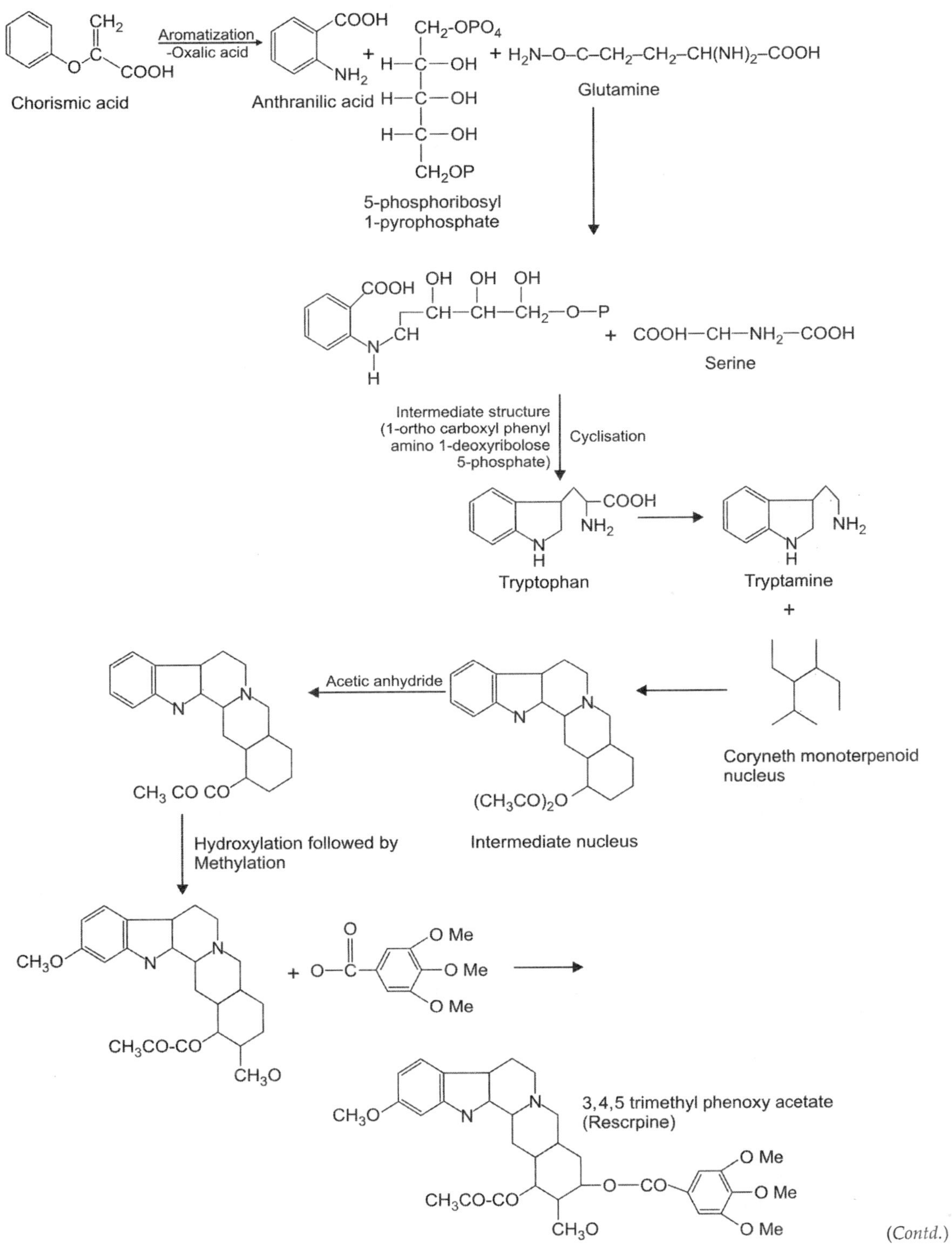

Medicinal Plant Biotechnology

Chorismic acid →(Aromatization, -Oxalic acid) Anthranilic acid + 5-phosphoribosyl 1-pyrophosphate + Glutamine

↓

Intermediate structure (1-ortho carboxyl phenyl amino 1-deoxyribolose 5-phosphate) + Serine

↓ Cyclisation

Tryptophan → Tryptamine

+ Coryneth monoterpenoid nucleus

↓

Intermediate nucleus $(CH_3CO)_2O$

←(Acetic anhydride)

↓ Hydroxylation followed by Methylation

+ 3,4,5 trimethyl phenoxy acetate (O Me, O Me, O Me)

→ Rescrpine

(Contd.)

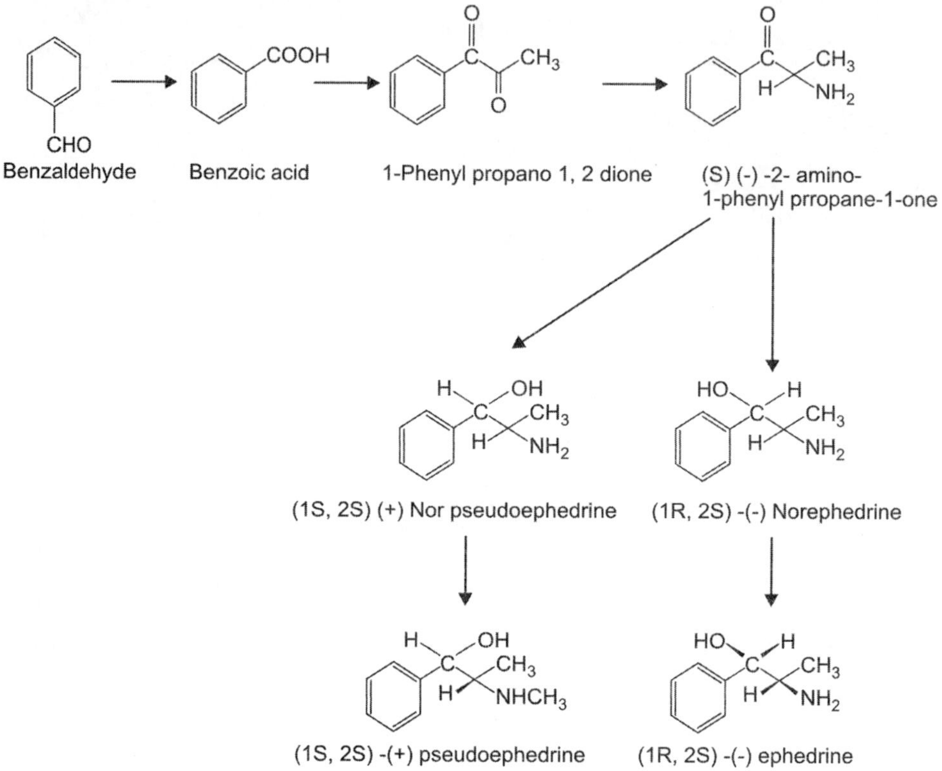

Fig. 2.7: Biosynthesis of ephedrine

Pharmacology

- Atropine is anticholinergic or parasympatholytic drug, which inhibits the parasympathetic nervous system.
- Atropine has been used in the treatment of peptic ulcer, it ameliorates by reducing acid secretions in the stomach when it is empty and by decreasing the strength of smooth muscle contractions. It is also used to treat some other GI disturbances. It also relieves cystitis (bladder inflammation) by relaxing smooth muscles of the bladder.
- It is used in the eye to dilate it and to paralyze accommodation (i.e. temporarily prevents the eye from focusing).
- It acts as a competitive antagonist of acetylcholine at muscarinic receptors, blocking stimulation of muscles and glands by parasympathetic and cholinergic sympathetic nerves. It is used as the sulfate salt, as a smooth muscle relaxant, as an antiarrhythmic, as a preanesthetic to reduce secretions, as an antidote to poisoning by organophosphorus compounds, cholinesterase inhibitors, or muscarine, and as a mydriatic and cycloplegic (Fig. 2.9).

RESERPINE

(Methyl(3β,16β,17α,18β,20α)-11,17 dimethoxy-18-[(3,4,5 trimethoxybenzoyl)oxy] yohimban-16 carboxylate)

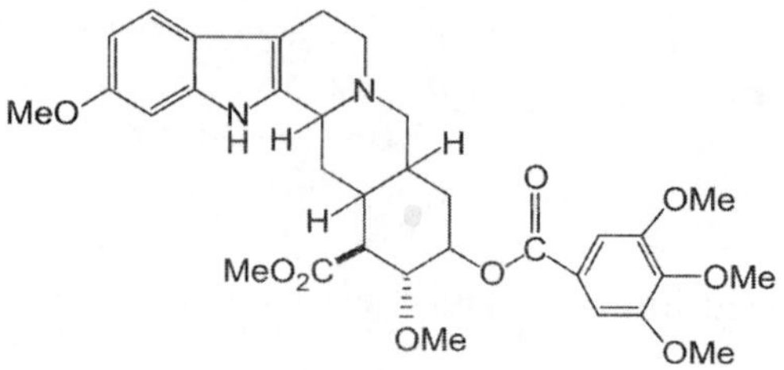

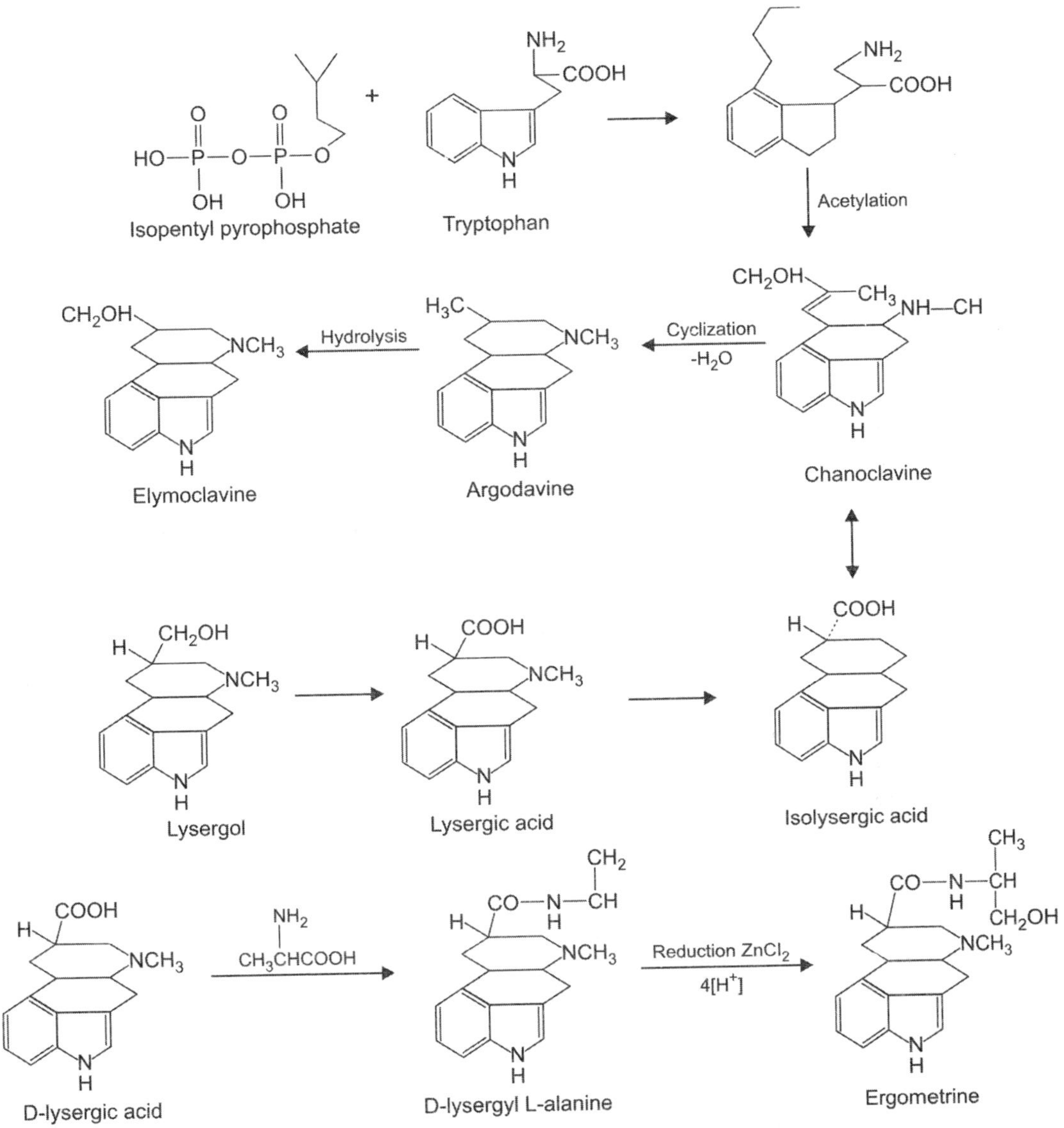

Fig. 2.8: Biosynthesis of ergometrine

Chemistry

Reserpine is indole alkaloid with molecular formula $C_{33}H_{40}N_2O_9$. Reserpine, a pure crystalline alkaloid of rauwolfia, is a white or pale buff to slightly yellowish, odorless crystalline powder. It darkens slowly on exposure to light, but more rapidly when in solution. It is insoluble in water, freely soluble in acetic acid and in chloroform, slightly soluble in benzene, and very slightly soluble in alcohol and in ether. Its molecular weight is 608.69.

Biological Source

It is obtained from dried roots and rhizomes of *Rauwolfia serpentina* belonging to family Apocynaceae.

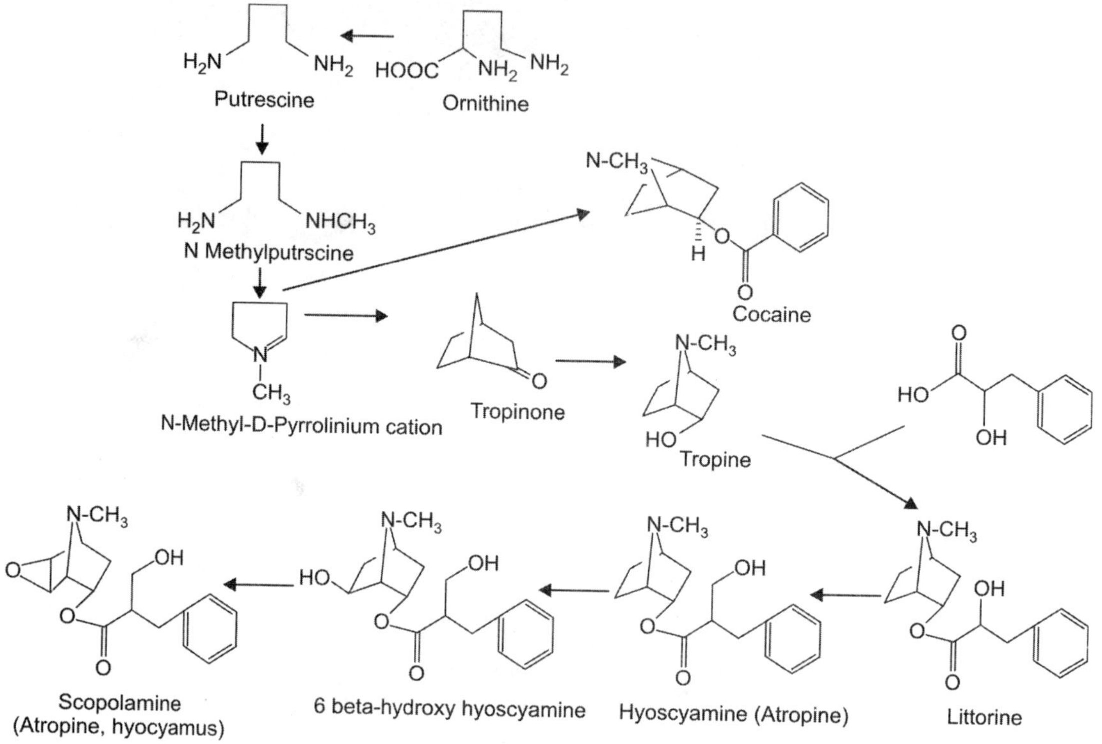

Fig. 2.9: Biosynthesis of atropine

Pharmacology

Reserpine depletes stores of catecholamines and 5-hydroxytryptamine in many organs, including the brain and adrenal medulla. It has sedative and tranquilizing properties. Reserpine, like other rauwolfia compounds, is characterized by slow onset of action and sustained effects. Both cardiovascular and central nervous system effects may persist for a period of time following withdrawal of the drug.

Reserpine has several complementary actions of benefit to the hypertensive patient, including a calming effect and a slowing of the pulse rate (Fig. 2.10).

STRYCHNINE (Strychnidin-10-one)

Chemistry

Strychnine is an alkaloid derivative with molecular formula $C_{21}H_{22}N_2O_2$. Strychnine is a base and forms water-soluble salts with acids. It is a white, odorless, bitter crystalline powder.

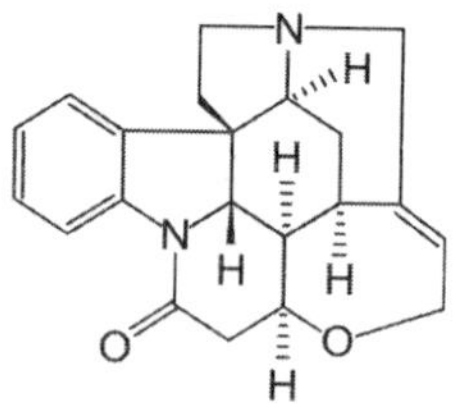

Biological Source

It is obtained from seeds of *Strychnos nux-vomica* L. belonging to family Loganiaceae.

Pharmacology

- Strychnine is an antagonist of glycine and acetylcholine receptors. It primarily affects

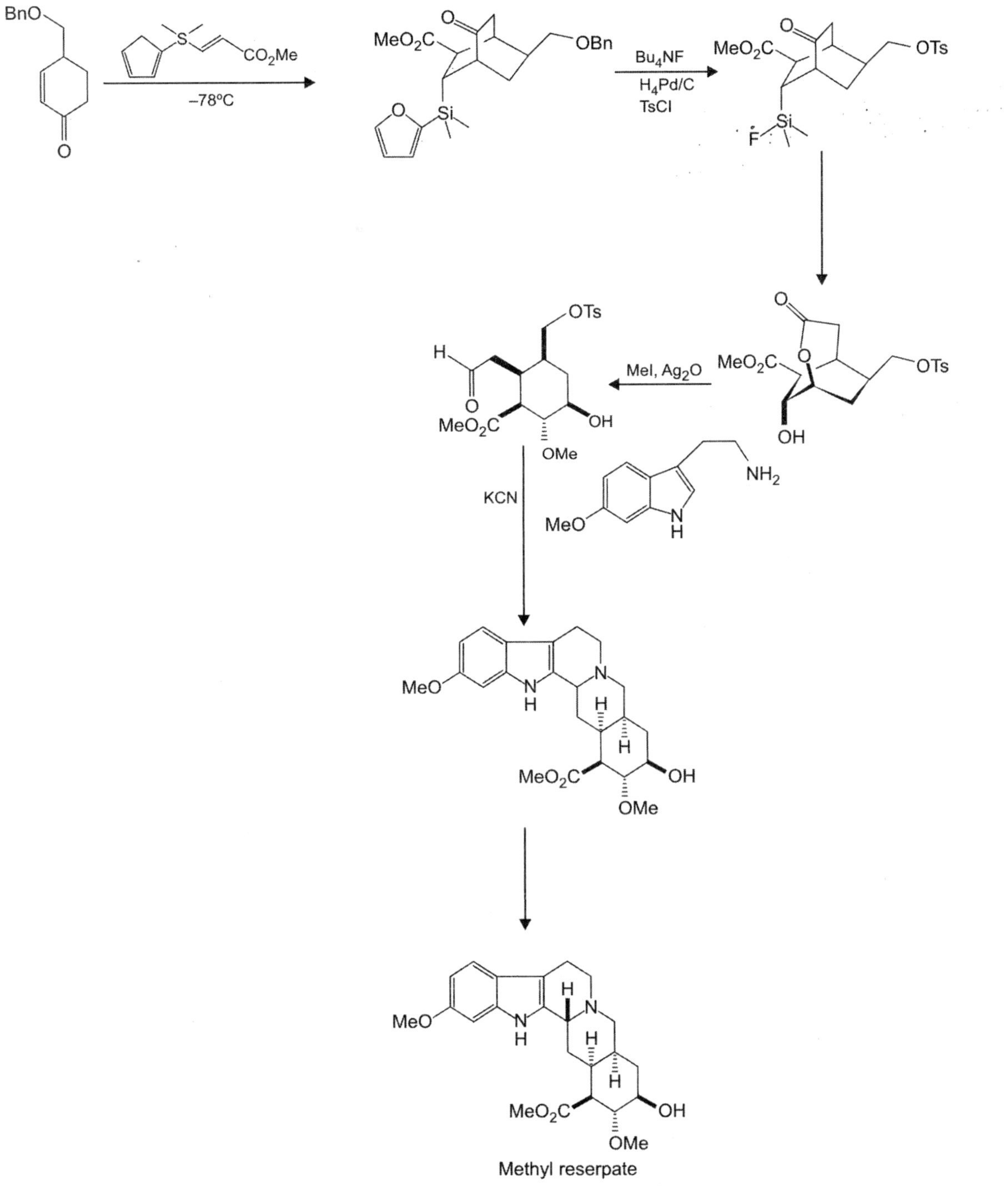

Fig. 2.10: Biosynthesis of reserpine

the motor nerves in the spinal cord which control muscle contraction.
- It can act as a stimulant and has been used by athletes to enhance their performance.
- It has been used as an analeptic, in the treatment of nonketotic hyperglycinemia and sleep apnea.
- Strychnine can act as a stimulant and has been used by athletes to enhance their performance (Fig. 2.11).

QUININE

(R)-[(2S,5R)-5-ehtenyl-1-azabicyclo[2,2,2]octan-2-yl]-(6-methoxyquinoline-4-yl) methanol.

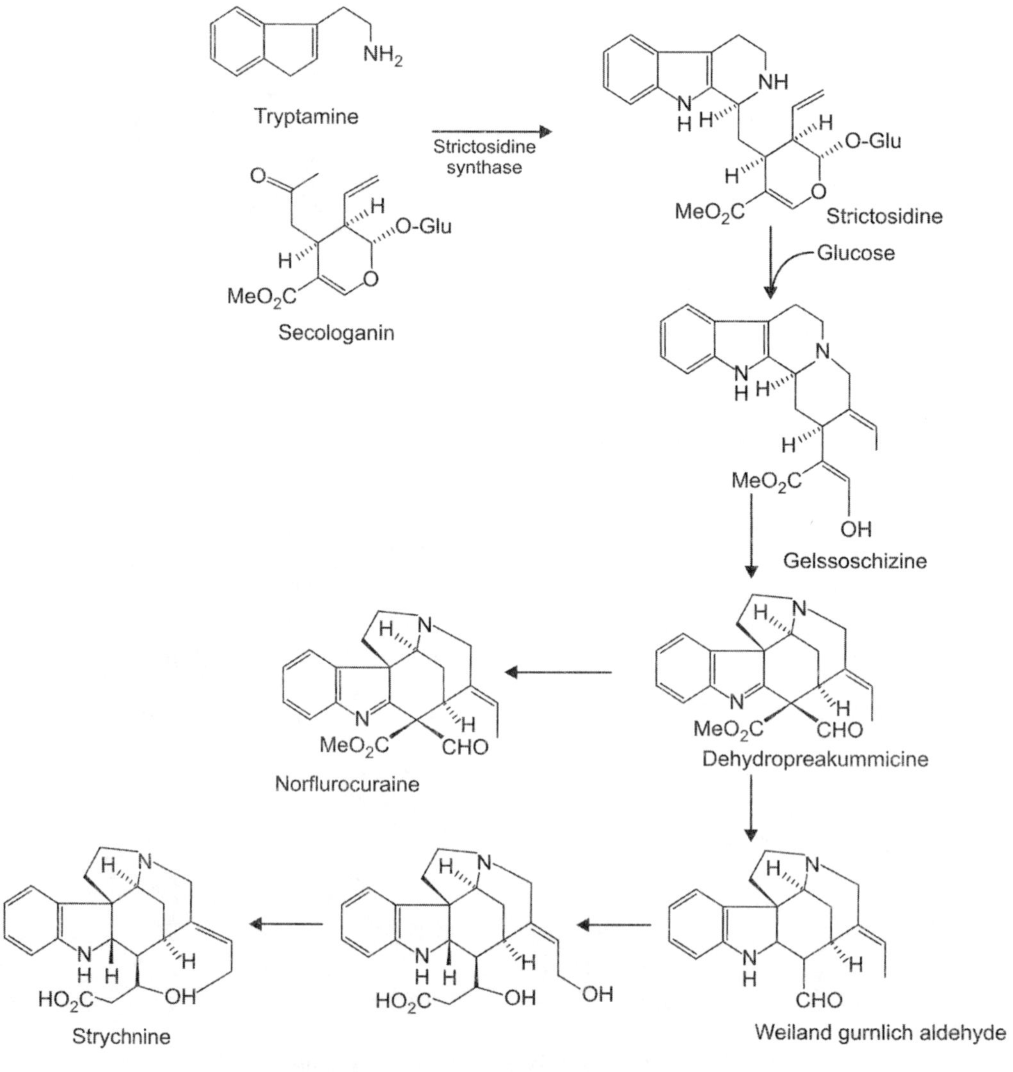

Fig. 2.11: Biosynthesis of strychnine

Chemistry

- Its molecular formula is $C_{20}H_{24}N_2O_2 \cdot 3H_2O$. It has methoxy group attached to the quinoline heterocyclic ring and specific rotation of 165° at 20°.
- Quinine forms two series of quarternery salts by absorbing two moles of CH_3I. It is mono-acetylated, monobenzylated and converted to monochloro derivative indicating presence of hydroxyl group.

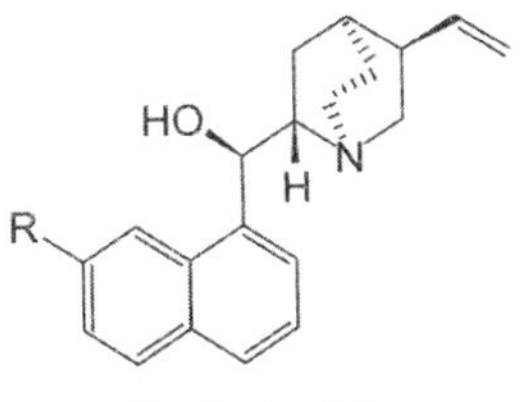

R= H, cinchonidine
R= OMe, quinine

Biological Source

Quinine is obtained from dried bark of the stem or of the root of *Cinchona succirubra, Cinchona calisaya, Cinchona ledgeriana* or *Cinchona officinalis* belonging to family Rubiaceae.

Pharmacology

Quinine is a mild antipyretic and analgesic and has been used in common cold preparations. It is used commonly as a bitter and flavoring agent, and is useful for the treatment of babesiosis. Quinine is also useful in some muscular disorders, especially nocturnal leg cramps and myotonia congenita, because of its direct effects on muscle membrane and sodium channels (Fig. 2.12).

MENTHOL (1R, 2S, 5R)-2-Isopropyl-5-methylcyclohexanol

Chemistry

Menthol is a waxy, crystalline substance, clear or white in color, which is solid at room temperature and melts slightly above. The

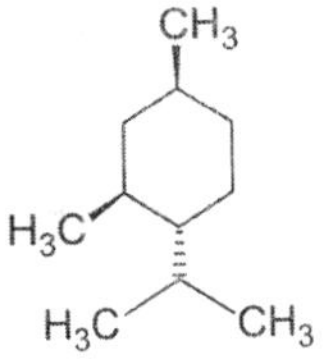

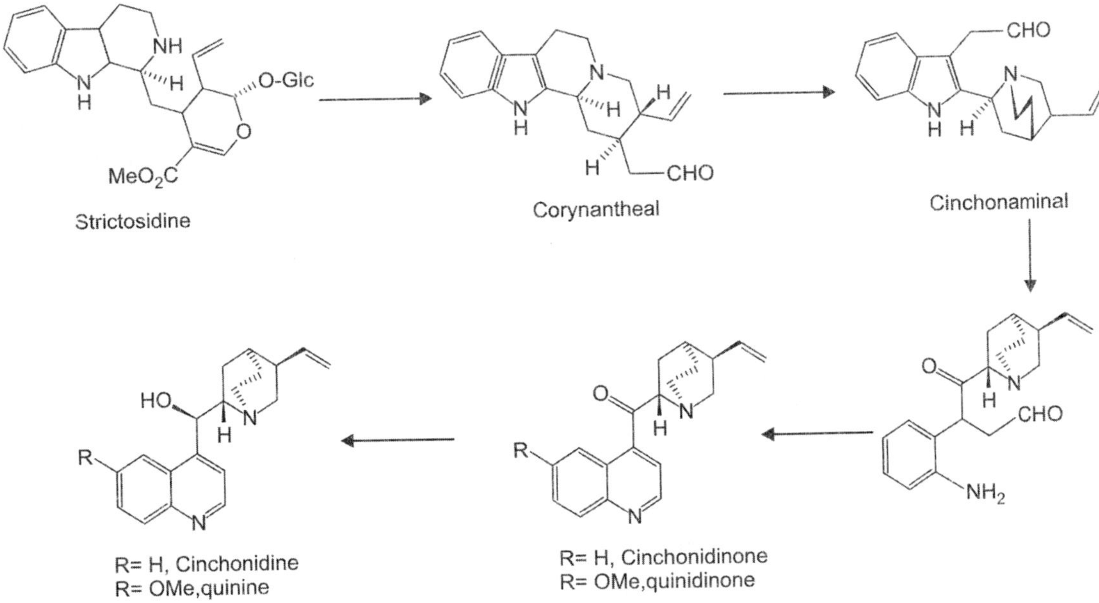

Strictosidine → Corynantheal → Cinchonaminal

R= H, Cinchonidine
R= OMe, quinine

R= H, Cinchonidinone
R= OMe, quinidinone

Fig. 2.12: Biosynthesis of quinine

main form of menthol occurring in nature is (–) menthol, which is assigned the (1R, 2S, 5R) configuration. Its molecular formula is $C_{10}H_{20}O$ and levorotatory in nature.

Biological Source

It is obtained by steam distillation of fresh flowering tops of *Mentha piperita* belonging to family Labiatae.

Pharmacological Activity

- Menthol helps to relieve pain, stress, and bacteria. When menthol is used topically, its analgesic properties can be used for muscle cramps, sprains, and headaches.
- It is used internally to alleviate nausea and motion sickness.
- Menthol is used as toothpaste and sunburn relief gels (Fig. 2.13).

CITRAL (3, 7-dimethyl-2, 6-octadienal).

Chemistry

Citral is a mixture of a pair of terpenoids with the molecular formula $C_{10}H_{16}O$. The two compounds are double bond isomers. The E-isomer is known as **geranial** or citral A. The Z-isomer is known as **neral** or citral B. Geranial has a strong lemon odor. Neral's lemon odor is less intense, but sweeter.

Biological Source

Citral is obtained from steam distillation of leaves and aerial parts of *Cymbopogon flexuousus* belonging to family Graminae.

Pharmacological Activity

- Citral is an aroma compound used in perfumery for its citrus effect.
- It is also used as a flavor and for fortifying lemon oil.
- It also has strong antimicrobial qualities, and pheromonal effects in insects.
- It is stimulant and carminative in action (Fig. 2.14).

TAXOL ($C_{47}H_{51}O_{14}N$)

Chemistry

Taxol (paclitaxel) is one of natural diterpenoid alkaloids.

Taxol biosynthetic pathway is considered to require 19 enzymatic steps from the universal diterpenoid precursor geranylgeranyl diphosphate.

The structural elements of taxol A, B and C rings, include the oxetane ring (D ring), the N-benzoyl-3-phenyl isoserine side chain appended to C13 of the A-ring, and the benzoate group at C2 of the B-ring.

Biological Source

Taxol is obtained from *Taxus brevifolia, Taxus cuspidate, Taxus Canadensis* and *Taxus baccata* belonging to family Taxaceae.

Pharmacological Activity

1. Taxol induces apoptosis and has anti-angiogenic property.
2. Paclitaxel is a chemotherapy drug usually given to treat ovarian, breast and non-small cell lung cancers.

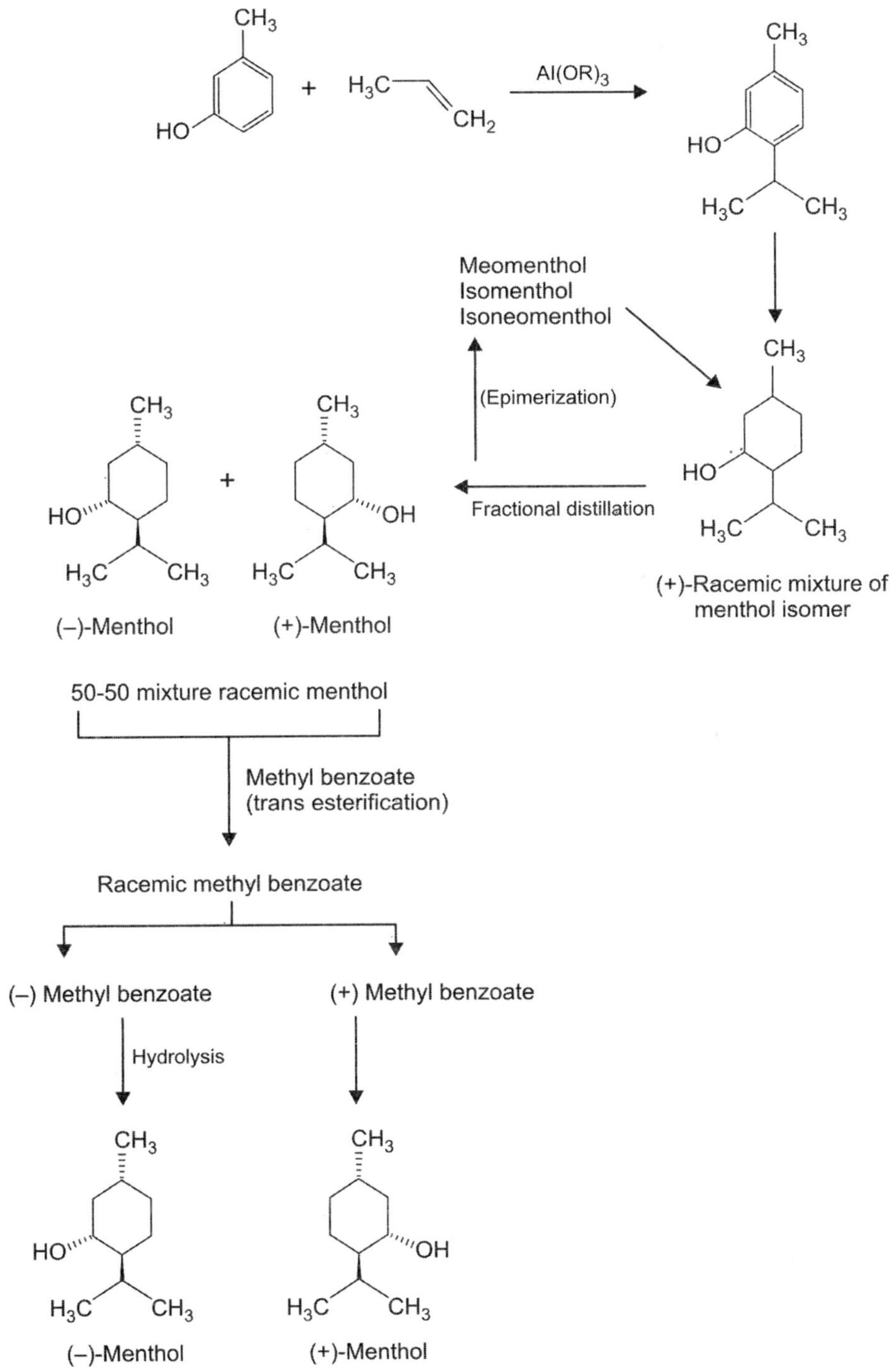

Fig. 2.13: Biosynthesis of menthol

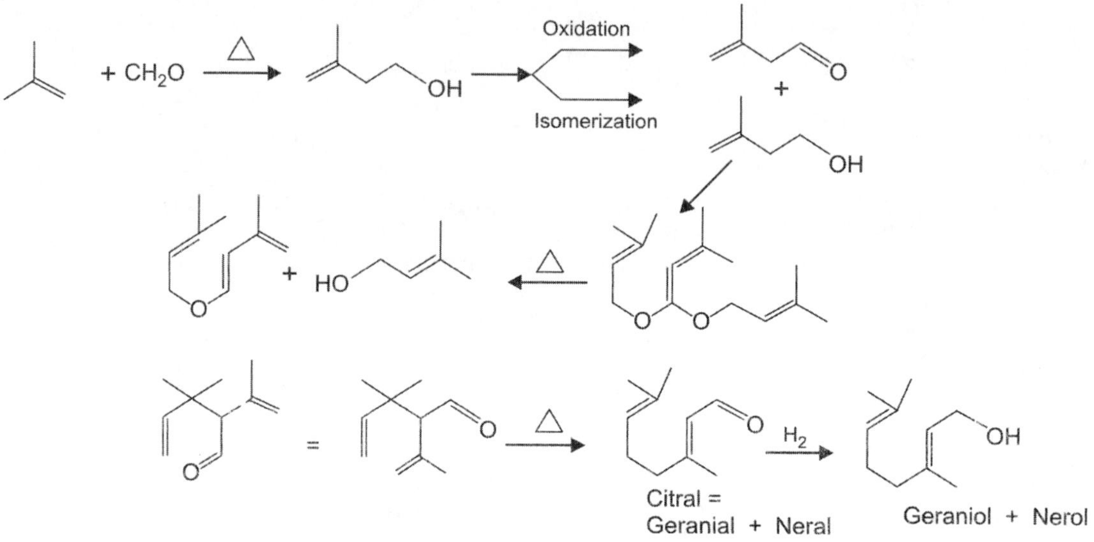

Fig. 2.14: Biosynthesis of citral

3. It has potential to treat lung, neck and head cancers.
4. Paclitaxel is a novel antimicrotubule agent that promotes the assembly of microtubules from tubulin dimers and stabilizes microtubules by preventing depolymerization (Fig. 2.15).

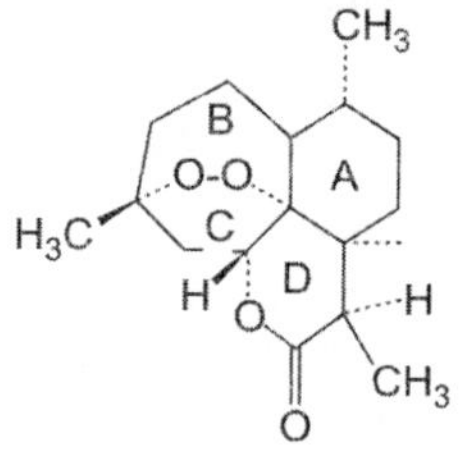

ARTEMISININ

(1R,4S,5R,8S,9R,12S,13R)-1,5,9-Trimethyl-11,14,15,16 tetraoxatetracyclo [10.3.1.0^{4,13}.0^{8,13}] hexadecan-10-one

Chemistry

- Chemically, artemisinin is a sesquiterpene lactone containing an unusual peroxide bridge.
- Artemisinin has poor solubility in either water or oil, and instead, it is soluble in many aprotic solvents.
- It is thermostable: even when the temperatures reaches its melting point at about 156–157°C, no obvious decomposition is observed.
- Artemisinin is unstable in the presence of alkali or acid, resulting in the generation of mixed products.

Biological Source

Artemisinin is obtained from leaves and aerial parts of *Artemisia annua* belonging to family Asteraceae.

Pharmacological Activity

- Artemisinin has become essential antimalarial drug for increasingly widespread drug-resistant malaria strains.
- It is anti-gametocyte and blocks sporogony.
- Antimalarial mechanism includes alkylation of heme by carbon-centered free

radicals, interference with proteins, such as the sarcoplasmic/endoplasmic calcium ATPase, as well as damaging of normal mitochondrial functions (Fig. 2.16).

RUTIN (quercetin-3-O-rutinoside).

Chemistry

- Rutin is rhamnoglucoside of quercetin which contains at C-3 position, the sugar rutinase.
- On hydrolysis, it yields quercetin, rhamnose and glucose.
- Microcrystalline greenish yellow tasteless powder, soluble in methanol, isopropyl alcohol, pyridines and solutions of alkali hydroxides.

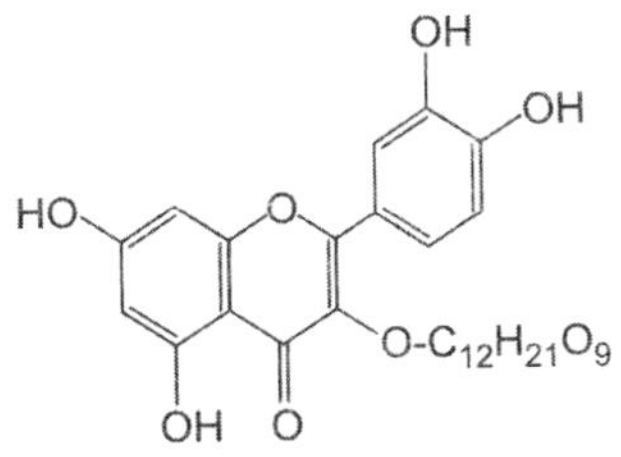

Biological Source

Rutin is obtained from *Fagopyrum esculentum* belonging to family Polygonaceae.

Pharmacological Activity

- Rutin inhibits platelet aggregation, as well as decreases capillary permeability, making the blood thinner and improving circulation.
- It shows anti-inflammatory activity in some animal and *in vitro* models.
- It inhibits aldose reductase activity. Aldose reductase is an enzyme normally present in the eye and elsewhere in the body. It helps change glucose into the sugar alcohol sorbitol.
- It also strengthens the capillaries and, therefore, can reduce the symptoms of hemophilia. It also may help to prevent a common, unpleasant-looking, venous edema of the legs; however, a double-blind clinical study on the effect of buckwheat tea containing rutin did not show a significant effect above placebo.
- It is also an antioxidant compared to quercetin, acacetin, morin, hispidulin, hesperidin, and naringin, it was found to be the strongest (Fig. 2.17).

DIGITOXIN

(3β,5β)-3-{[2,6-Dideoxy-α-D-ribo-hexo-pyranosyl-(1->4)-2,6-dideoxy-α-D-arabino-

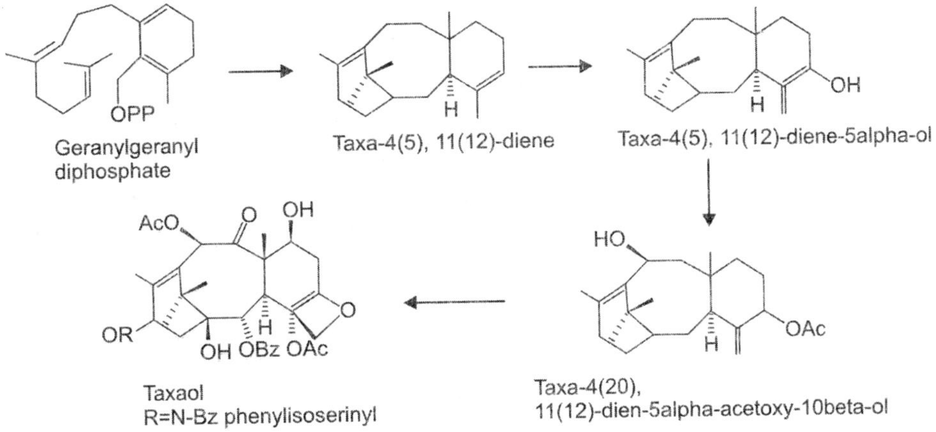

Fig. 2.15: Biosynthesis of taxol

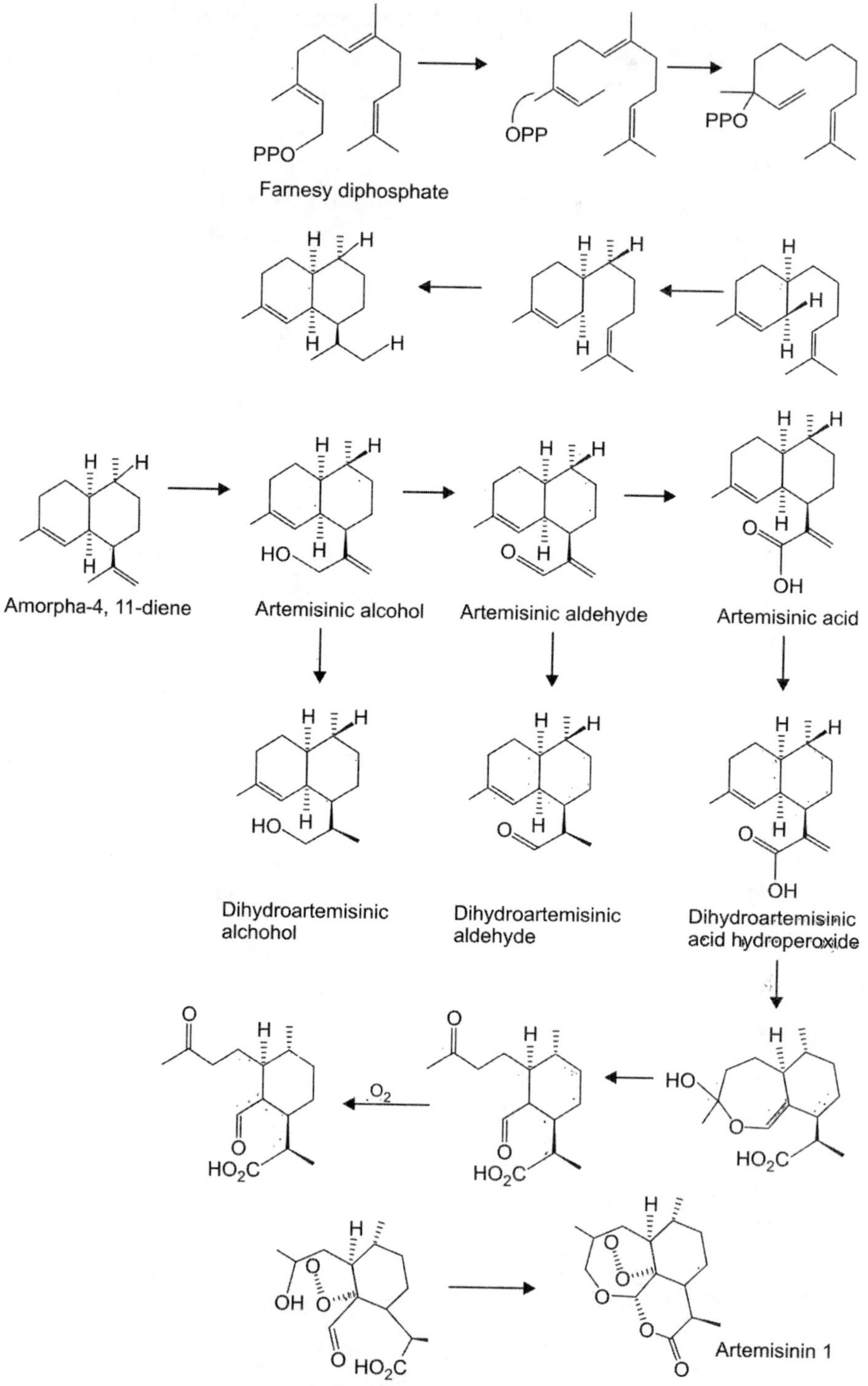

Fig. 2.16: Biosynthesis of artemisinin

hexopyranosyl-(1->4)-2,6-dideoxy-β-D-ribo-hexopyranosyl]oxy}-14-hydroxycard-20(22)-enolide.

Chemistry

- Its molecular composition is $C_{41}H_{64}O_{13}$.
- Digitoxin, glycosides on acid hydrolysis results in separation of aglycone/genin called as degitoxigenin and a sugar, digitoxose.
- The structure contains hydroxyl group at 14β carbon atom and unsaturated lactone ring at C-17β.
- Digitoxin contains basic structure of cardenolides, which contain sugar residues on 3β hydroxyl group (Fig. 2.18).

Biological Source

Digitoxin is obtained from leaves of *Digitalis purpurea* belonging to family Scorphulariaceae.

Pharmacological Activity

Digitoxin strongly stimulates the contraction of the heart. It is used in treatment of congestive heart failure. It produces inotropic effects and increases rapidity and force of systolic contraction of heart muscles, thus increasing cardiac output. The primary effect of digitoxin on heart is inhibition of sodium–potassium ATPase pump in the cell membranes of heart muscles. It produces anorexia, nausea and vomiting and diarrhea due to stimulation of chemoreceptor trigger zone (Fig. 2.19).

SENNOSIDES

(9R,9′R)-5,5′-Bis(β-D-glucopyranosyloxy)-4,4′-dihydroxy-10,10′-dioxo-9,9′,10,10′-tetrahydro-9,9′-bianthracene-2,2′-dicarboxylic acid.

Chemistry

- Sennosides are an anthracene derivative having molecular composition $C_{42}H_{38}O_{20}$.
- Aglycone of sennoside A is dextrorotatory while sennoside B is meso-form.
- The sugar moiety of glycosides also acts as a protector which prevents oxidation of aglycone.

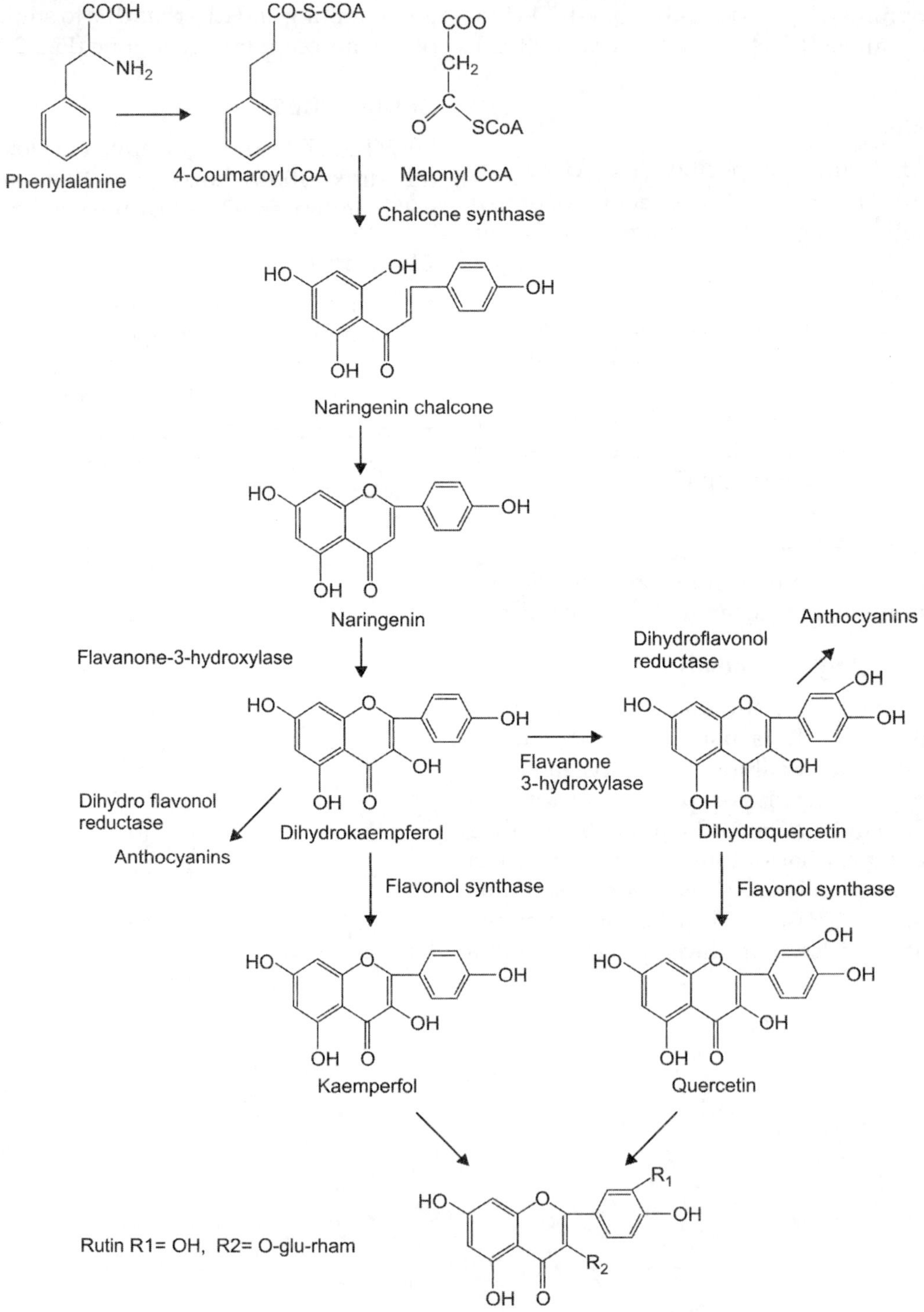

Fig. 2.17: Biosynthesis of rutin

Biological Source

Sennosides are obtained from leaves of *Cassia angustifolia* belonging to family Leguminosae.

Pharmacological Activity

- Sennosides are cathartic, with a similar mode of action as cascarosides. They are used as a febrifuge, anemia, typhoid, cholera, biliousness, jaundice, gout, rheumatism, tumors and probably in leprosy.
- They are employed in treatment of amoebic dysentery, and are used in constipation, abdominal disorders, leprosy, skin disorders, leuoderma, cough and bronchitis (Fig. 2.19).

SARSASAPOGENIN (3β,5β,25S)-23-Oxospirostan- 3-yl acetate

Chemistry

Sarsasapogenin is a steroidal sapogenin, that is the aglycosidic portion of a plant saponin. Sarsasapogenin has a *cis*-linkage between rings A and B of the steroid nucleus, as opposed to the more usual *trans*-linkage found in other saturated steroids. This 5β configuration is biologically significant, as a specific enzyme sarsasapogenin 3β-glucosyltransferase is found in several plants for the glycosylation of sarsasapogenin. The (S)-configuration at C-25 is also in contrast to other spirostan sapogenins: the epimer with a (25R)-configuration is known as smilagenin.

Biological Source

Sarsasapogenin obtained from plant of *Smilax aristolochiaefolia* belonging to family Liliaceae.

Pharmacological Activity

- Sarsaparilla is used to treat venereal diseases, herpes, arthritis, gout, epilepsy, insanity, chronic nervous diseases, abdominal distention, intestinal gas, debility, impotence and turbid urine.
- Sarsaparilla has been used worldwide for treating gout, syphilis, gonorrhea, wounds, fever, cough, scrofula, hypertension, digestive disorders, and cancer.
- The plant root is one of the ingredients in a range of herbal remedies prepared for skin disorders, libido enhancement, hormone balancing, and sports nutrition formulas (Fig. 2.20).

DIOSGENIN

(3β,25R)-Spirost-5-en-3-ol

Chemistry

Diosgenin, a steroid sapogenin, is the product of hydrolysis by acids, strong bases, or enzymes of saponins

Hydrolysis of this saponin leads to scission of the trisaccharide at the 3-position and the formation of the aglycone, diosgenin.

Oxidation by means of chromium trioxide leads to preferential attack at the electron-rich enol ether double bond. In effect, this transformation converts the side chain at C-17 in diosgenin to the acetyl group required for many steroid drugs.

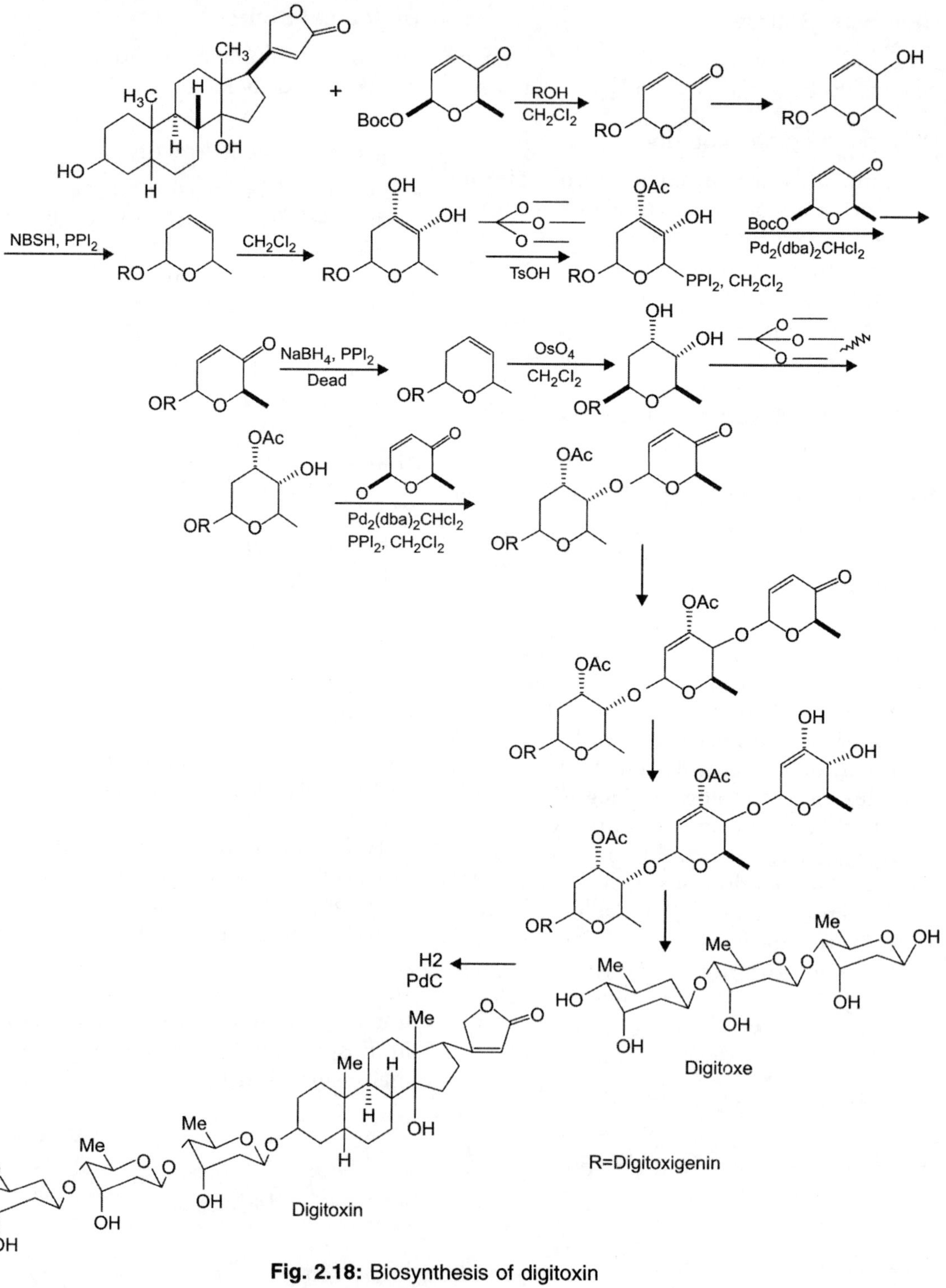

Fig. 2.18: Biosynthesis of digitoxin

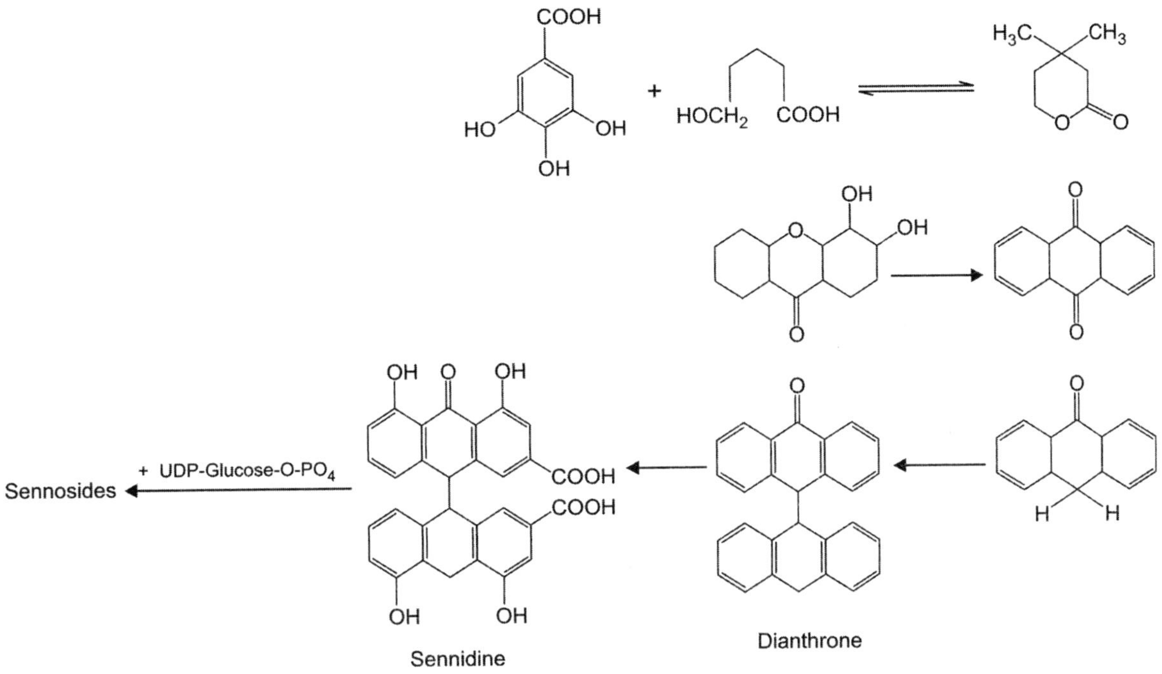

Fig. 2.19: Biosynthesis of sennosides

Biological Source

Diosgenin is obtained from dried tubers of *Dioscorea deltoidea* and *Dioscorea composita* belonging to family Dioscoreaceae.

Pharmacological Activity

- Diosgenin is used in treatment of rheumatic arthritis.
- It produces synergistic effect on the body and increases activity of ciliary epithelium.
- It is a precursor to progesterone, and was once used to make birth control pills.
- It improves immune system and reduces autoimmune disorders.
- It stops illness or death from coronary artery diseases.
- It reduces the symptoms of menopause (Fig. 2.21).

RADIOACTIVE TRACER TECHNIQUE

Biosynthesis: Biosynthesis is an enzyme-catalyzed process in cells of living organisms by which substrates are converted to more complex products. It is a phenomenon where chemical compounds are produced from simpler reagents. Biosynthesis, unlike chemical synthesis, takes place within living organisms and is generally catalysed by enzymes. The synthesis generally consumes energy, usually in the form of ATP. The process is vital part of metabolism.

Biogenesis: Biogenesis is a process in which life forms arise from similar life forms. It asserts that living things can only be produced by another living thing, and not by a non-living thing.

The various biosynthetic reactions occurring in plant cells are enzyme-dependent, wherein, enzymes act as catalysts of metabolism and through the control of enzymatic activity that plant metabolite is directed into specific

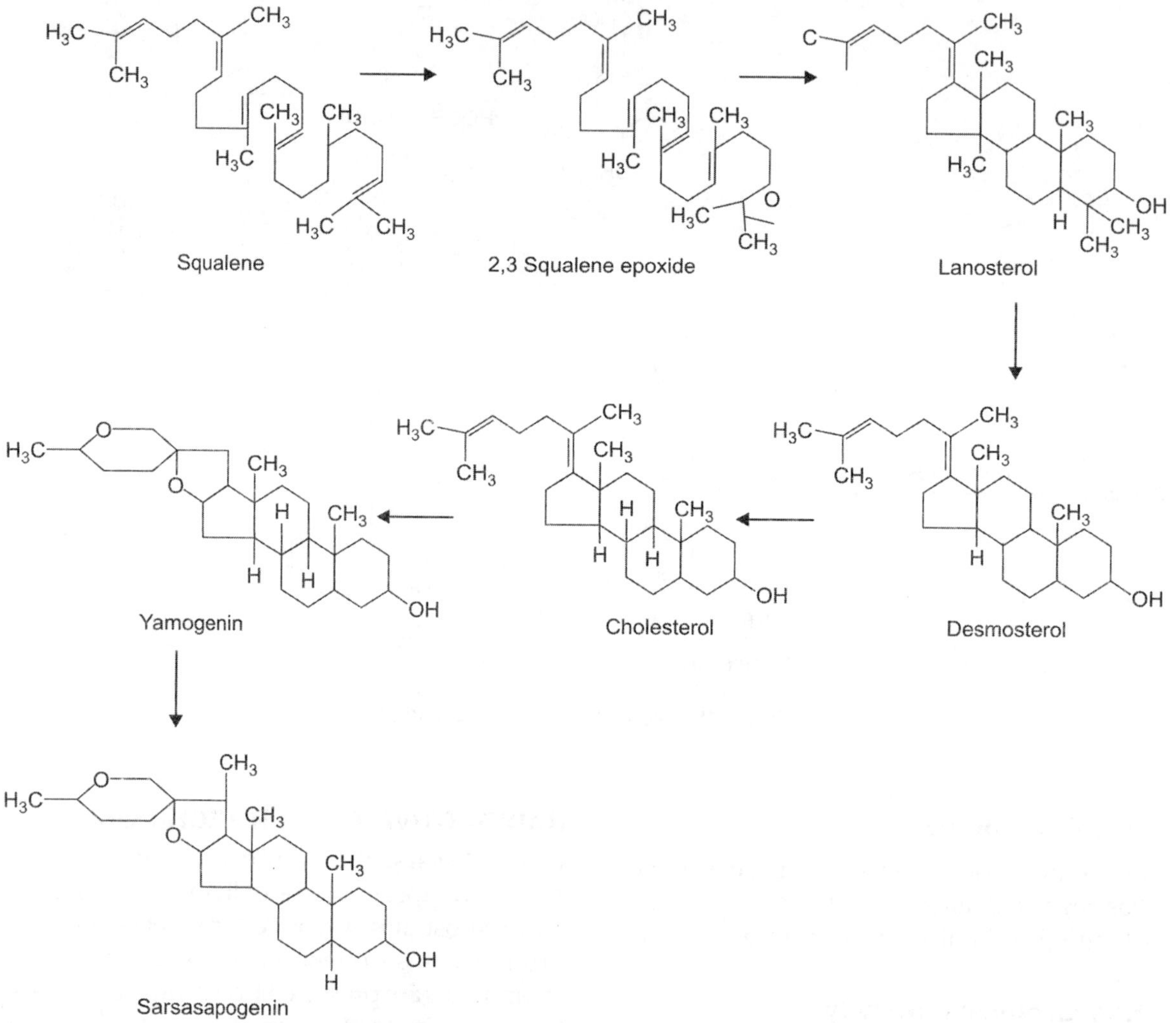

Fig. 2.20: Biosynthesis of sarsasapogenin

biosynthetic pathways. The enzyme reactions are reversible and in plants, many a time, the secondary metabolites are synthesized and hydrolyzed under the influence of more or less specific enzymes. The **biosynthetic pathways** are sequence of enzymatic reactions occurring in plants to finally synthesize secondary metabolites. Therefore, the production of secondary metabolites can be improved by studying biosynthetic pathway.

Thus by knowing the precursor (starting materials) for the synthesis of secondary metabolites and feeding the same precursor may lead to increase in final concentration of that particular secondary metabolites, e.g. ornithine (amino acids) is the precursor for the synthesis of tropan alkaloids (e.g. atropine, hyoscine, etc.) thus the yield can be increased by either feeding ornithine by any other intermediate formed in biosynthesis.

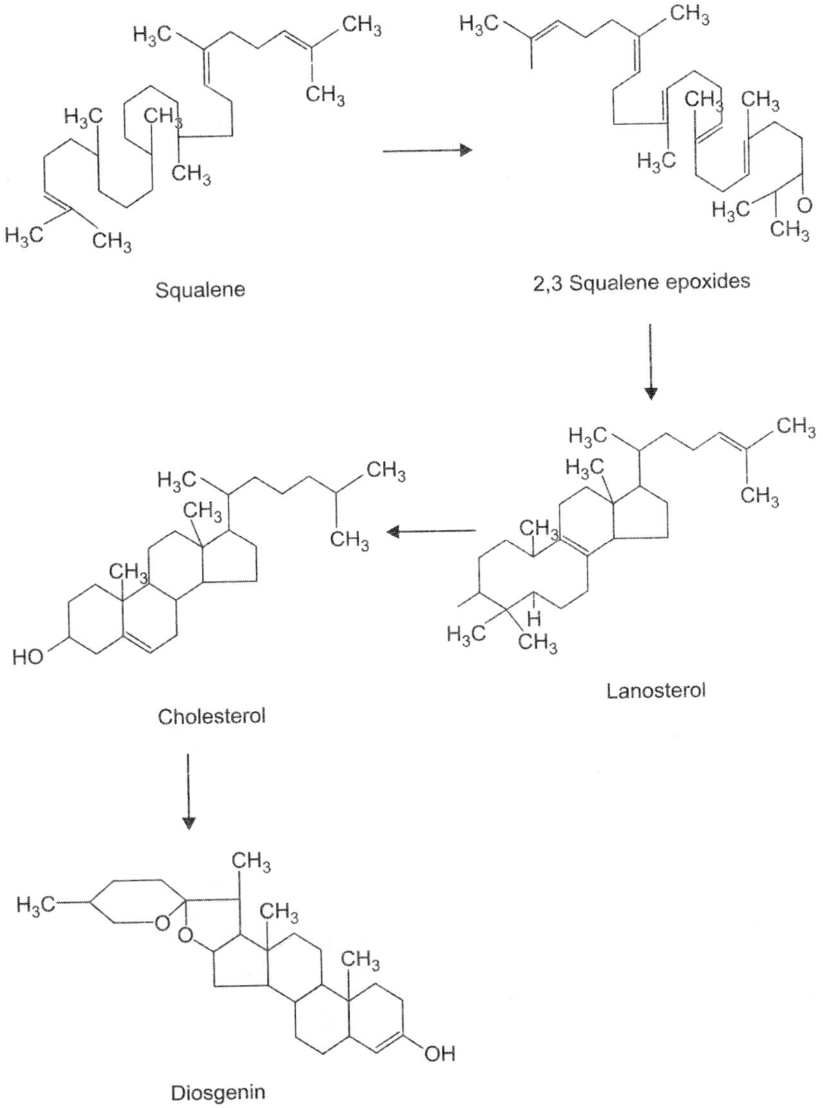

Fig. 2.21: Biosynthesis of diosgenin

Techniques used for investigation of biosynthetic pathway are:

- Tracer technique
- Use of isolated organ and tissue
- Grafting method
- Use of mutant strain
- Enzymatic studies

Tracer techniques: Tracer technology now widely employed in all branches of sciences. This technique exists with the concept of element with same chemical proportion, i.e. same atomic number but different atomic weight called isotopes.

Application of tracer techniques

- This technique uses the labeled compound to trace the different intermediates and

various steps in biosynthetic processes in plant at given rate and given time.
- Location and quantity of compound can be determined.
- Nitrogen atom is used for studies of alkaloids, amino acids and protein.
- O, N, S and C atoms for glycosidic linkage.
- O atom for study of terpenoids.

Various methods involved in tracer technology
- Radioactive tracers
- Detection and assay of radio actively labeled compounds.
- Autoradiography
- Precursor product sequences
- Competitive feeding
- Administration of precursor
- Sequential analysis
- Use of stable isotopes.

Basic steps involved in tracer techniques
- Preparation of labeled compound
- Incorporation of labeled compound to tissue system
- Separation and isolation of labeled compound from tissue system.
- Detection and assay of radioactive labeled compounds.

Preparation of labeled compound/radioactive tracer

The labeled compound may prepared by use of radioactive isotopes and stable isotopes. Radioisotopes are unstable isotopes which decay and give out radioactive emissions. Isotopes are either stable or unstable.

Stable: ^2H, ^{13}C, ^{15}N, ^{18}O

Unstable: ^1H, ^{14}C (decay with the emission of radiations).

Advantages of using radioactive tracer
- Radioactive tracers are easy to detect and measure the high precision to sensitive of 10^{-16} to 10^{-6} g.
- Radioactivity is independent of temperature, pressure, chemical and physical state.
- Radiotracers do not affect the system and can be used in non-destructive techniques.
- If the tracer is technically pure, then interference from other elements is of no concern.
- For most radioisotopes, the radiation can be measured independently of the matrix, eliminating the need of calibrating curves.

Applications of Radioactive Isotopes

Radioisotopes have a wide range of applications including medicine, agriculture, archeology and industry.

Medicine: A radioisotope is taken in by the patient through the digestive system, by inhalation or through the blood vessels by injection. The radiation emitted enables organs, such as the thyroid, bones, heart or liver to be easily imaged by imaging equipment. Disorders in their function can then be detected.

Agriculture: Radioisotopes have many uses in the field of agriculture. By measuring the radioactivity of the stem and leaves, scientists can find out how much fertiliser has been absorbed by the plant. Radioisotopes are also used to kill pests and parasites and to control the ripening of fruits.

Archeology: The amount of carbon-14 left in a decayed plant or animal can be used to tell its age. One of the most important uses of radioisotopes in archeology is carbon-14 dating. Carbon-14 is a radioisotope with a half-life of 5730 years and decays by emitting α-particles.

Industries: Industries have found many uses for radioisotopes. γ-rays can be used to penetrate deep into weldings to detect faults. Water can be made radioactive by dissolving some radioactive salt which contains sodium-24. The β-particles emitted are detected by a GM tube. The α-particles from polonium-210 is used to neutralise static charge in photographic plates and other materials.

Introduction of labeled compound to tissue system

The six methods are used to labeled compound to tissue systems are:
- Root feeding
- Stem feeding
- Direct injection
- Infiltration
- Floating method
- Spraying technique

Separation and isolation of labeled compounds

The method of extraction employed depends on nature of drug (Table 2.7).

Type of solvent depends on the chemical nature of the drug

Fat and oil: Non-polar solvents.

Alkaloids, glycosides and flavonoids: Slightly polar solvents.

Plant phenol: Polar solvents.

The separation techniques used are column chromatography, partition and fractional crystallization.

Detection and assay of radioactive labeled compounds

When the radioactive tracers are used in biogenetic studies, depending on nature of isotopes, various instrumentation methods for detection and estimation of label are essential (Table 2.8).

The liquid scintillation counter is used for soft and easily absorbed radiation. The advantage of detector is tremendous due to development of photomultiplier tube. In scintillation counting, the sample is mixed with a material that will fluoresce upon interaction with a particle emitted by

Table 2.6: Properties of some radioactive isotopes

Natural	Radioactive	Toxicity	Radiation	Half life
C^{12}	C^{14}	Medium	Beta	5760 yrs
I^{127}	I^{131}	Medium	Beta, gamma	8.04 days
H^1	H^3	Low	Beta	12.43 years
S^{32}	S^{35}	Medium	Beta	87.4 days
P^{31}	P^{32}	Medium	Beta	14.3 days

Table 2.7: Extraction method for plant materials

Type of plant material	Extraction method
Soft and fresh tissue	Infusion and decoction
Hard tissue	Decoction and hot percolation
Unorganized drug	Maceration

Table 2.8: Instrumentation methods for isotopes

For radioactive isotopes	For stable isotopes
Liquid scintillation counter	Mass spectroscopy
Ionization chamber	NMR
GM-counters	

radioactive decay. The scintillation counter quantifies the resulting flashes of light. The principle of this method is to convert the radioactive emissions from a sample to photons of visible light that a photomultiplier tube can detect.

GM tube and an ionization chamber work on similar principles but there are some important differences. GM tubes can detect single particles but take time to recover after each count so cannot measure very high activities. Ionization chambers are not good at measuring very low levels of radioactivity but will cope with very high levels.

Methods in Tracer Techniques

1. Autoradiography: Autoradiography records the distribution of radioactive materials in botanical and histological specimens placed in contact with a photographic emulsion. This technique has been applied to the study of metabolism of plants and animals; it records the activity of organic compounds of radioactive isotopes introduced into the biological system.

Advantages: Highly specific technically easy tool to pharmacologically characterize receptors in tissue (unlike tissue bath preparations); provides location of receptor (etc.) in tissue; enables characterization of receptors in different tissues between different animals or brain regions.

Disadvantages: There is no biochemical or physiological criteria to assess the binding specificity (i.e. to determine whether the binding site really corresponds to an actual receptor), the presence of a high-affinity radiolabeled receptor does not necessarily imply that the receptor has physiological significance and ligands are not always very specific.

Autoradiography Method

- Living cells are briefly exposed to a 'pulse' of a specific radioactive compound.
- The tissue is left for a variable time.
- Samples are taken, fixed, and processed for light or electron microscopy.
- Sections are cut and overlaid with a thin film of photographic emulsion.
- Left in the dark for days or weeks (while the radioisotope decays). This exposure time depends on the activity of the isotope, the temperature and the background radiation (this will produce with time a contaminating increase in 'background' silver grains in the film).
- The photographic emulsion is developed (as for conventional photography).
- Counterstaining, e.g. with toluidine blue, shows the histological details of the tissue. The staining must be able to penetrate, but not have an adverse effect on the emulsion.
- Alternatively, pre-staining of the entire block of tissue can be done (e.g. with osmium on plastic sections coated with stripping film [or dipping emulsion] as in papers by McGeachie and Grounds) before exposure to the photographic emulsion. This avoids the need for individually (post-) staining each slide.
- It is not necessary to coverslip these slides.
- The position of the silver grains in the sample is observed by light or electron microscopy. *Note:* The grains are in a different plane of focus in the emulsion overlying the tissue section. Often oil with a × 100 objective is used for detailed observation with the light microscope.
- These autoradiographs provide a permanent record.

Uses

- Map anatomical location of radiolabelled ligands to visualize and quantify receptors in tissue.

- Trace neurons by axonal transport of radioactively labelled amino acids, certain sugars, or transmitter substances.
- Measure DNA production (e.g. 3H-thymidine).

2. Precursor product sequence: This method is used for the elucidation of biosynthetic pathways in plants by means of labeled compounds.

Procedure: In this method, precursor of constituents under investigation in labeled form is fed to plants. After suitable time, constituent is isolated and purified and radioactivity is determined.

Application: This method is extensively employed for biogenesis of morphine and ergot alkaloids.

3. Competitive feeding: Competitive feeding is normally used to determine two possible intermediates in plants. If the incorporation is obtained, it is still necessary to consider the fact that is normal route of synthesis of plant not a subsidiary pathway (Fig. 2.22).

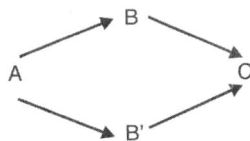

Fig. 2.22: Competitive feeding

Competitive feeding could distinguish whether B or B' was the normal intermediate in formation of C from A.

4. Sequential analysis: The main principle of this method is investigation of plant grown in $^{14}CO_2$ atmosphere and by analysis of the plant at given time interval, to obtain the sequence in various related compound become labeled.

Application: It is used in elucidation of the path of carbon in photosynthesis and also for determined the sequential formation of the opium, hemlock and tobacco alkaloids. Some variation of intermediates can be obtained from this method.

5. Use of stable isotopes: The stable isotopes like ^2H, ^{13}C, ^{15}N and ^{18}O which have a low natural occurrence can also be used as other radioactive isotopes for labeling compounds to be used as possible intermediates in biosynthetic pathways.

The usual methods of detection are:
- Mass spectroscopy (^{15}N, ^{18}O)
- NMR spectroscopy (^2H, ^{13}C).

6. Isolated organs tissue and cells: Isolated organs tissue and cells are grown on nutrient media aseptically are being utilized for elucidation of biosynthetic pathways of secondary metabolites.

Advantages and disadvantages: Isolated cells generally more closely mimic intact animal systems. Isolated cells are potentially very useful in metabolism studies because: (1) they retain the various metabolizing enzymes; (2) they contain coenzymes and cosubstrates at physiological concentrations; and (3) they have intact cell membranes and intracellular particles. Disadvantages include the difficulty of preparation, the short period of viability and difficulties in cryopreservation.

Uses: It is used in feeding experiments in conjugation with labeled compounds and is useful for determination of site and synthesis of particular compounds.

7. Grafting: This technique is used in biosynthetic studies, particularly for determination of the sites of primary and secondary metabolism of some secondary plant products.

Examples: Tomato scions in Datura stocks (accumulate tobacco alkaloids). Datura scions on tomato stocks (only small amount of tropane alkaloids).

8. Mutant strains: The use of mutant strains is useful in biosynthetic studies and has proved to be important in investigations. The mutant strains are produced by either chemical or physical means.

Physical: Radiations and; *Chemical:* Colchicin.

Example:
- UV-induced mutant of ergot which number of amino acids have been produced.
- A mutant of Lactobacillus acidophilus has ability to utilize constituents of brewer soluble but not acetal led to isolation of melvonic acid an important intermediate of Isopremoid compound pathway.

3

Medicinal and Aromatic Plant Substances

CULTIVATION OF MEDICINAL PLANTS

The principle of cultivation is to turn the soil into a fine tilth to provide the ideal environment for seeds to germinate. Cultivation was also a traditional form of weed control. Cultivation may be used in crusted soils to increase soil aeration and infiltration of water; it may also be used to move soil to or away from plants as desired. Cultivation among crop plants is best kept at a minimum; excessive cultivation can be harmful as it may cause root pruning and loss of soil water due to increased evaporation. Most of medicinal plants, even today, are collected from wild. The continued commercial exploitation of these plants has resulted in receding the population of many species in their natural habitat. It is necessary to initiate systematic cultivation of medicinal plants in order to conserve biodiversity and protect endangered species. In the pharmaceutical industry, where the active medicinal principle cannot be synthesized economically, the product must be obtained from the cultivation of plants. Systematic conservation and large scale cultivation of the concerned medicinal plants are thus of great importance. Efforts are also required to suggest appropriate cropping patterns for the incorporation of these plants into the conventional agricultural and forestry cropping systems. Cultivation of this type of plants could only be promoted, if there is a continuous demand for the raw materials. In order to initiate systematic cultivation of medicinal and aromatic plants, high yielding varieties have to be selected.

Advantages and disadvantages of cultivation are described in Table 3.1.

Table 3.1: Advantages and disadvantages of cultivation

Advantages of cultivation Cultivation is conducted for a variety of good reasons.	Disadvantages of cultivation Cultivation has the potential to destroy soil structure and make soils more prone to other forms of degradation, such as erosion
• It roughens the soil surface thus it can help to retain moisture. • It is often a form of weed control. • It can play a part in pest management • It may be required to incorporate herbicides and soil ameliorants, such as lime. • It may reduce the incidence of soil-borne diseases like rhizoctonia. • It reduces soil strength. High soil strength is one reason for poor seedling vigour in direct-drilled crops on poorly structured soils.	• There may be a reduction in soil organic matter and, therefore, a decline in soil structure. • Cultivation that mixes surface soil with sub-surface soil will lead to a dilution of organic matter. • Cultivation can make hardsetting and crusting problems worse. Since soil organic matter and stable aggregates are destroyed. • Cultivation can bring sodic material to the soil surface. This can cause or increase soil crusting.

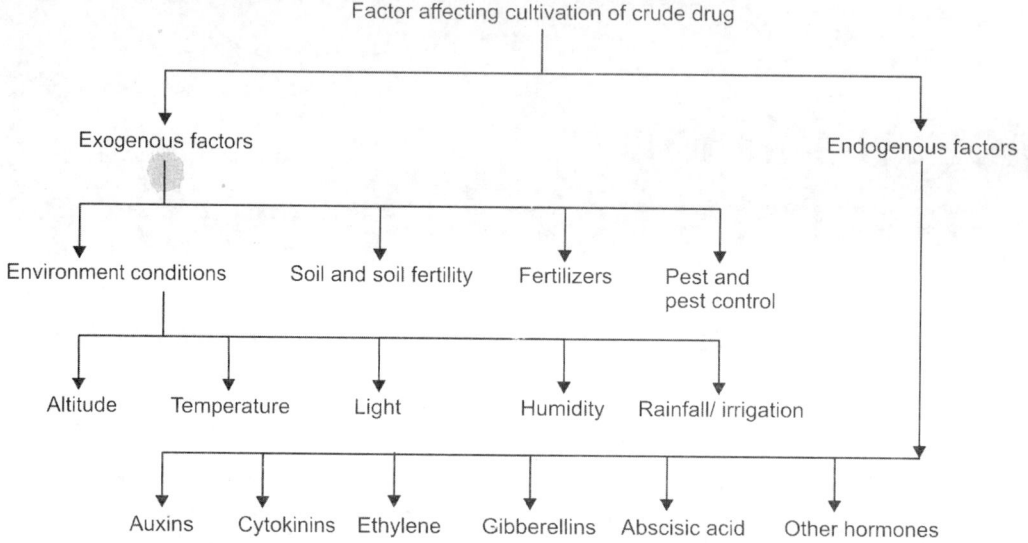

Fig. 3.1: Factor affecting cultivation of crude drug

FACTORS AFFECTING CULTIVATION

Cultivation of medicinal and aromatic plants takes cognizance of plants habitats and climatic requirements for favorable growth. The factor affecting are described in Fig 3.1

Environmental Conditions

The environmental conditions are the basic requirement to control plant growth and development. The type of vegetation, climatic conditions and environmental factors affect growth and development of the plants. The factors affecting plant growth altitude.

Light

The most important ecological factor affecting plant growth is light which is ultimate source of energy. Any variations in intensity, quality and duration affect plant growth. Light is necessary for photosynthesis, the process that converts light energy into chemical energy. Amount and intensity of light needed differs from herb to herb. The day length affects the amount of glycosides, alkaloids and volatile oils produced.

Example: Under long-day conditions, peppermint leaves contain menthone, menthol and traces of menthofuran; whereas under short-day conditions, contain menthofuran as a main component of volatile oil. Furthermore, a long photoperiod for young leaves activates the reduction pathway with conversion of menthone to menthol.

Example: Belladonna, stramonium and cinchona produce higher content of alkaloids in sunshine.

Light intensity varies greatly with season and time of day because of changes in the angle of incidence of the sun's rays and the distance light travels through the atmosphere. Light intensity also varies with the amount of humidity and cloud cover because atmospheric moisture absorbs and scatters light rays. However, the greatest variation in intensity of light received by range plants results from the various degrees of shading from other plants. Because most range plants require full sunlight or very high levels of sunlight for best growth, shading can reduce or limit growth of range plants. Duration of sunlight (day-length period

Table 3.2: Difference between long-day and short-day plants

Long-day plants	Short-day plants
Cool-season plants are long-day plants	Warm-season plants are short-day plants
Long-day plants reach the flowering stage after exposure to a critical photoperiod during the period of increasing daylight between the beginning of active growth and mid-June and usually flowering before 21 June	Short-day plants are induced into flowering by day lengths that are shorter than a critical length and that occur during the period of decreasing day-length after mid-June and usually flowering after 21 June
Long-day plants are technically responding to the increase in the length of the day period.	Short-day plants are technically responding to the increase in the length of night period rather than to the decrease in the day length.

or photoperiod) is one of the most dependable factor by which plants time their activities in temperate zones. The buds or leaves of a plant contain sensory receptors, specially pigmented areas that detect day-length and night-length and can activate one or more hormones and enzyme systems that bring about physiological responses.

Differences between long-day and short-day plants are described in Table 3.2.

Temperature

The important factor for plant biological activity and growth is temperature which is an approximate measurement of the heat energy. The growth occurs within only a narrow range of temperatures, between 32°F (0°C) and 122°F (50°C). High temperatures limit biological reactions because the complex structures of proteins are disrupted or denatured. Although respiration and photosynthesis can continue slowly at temperatures well below 32°F, if plants are physiologically "hardened", low temperatures limit biological reactions because water becomes unavailable when it is frozen and because available energy is inadequate. Low temperatures define the length of the active growing season. Perennial plants maintain physiological processes throughout the year. Winter dormancy in perennial plants is not total inactivity but reduced activity. Perennial grassland plants can grow actively beyond the frost-free period, if temperatures are above the level that freezes water in plant tissue and soil. Perennial plants begin active growth more than 30 days before the last frost in spring and continue growth after the first frost in fall; the growing season for perennial plants is considered to be between the first 5 consecutive days in spring and the last 5 consecutive days in fall with a mean daily temperature at or above 32°F (0°C), generally from mid-April through mid-October. Low air temperature during the early and late portions of the growing season and high temperatures after mid-summer greatly limit plant growth. Different plant species have different optimum temperature ranges. Cool-season plants, which are C_3 photosynthetic pathway plants, have an optimum temperature range of 50° to 77°F (10° to 25°C). Warm-season plants, which are C_4 photosynthetic pathway plants, have an optimum temperature range of 86° to 105°F (30° to 40°C).

Example: *Datura stramonium* produces lower alkaloids in cloudy/rainy weather (winter).

Volatile oils are produced more readily in warmer weather, yet very hot days lead to a physical loss of oil. Peppermint cultivation is done in shade rather than the sun.

Altitude

Altitude is the height of plant from the sea level. Altitude is very important factor in cultivation of medicinal plants. Vegetable plant growth is more under irrigated condition at lower altitude. Flower production is also affected by location (altitude). As altitude increases gentian (bitter constituents) increases. Thyme and peppermint constituents decrease with altitude. Fat/oil production may be influenced by latitudes (Table 3.3).

Example: Peanut and olive trees grown in the subtropics have a higher unsaturated fat content.

Table 3.3: Effect of altitude on cultivation of plants

Plant	Altitude (meters)
Saffron	Up to 1250
Clove	Up to 900
Coffee	1000–2000
Cinnamon	250–1000
Tea	1000–1500
Camphor	1500–2000

Humidity

Water, an integral part of living systems, is ecologically important because it is a major force in shaping climatic patterns and biochemically important because it is a necessary component in physiological processes. Water is the principal constituent of plant cells, usually composing over 80% of the fresh weight of herbaceous plants. Water is the primary solvent in physiological processes by which gases, minerals, and other materials enter plant cells and by which these materials are translocated to various parts of the plant. Water is the substance in which processes, such as photosynthesis and other biochemical reactions, occur and a structural component of proteins and nucleic acids. Water is also essential for the maintenance of the rigidity of plant tissue and for cell enlargement and growth in plants.

Plants in water stress have limited growth and reduced photosynthetic activity. Plant vigor is decreased, carbohydrate storage is reduced, and root biomass is reduced. Plant height and herbage biomass accumulation are reduced. Leaf senescence increases and, as a result, nutritional quality of forage decreases. The rate of sexual reproduction is diminished as a result of a decrease in seed stalk numbers and height and a reduction in numbers of seeds in the seed heads. Rate of vegetative reproduction is reduced because the number of axillary buds and the number of secondary tillers decrease (Table 3.4).

Table 3.4: Effect of climate on plants

Plant	Climate
Pyrethum	Dry weather
Saffron	Cold
Camphor and coffee	Cannot withstand frost

Rainfall and Irrigation

Plants use a tremendous amount of water. Water requirement for rice is 300 to 950 mm; for sorghum, it is 300 to 650 mm. Rains, to a major extent, provide this water through the soil for the development and growth of plants. Rainfall is the first source of water. Irrigation can supplement rainfall to supply crop water needs. Irrigation is a primary component in photosynthesis and respiration, it is needed for the physiological processes to complete plant life cycle, i.e. seed to seed. It is responsible for turgor pressure in cells and maintains temperature of plant body. The water helps in the uptake of nutrients from soil. It serves as a medium through which nutrients and other solutes move in the plants.

Thus, water from rainfall is vital for plant growth. Equally damaging is excess rainfall causes flooding of fields and water stagnation affects the growth processes. Continuous rain during flowering time affects fertilization,

Grain formation and filling, favors plant diseases and pests, interferes with many farming operations like: seedbed preparation, sowing, harvesting, threshing, and processing of crops. Lastly, it results in low crop yields.

Soil and its Fertility

Soil is the unconsolidated mineral or organic material on the immediate surface of the earth and serves as a natural medium for the growth of land plants. A soil consists of mineral matter, organic matter and pore space, which is shared by air, water and life forms. In addition to the above constituents, the soil also contains a large and varied population of micro-organism and macro-organisms. Soil is crucial for plant and life. It supports plant roots and provides essential nutrients for plant growth. All soils contain four major elements that are given in Table 3.5.

Table 3.5: Composition of soil with its volume

Components	Volume
Air	20–30%
Soil solution	20–30%
Mineral fraction	45%
Organic matter	5%

Soil fertility is a complex quality of soils that is closest to plant nutrient management. It is the component of overall soil productivity that deals with its available nutrient status, and its ability to provide nutrients out of its own reserves and through external applications for crop production. It combines several soil properties (biological, chemical and physical), all of which affect directly or indirectly nutrient dynamics and availability. Soil fertility is a manageable soil property and its management is of utmost importance for optimizing crop nutrition on both a short-term and a long-term basis to achieve sustainable crop production. Soil productivity is the ability of a soil to support crop production determined by the entire spectrum of its physical, chemical and biological attributes. Soil fertility is only one aspect of soil productivity but it is a very important one. For example, a soil may be very fertile, but produce only little vegetation because of a lack of water or unfavorable temperature. Even under suitable climate conditions, soils vary in their capacity to create a suitable environment for plant roots.

Types of soil

Depending on the size of the particles in the soil, it can be classified into following types (Table 3.6):

1. Sandy soil
2. Silty soil
3. Clay soil
4. Loamy soil
5. Peaty soil
6. Chalky soil

Fertilizers

Fertilizers are very important to plants. They are soil amendments applied to promote plant growth. The main nutrients present in fertilizers are nitrogen, phosphorus, and potassium (the 'macronutrients') and other nutrients ('micronutrients') are added in smaller amounts (Table 3.7). Aside from sunlight and water, fertilizer is essential to them. So fertilizers can be like plant "food." If the soil is well-loamed and rich, it is a good source of nutrients for the plants in the area. However, if the soil has gone through cycles of planting and harvesting already, then it has been stripped of all the nutrients it can give. Since the soils can no longer meet the adequate needs of the plants, "supplements" in the form of fertilizers would have to be given to meet the nutritional needs of plants for optimum growth and yield.

Table 3.6: Types of soil with their characteristics

Types of soil	Characteristics
Sandy soil	Sandy soil (0.05 to 2 mm) is good for plants. It is granular and consists of rock and mineral particles. The texture is gritty and is formed by the disintegration and weathering of rocks, such as limestone, granite, quartz and shale. Sandy soil retains moisture and nutrients.
Silty soil	Silty soil (0.002 to 0.05 mm) is considered to be one of the most fertile of soils. It is composed of minerals like quartz and fine organic particles. It is granular like sandy soil but it has more nutrients than sandy soil and it also offers better drainage.
Clay soil	Clay soil (less than 0.002 mm) is formed after years of rock disintegration and weathering. It is also formed as sedimentary deposits after the rock is weathered, eroded and transported.
Loamy soil	This soil is the ideal for cultivation, consists of sand, silt and clay to some extent. It is considered to be the perfect soil. The texture is gritty and retains water very easily, yet the drainage is well.
Peaty soil	It is basically formed by the accumulation of dead and decayed organic matter and naturally contains much more organic matter than most of the soils. It is generally found in marshy areas. Peaty soil is blocked by the acidity of the soil.
Chalky soil	Chalky soil is very alkaline in nature and consists of a large number of stones. Chalky soil, apart from being dry, also blocks the nutritional elements for the plants, like iron and magnesium. The fertility of this kind of soil depends on the depth of the soil that is on the bed of chalk. This kind of soil is prone to dryness and in summers, it is a poor choice for plantation.

Table 3.7: Essential plant nutrients

	Essential plant nutrients		
Nutrient supplied by air and water	Nutrient supplied by soil system with help of fertilizers		
Non-mineral	Primary macronutrients	Secondary micronutrients	Macronutrients
Carbon	Nitrogen	Calcium	Boron, chlorine, manganese
Hydrogen	Phosphorus	Sulfur	Iron, zinc, copper
Oxygen	Potassium	Magnesium	Molybdenum and selenium

Chemical fertilizers typically provide, in varying proportions (Table 3.8).

Pest and Pest Control

Pests are organisms, such as insects, rodents, nematodes, fungi, weeds, birds, bacteria, viruses, etc., which damage the crops and reduce yield. Pests are injurious to human health and/or farmers economic efforts.

Pest control refers to the regulation or management of a species defined as a pest, usually because it is perceived to be detrimental to a person's health, the ecology or the economy.

Pesticides are chemicals or mixtures of chemicals that are used for killing, repelling, mitigating or reducing pest damage.

Classification of Pesticides

Pesticides may be classified according to:
 a. The target pest species.
 b. Their chemical constitution
 c. Their site of action

Table 3.8: Major types of fertilizers

Types of fertilizers	Description
Inorganic fertilizers	Inorganic fertilizers are actually artificial or synthetic fertilizers. Inorganic fertilizers immediately produce ammonia as a by product.
Plant-specific fertilizers	Plant-specific fertilizers are special formulas designed to meet the adequate nutrient needs of a particular plant in order to grow optimally.
Liquid fertilizers	Liquid fertilizers are great in delivering nutrients to the plants since the liquids seep right into the roots where plants may immediately take up the necessary nutrient needed.
Time release fertilizer	Time release fertilizer usually releases the fertilizer slowly over a certain period, usually around 2–6 months. The release of nutrients is accelerated in the presence of water and moisture. This type of fertilizer is also more expensive than the conventional ones.
Fertilizer with pesticide	The plants get their nourishment and they are also protected from pests that may damage them. This even comes a whole lot cheaper than getting the two separately

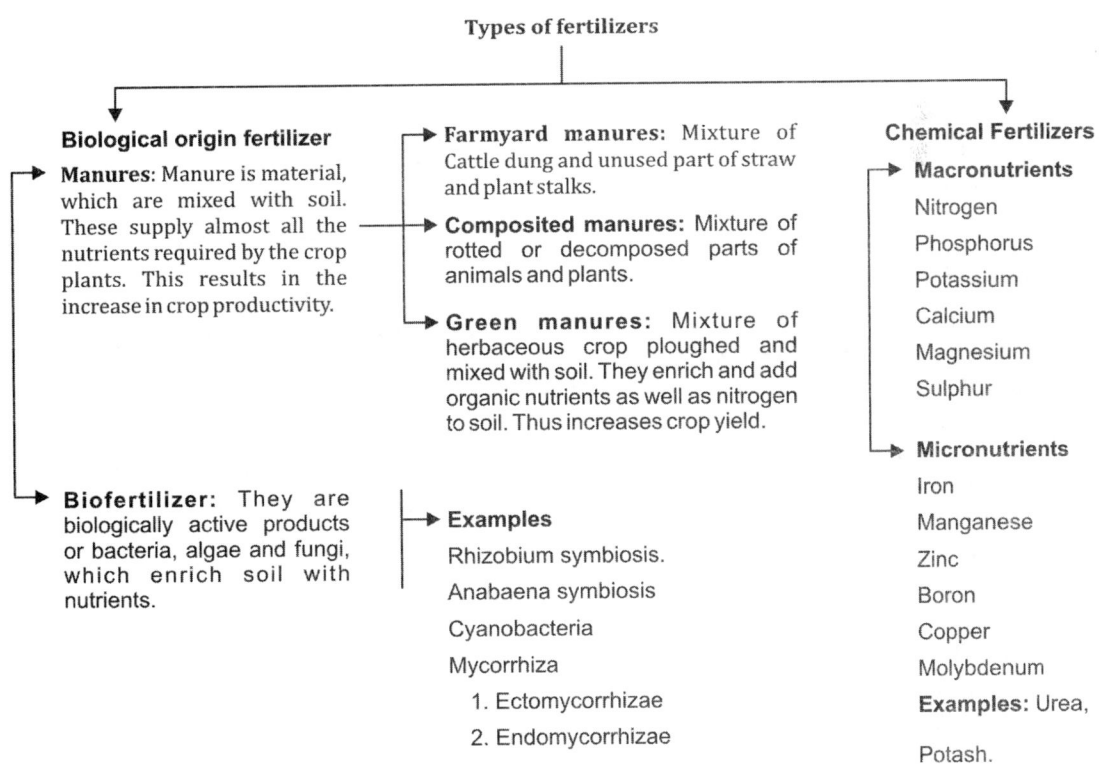

Fig. 3.2: Fertilizers and its types

Classification based on Target Pest Species

The following explains the classification of pesticides based on target organisms. For certain organisms, sub-classifications are also made.

Microorganisms
- Fungi—Fungicides
- Algae—Algaecides
- Bacteria—Bactericides
- Archanids—Acaricides
- Insects—Insecticides
- Rodents—Rodenticides
- Birds—Avicides
- Plant—Weedicides, Herbicides

Classification based on Chemical Nature

The classification of pesticides based on their chemical nature is rather complex. Modern pesticides are, in general, organic chemicals (compounds with carbon). However, some inorganic compounds are also used as pesticides. The organic pesticides can be sub-divided into classes based on their molecular structure. These classes are organochlorines, organophosphates, carbamates, organomercurials, thiocarbamates, acetamides, ureas, etc.

Classification based on Site of Action

By segmenting insecticides/acaricides and fungicides separately, insecticides/acaricides can be classified on the basis of their routes of entry into the body system of the target pest. They can be grouped as follows:
   i. Stomach poisons.
   ii. Contact poisons.
   iii. Systemic poisons.
   iv. Fumigants.

METHODS OF PEST CONTROL

The different methods for an approach to control pests are briefly summarized as under:

a. **Mechanical Method:** This method involves manual labour with different devices for collection and destruction of pest. The method employs different approaches like to collect and destruct eggs, larvae, pupae and adults of insects, to construct concrete warehouses of metal reinforcement corners on window frames for rodents like rats, to trap flying insects with flavored attractants placed in funnel shaped container, which are formulated with rose oil, anise oil, etc. mixed with saw dust. Other simple techniques used are hand-picking, pruning, burning and trapping of pests.

b. **Agricultural Method:** This method employs advanced plant breeding techniques to induce genetic manipulations for the production of pest-resistant species. The method involves production of hybrid varieties, which are resistant to fungal and bacterial attack. The mechanisms of systemic insecticides are that they get absorbed through the roots and reach to leaves by which all the foliage portion becomes distasteful for insects. Other approach is ploughing, which should be sufficiently deep so as to eradicate weeds, as well as, early stages of insects. If a plant is found to favor insects for food, such cultivated lands should be subjected to crop rotation.

c. **Biological Control:** This method is practiced by combating the pests, mostly the insects, with other living organisms. The chemical substances produced and released by some female insects are capable of eliciting a sexual response from the opposite sex, which could be properly exploited for biological control of pests. Such substances are called as sex pheromones, e.g. 7,8-epoxy – 2 methyloctadecane from gypsy-moth. If it is properly designed, it may evolve as an effective, safe and economic method of pest control.

d. **Chemical Control:** The chemical control is done by use of chemical pesticides, which includes insecticides, fungicides, herbicides and rodenticides. Although pesticides are toxic in nature, their use is regulated by the Insecticides Act in India; Federal Insecticide, Fungicide and Rodenticide Act in United States and the Agriculture (Poisonous substances) Regulations in U.K. The pesticides are classified as rodenticides, insecticides, acaricides, fungicides, herbicides, predacides, ovicides, bactericides, arboricides, etc.

   i. **Rodenticides:** Arsenic trioxide, warfarin, strychnine, etc.
   ii. **Insecticides:** D.D.T, gammaxine, methoxychlor, parathion, etc.
   iii. **Fungicides:** Chlorophenols, quaternary ammonium compounds, etc.
   iv. **Herbicides:** 2, 4-dichlorophenoxy acetic acid, calcium arsenate, sulphuric acid.

ENDOGENOUS FACTORS

Plant hormones, referred to as 'phytohormones', are a group of naturally occurring, organic substances which influence physiological processes at low concentrations. Plant hormones play a crucial role in controlling the way in which plants grow and develop as well as differentiate. In addition they control the processes of reproduction. A plant hormone or phytohormone is a chemical substance produced naturally in plants which is translocated to another region for regulating one or more physiological reactions when present in low concentration.

"All phytohormones are growth regulators but all growth regulators are not phytohormones".

Plant hormones shape the plant, affecting seed growth, time of flowering, sex of flowers, senescence of leaves and fruits. They affect gene expression and transcription levels, cellular division and growth.

Characters of Plant Hormones

- They are chemical messengers, influence cell division, enlargement and differentiation.
- They often diminish or amplify the effects of other hormones.
- They are involved in all aspects of development and often synthesized long distances from their sites of action.
- They are not directly involved in the chemistry of synthesis of plant compounds, like roots synthesize most hormones although hormones are not made exclusively by the roots.
- Same hormones can produce a different response in different organs, e.g. auxin concentration promotes shoot growth but inhibits root growth.

Classes of Plant Hormones

It is generally accepted that there are five major classes of plant hormones. Each class have positive as well as inhibitory functions and they often work in tandem with each other, with varying ratio of one or more interplaying to affect growth regulation. Five major classes are auxin, gibberellins, cytokinins, abscisic acid and ethylene (Table 3.9).

AUXINS

Auxins are a general term used to indicate substances that promote elongation of coleoptile tissues. They are either natural auxins which are produced by plants themselves or synthetic auxins, which have the same action as natural auxins. IAA is the principle auxin and other natural auxins are indole-3-acetonitrile (IAN), 4-chloroindole 3-acetic acid and phenyl acetic acid. The synthetic auxins are indole-3-butyric acid (IBA),

Table 3.9: Phytohormones with their description

Phytohormones	Nature and precursor	Transport	Bioassay	Site of biosynthesis	Effects
Auxins CH_2-COOH (indole structure) 4-chloro-indole-3 acetic acid. Phenylacetic acid Synthesized auxins are: Indole-3-butyric acid (IBA). Napthelene acetic acid (NAA).	Occur in cell in concentration of $10^{-8}–10^{-6}$ Mol/litre. Tryptophan is the precursor of IAA & Zn is required for synthesis.	Basipetal in stem & acropetal in roots	Avena curvature test. Split pea stem curvature test.	IAA transport is cell to cell mainly in the vascular cambium and epidermal cells.	Induce cell enlargement and stem growth. Enhance cell division by inducing meristematic activity and Cambium cell activity. Vascular tissue differentiation (xylem and phloem). Root initiation (stem cuttings) and differentiation (tissue culture). Tropistic responses of shoots and roots to gravity and light. Growth of flower parts and delay fruit ripening. Leaf and fruit abscission (inhibit or promote via ethylene). Fruit setting and growth. Auxin delays leaf senescence ripening. Apical dominance. IAA promotes formation of female flowers (feminization).
Gibberellins (GAs) Weakly acidic plant growth hormone (structural diagram)	The gibberellins (GAs) are a family of compounds based on the entgibberellane structure	They are probably transported in the phloem and xylem	Dwarf pea elongation technique. Barley endosperm digestion technique.	Synthesized from glyceraldehyde-3-phosphate, via isopentenyl diphosphate, in young tissues of the shoot and developing seed.	Enhances seed germination by enhancing amylase synthesis (enzyme production). Overcome dormancy. GA1 causes hyperelongation of stems by stimulating both cell division and cell elongation. Induction of seed germination. GAs cause stem elongation in response to long days. Fruit setting and growth. GA produces male flower production in cannabis. GA causes etiolation in plants when kept in dark.

(Contd.)

Table 3.9: Phytohormones with their description (Contd.)

Phytohormones	Nature and Precusor	Transport	Bioassay	Site of Biosynthesis	Effects
Cytokinins (CKs) Mildly basic growth hormones

Kinetin (6-furfuryl aminopurines).
6-Benzyl aminopurine. | CKs are adenine derivatives characterized by an ability to induce cell division. Chemically precursor of CK is adenine or adenosine | CK transport is via the xylem from roots to shoots. | Chlorophyll preservation test or delay in senescence test. Tobacco pith culture test. | CK biosynthesis is through the biochemical modification of adenine. | It occurs in root tips and developing seeds. Cell division and cell enlargement are enhanced by CKs. Morphogenesis. CKs delay leaf senescence. CKs may enhance stomatal opening in some species. CK leads to an accumulation of chlorophyll and promotes the conversion of etioplasts into chloroplasts. In turn leads to chloroplast development. Growth of lateral buds. CKs are quite effective in breaking dormancy of seeds. It counteracts the phenomenon of apical dominance. Kinetins are reported to play the role in nucleic acid metabolism and protein synthesis. Increases the self-life of vegetables and improves yield and quality of fruit. |
| **Abscisic acid (ABA)** Terpene derivatives. | It is mainly a 15-C sesquiterpenes, act as a inhibitor because it opposes the growth promotion effect of auxins, GA, CKs | ABA is exported from roots in the xylem and from leaves in the phloem | Rice seedling growth inhibition test. Inhibition of α-amylase synthesis in barely endosperm. | Biosynthesis of ABA take place through mevalonic acid or xanthophylls. | Induces dormancy in buds. It is also known as antigibberellin as it counters effects of gibberellins like induction of hydrolases, α-amylase in barely seedlings. It is known as stress hormone and leads to stomatal closure thus acts as a antitranspirant. ABA inhibits shoot growth. ABA induces storage protein synthesis in seeds. ABA affects the induction and maintenance of some aspects of dormancy in seeds. Increase in ABA in response to wounding induces gene transcription, notably for proteinase inhibitors. |

(Contd.)

Table 3.9: Phytohormones with their description (*Contd.*)

Phytohormones	Nature and precusor	Transport	Bioassay	Site of biosynthesis	Effects
Ethylene $CH_2 = CH_2$ Naturally occurring volatile hormone.	It is gaseous hormone.	Ethylene moves by diffusion from its site of synthesis.	Triple pea test. Pea stem swelling test.	It is produced from L-methionine. Ethylene is synthesized by most tissues in response to stress like tissue undergoing senescence or ripening.	Maintenance of the apical hook in seedlings. Stimulation of numerous defense responses in response to injury or disease. Release from dormancy. Shoot and root growth and differentiation. Adventitious root formation. Leaf and fruit abscission. Flower induction in some plants. Induction of femaleness in dioecious flowers. Flower opening. Flower and leaf senescence. Fruit ripening.

2-napthyloxyacetic acid(NOA), α-napthyl acetic acid (NAA), 1-napthyl acetamide (NAD)[2], 4-dichlorophenoxy acetic acid (2, 4-D), 2, 4, 5 trichlorophenoxy acetic acid and 5-carboxymethyl-N, N-dimethyl dithiocarbamate. The proposed mechanism of action of IAA is its interaction with one or more components of biochemical systems involved in the synthesis of proteins. The other hypothesis suggested is the role of IAA to alter the osmotically active contents of cell vacuole during cell expansion or cell wall extension.

Gibberellins

The research has shown that gibberellins A is actually a mixture of atleast 6 gibberellins referred to as GA_1, GA_2, GA_3, GA_4, GA_7, GA_9. GA_3 is termed as gibberellic acid. All of them are the derivatives of gibbane ring skeleton. In addition to free gibberellins, they are also present in conjugated forms. The mechanism of action of gibberellic acid is mainly to induce activity of gluconeogenic enzymes during early stages of seed germination and this specificity ensures a rapid conversion of lipid to sucrose, which is further used in supporting growth and development of the embryonic axis to a competent root and shoot system. It is also found that gibberellins induce the synthesis of α-amylase and other hydrolytic enzymes during germination of monocot seeds. They are also involved in mobilizing seed storage reserves during germination and seedling emergence.

Cytokinins

These are either natural (zeatin) or synthetic (kinetin) compounds with significant growth regulating activity. Zeatin has effect on cell division and leaf senescence and synthetic cytokinins are useful in promoting lateral bud development and inhibition of senescence. The naturally occurring cytokinins are zeatin, N^6 dimethyl amino purine, and N^6-A^2- isopentenyl aminopurine. The synthetic cytokinins are kinetin, adenine, 6-benzyl adenine benzimidazole and N. N^1-diphenyl urea.

Ethylene

It is a simple organic molecule present in the form of volatile gas and shows profound physiological effects. Ethylene shows a broad array of growth responses in plants, which include fruit ripening, leaf abscission, stem swelling, leaf bending, flower petal discoloration, and inhibition of stem and root growth. It is commercially used for promotion of flowering and fruit ripening, induction of fruit abscission, breaking dormancy and stimulation of latex flow in rubber trees.

Abscisic Acid (ABA)

A diffusible abscission-accelerating substance was found by Osborne (1955) in senescent leaves. Carns et al. isolated several abscission accelerating substances from cotton plants and named them as abscisin I and abscisin II.

In an inhibitory way, ABA interacts with other plant growth substances. It inhibits the GA-induced synthesis of α-amylase and other hydrolytic enzymes. During maturation, ABA accumulates in many seeds and helps in seed dormancy. ABA concentrations are found to be enhanced in stress conditions, like mineral deficiency, injury, drought and flooding. ABA serves an important role as potential antitranspirant by closing the stomata, when applied to leaves.

Miscellaneous Hormones

Polyamines

$H_2N — (CH_2)_3 — NH — (CH_2)_4 — NH_2$

Spermidine

Polyamines are a group of aliphatic amines. The main compounds are putrescine, spermidine and spermine. They are derived from the decarboxylation of the amino acids arginine or ornithine. They are widespread in all cells and can exert regulatory control over growth and development at micromolar concentrations. Polyamines have a wide range of effects on plants and appear to be essential for plant growth, particularly cell division and normal morphologies. It appears that polyamines are present in all cells rather than having a specific site of synthesis.

Brassinosteroids (BAs)

Brassinosteroids are plant steroids, typified by the compound brassinolide that was first isolated from *Brassica* pollen. They produce effects on growth and development at very low concentrations and play a role in the endogenous regulation of these processes.

Effects

- Cell division, cell elongation, vascular differentiation and they are needed for fertility.
- Inhibition of root growth and development.
- They help in promotion of ethylene biosynthesis and epinasty.

Jasmonates (JA)

Jasmonates are represented by jasmonic acid (JA) and its methyl ester. Jasmonic acid is synthesized from linolenic acid, while jasmonic acid is most likely the precursor of tuberonic acid.

Jasmonic acid

Effects

- Jasminates play an important role in plant defense and inhibit many plant processes, such as growth and seed germination.
- They promote senescence, abscission, tuber formation, fruit ripening, pigment formation and tendril coiling.
- JA is essential for male reproductive development of arabidopsis.

Salicylic Acid (SA)

Salicylates have been known for a long time to be present in willow bark, but have only recently been recognized as potential regulatory compounds. Salicylic acid is biosynthesized from the amino acid phenylalanine.

Salicylic acid (SA)

Effects

- Salicylic acid plays a main role in the resistance to pathogens by inducing the production of 'pathogenesis-related proteins'.
- SA is the calorigenic substance that causes thermogenesis in *Arum* flowers.
- It has also been reported to enhance flower longevity, inhibit ethylene biosynthesis and seed germination, block the wound response, and reverse the effects of (ABA) Absicic acid.

Collection and Processing of Crude Drugs

After collection of the crude drugs, before marketing there is intense need of processing a drug. The reasons for processing are to stabilize them during transport and storage and to ensure the absence of foreign organic matter and substitutes. Generally, these methods include proper methods of collection, harvesting, drying and garbling. Sometimes, coating and bleaching are also necessary for converting the drug into suitable form for the market. While performing these activities, it should be noted that neither the potency of the drug is lowered down nor it is adulterated, due to additives and substituent's used in the process.

Collection

The existing environmental conditions are taken into consideration while collection of the crude drugs. The collection techniques are discussed below:

1. In case of drug containing Leaf and flowering tops of plants. They are collected just before they reach their maturity in flowering stage; e.g. senna, vinca, belladonna, etc. although aloe leaves are collected when they are sufficiently thick.
2. Flowers need to be collected in dry weather and preferably during morning hours and many a times, before their full expansion, e.g. saffron, chamomile, clove buds, etc.
3. While collecting barks, they are collected in spring or early summer when cambium is active as well as it is easy to remove them from the stem. Otherwise, they are collected in autumn (wild cherry) or in rainy season (cinnamon). Three different methods for collecting barks are:
    i. Felling,
    ii. Uprooting, and
    iii. Coppicing.
        In felling method, the trees are cut at base and bark is peeled out. In uprooting technique, the roots are dug out and bark is stripped off from roots and branches. In coppicing method, the plant is allowed to grow for a definite period and then it is cut off at specific distance from soil.
4. Collection of fruits depends upon the part of the fruits used, collected either ripe of half ripe, but fully grown. For example, cardamom fruits are collected just before their dehiscence; bael and tamarind, after their, full maturity, while caraway, fennel and coriander are collected, when they are fully ripe.
5. The roots are collected in spring, and they are sliced transversely or longitudinally to facilitate drying.
6. Rhizomes are collected, when they store ample of reserve food material and also contain maximum content of chemical constituents.
7. The unorganized drugs such as resins, gums, latices are collected, as soon as, they ooze out of the plant. Acacia gum is collected 2–3 weeks after making incisions on the bark of the tree and when it is sufficiently hard. Opium and papaya lattices are collected after coagulation of latex. Turpentine oleoresin and balsam of peru are collected when the plant is about 8–10 years old.

Harvesting

Harvesting reflects upon economic aspects of the crude drugs. The roots, rhizomes and tubers are harvested by diggers or lifters known as mechanical device. These parts are thoroughly washed in water to get rid of earthy-matter. The aerial parts of plant, flowers, seeds and small fruits are harvested by a special device known as seed stripper. Peppermint and spearmint are harvested by normal method with mowers, whereas fennel, coriander and caraway plants are uprooted and dried. After drying, either drugs are thrashed or beaten or the fruits are separated by winnowing.

Drying

Before making a crude drug, it is necessary to process it properly, so as to preserve it for a longer time and also to acquire better pharmaceutical elegance. Drying consists of removal of sufficient moisture content of crude drug, so as to improve its quality and make it resistant to the growth of microorganisms. Drying inhibits partially enzymatic reactions. Drying also facilitates pulverizing or grinding of a crude drug. Depending upon the type of chemical constituents, a method of drying can be used for a crude drug. Drying can be of two types—(1). natural (sun drying) and 2. artificial.

1. Natural Drying (Sun-drying)

Natural drying may be either sun-drying or in the shed. Drying in shed is preferred for retaining natural colour of the drug example digitalis, clove and senna and for volatile principles example peppermint. If the contents of the drugs are quite stable to the temperature and sunlight, the drugs can be dried directly in sunshine (gum acacia, seeds and fruits).

2. Artificial Drying

The artificial drying includes drying the drugs in (a) an oven; i.e. tray-dryers, (b) vacuum dryers, and (c) spray dryers.

- a. **Tray dryers:** Especially for drugs which do not contain volatile oils and are heat stable or which need deactivation of enzymes are dried in tray dryers. In tray-dryers, hot air at desired temperature is distributed through the dryers and this helps in removal of water content of the drugs. *Example:* Belladonna roots, cinchona bark, tea and raspberry leaves and gums.
- b. **Vacuum dryers:** The drugs which are sensitive to higher temperature are dried by this process, e.g. tannic acid and digitalis leaves.
- c. **Spray dryers:** Especially for highly sensitive drugs to atmospheric conditions. The technique is quick for drying plant or animal constituents, rather than the crude drugs.
  Examples: papaya latex, pectin, tannins, etc.

Garbling (Dressing)

The next step is garbling, that is removal of sand, dirt and foreign organic parts of the same plant. This foreign organic matter (extraneous matter) is permitted in crude drugs, the quality of drug suffers and, it does not pass pharmacopoeial limits. Excessive stems in case of lobelia and stramonium need to be removed, while the stalks, in case of cloves are to be removed. Drugs constituting rhizomes need to be separated carefully from roots and rootlets and also stem bases. Pieces of iron must be removed with the magnet in case of castor seeds before crushing and by shifting, in case of vinca and senna leaves. Pieces of bark should be removed by peeling as in gum acacia.

Packing

While packing the drugs the following parameters are taken into consideration like morphological and chemical nature of drug, its use and effects of climatic conditions during transportation and storage.

Requirement of Packaging Materials

The general requirements of packaging materials are the following (Kraisintu, 1997):

1. Economical or low cost.
2. Impermeable as glass or metal or of acceptable permeability to moisture, gases, volatile solvents, etc.
3. Non-reactive—relatively inert with no extraction, exchange or interaction.
4. Easy to manufacture in a wide range of shapes, preferably by a number of manufacturing processes.
5. Easy to decorate and/or print by a range of processes.
6. Good production line efficiency-performance, with the minimum of rejects or wastage.

Table 3.10: Packaging material of drugs

S. No.	Packaging material	Drug
1.	Goat skin	Aloe
2.	Kerosene tins	Colophony and balsam of tolu
3.	Well closed containers	Asafoetida (to prevent loss of volatile oil)
4.	Suitable container not affected by sunlight	Cod liver oil
5.	Well closed containers	Digitalis, Ergot and Squill (protect from microbial count and decomposition).
6.	Packed in big masses	Colophony (control auto-oxidation)
7.	Bags are coated with polythene	Indian opium

7. Effective as a pack (container and closure), i.e. easy to open and reclose and use if multidose; or open if single dose, whilst meeting any special requirements, such as child resistance, tamper evidence or resistance, etc.
8. Easy to produce and maintain clean.
9. Preferably readily available both in terms of source of supply for raw materials and as a converted item component from several suppliers.
10. Environment friendly.
11. Able to optimise use of space when stacked or during transportation.

Types of Packing Materials

The common types of packaging materials currently available are:

1. **Glass:** It can be found as several variants such as treated soda glass, soda glass and non-parenteral.
2. **Metals:** A variety of metals including tin plate (tin-coated mild steel), tin free steel, aluminum, aluminum alloys are widely used in packaging, being found as rigid containers, collapsible containers, aluminum foils, metalized coatings, etc.
3. **Plastics:** There are five economical materials for rigid type of containers, i.e. those based on polyethylene (PE), polypropylene(PP), polystyrene(PS), PVC and polyester.
4. **Elastomeric materials:** Elastomers can be found as a wide range of basic materials (i.e. natural rubber, synthetic polyisoprene, neoprene, nitryl, butyl, including bromo- and chlorobutyl, ethylene propylene diene modified (EPDM), acid silicone elastomers).

Storage of Crude Drugs

Preservation of crude drugs needs sound knowledge of their physical and chemical properties. A good quality of the drugs can be maintained, it they are preserved property. All the drugs should be preserved in well closed and, possibly, in the filled containers. Environment where they are stored should be waterproof, fireproof and rodent-proof.

1. Many of the drugs absorb moisture and become susceptible to the microbial growth. The moisture increase weight of the drug as well as deteriorate the quality as well. The excessive moisture content favors the growth of enzymes and result in deterioration of active constituents, e.g. Mold Infestation due to moisture in many drugs like Ergot, Wild cherry bark and Digitalis leaves.

2. Destruction of active chemical constituents can be due to effect of radiation from sunlight, e.g. Digitalis and Cod Liver oil.
3. The important role is also played by shape of drug in which it should be stored like Colophony stored in the entire form of big masses is preserved nicely, but if kept in powdered form, gets oxidized or loses its solubility in petroleum ether. Squill, stored in powdered form becomes hygroscopic and forms rubbery mass on prolonged exposure to air.
4. The costly phytopharmaceuticals are required to be preserved at refrigerated temperature in well closed containers. Small quantities of crude drugs could be readily stored in airtight, moisture proof and light proof containers such as tin, cans, covered metal tins, or amber glass containers. Wooden boxes and paper bags should not be used for storage of crude drugs.

Quality and Evaluation

Quality control of the phytoproducts for human consumption and world market can be ensured by maintaining the quality of raw material adequacy of processing technology and quality of the finished products. Thus, the quality concept commences right from the choice of authentic and improved seeds (varieties) to the post-harvest treatment of the raw material and to the process control for avoiding contamination. As such for developing phytoproducts, WHO's Good Manufacturing Practice (GMP) must be followed to satisfy the ISO 9000 certification. Recently, ISO 14000 certification has also become necessary to safeguard the environment. This means certifying that the product has been developed without inflicting ecological damage whatsoever.

(GAP) Good Agrotechnological Practices. Large cultivation of medicinal plants relies upon strong and continuing research. Plant varieties with an abundance of desired constituents can be reproduced and improved upon under cultivation even in an entirely different area, e.g. cultivation of American ginseng (*Panax quinquefolia*) in China. Attempt should be made to select appropriate region based on similar ecological conditions to introduce good cultivated variety, improve yield of the desired secondary metabolite and reduce the undesirable constituents.

Non-polluted cultivation: In order to protect the environment, to sustainably utilise the resources and to get a good quality of crude drug, non-polluted agrotechnology is rapidly developed in recent years. These products are commonly called as "green crude drugs". These involve biological control of insects and pathogens and use of botanical pesticides for the control of pest and diseases.

Post harvest technology: Right time harvesting, good processing, good storage, extraction or distillation, quality control.

4

Phytopharmaceuticals and Marker Constituents

Phytochemistry deals with study of chemical composition of the plant material (Phyto refers to plant). Plants are used in various forms varying from powders to extracts. Powder represents the drug in ground from and these types of preparations are considered to be crude. The standardized herbal extracts are considered to be more scientific than crude drugs. The commonly employed technique for removal of active substance from the crude drug is called extraction.

Biological source of the drug has great impact on finished product in herbal drug preparation. Proper identification of the drug is significant for phytochemical screening, which further exerts importance on therapeutic activity of the medicinal herb. Thus presence of identification standard is must in finished product of an herbal drug preparation. The latest method of preparing herbal extracts is by successive macerating of the powdered drug in order of increasing polarity. This process is known as successive solvent extraction and carried out in special assembly known as Soxhlet apparatus (Table 4.1).

Selection of the solvent is very critical in preparing the extracts, because the active constituents of the plants have affinity for solvents.

The concept of standardization has great impact on quality of herbal products. Standardization helps in adjusting the herbal drug formulation to a defined content of a constituent or constituents with therapeutic activity.

Table 4.1: Phytopharmaceuticals with their solvents

Extracts are prepared by application of a suitable solvent so that soluble matter can be separating from vegetable tissues. The resultant liquid is concentrated by evaporation to dryness to obtain solid extract. The active constituent of plant has affinity for solvents so selection of solvent is critical. The extracts are classified as alcoholic, etheral or aqueous.

Phytopharmaceuticals	Solvents
Alkaloids	Chloroform and ether
Tannins and phenols	Alcohol and ethyl acetate
Glycosides	Water and alcohol
Fixed and essential oils	Water and petroleum ether

A constituent of a medicinal herb, which is used for quality control and assurance of herbal product, is known as *marker compound*. According to WHO, a marker compound is "any characterizing physiological constituent of crude drug, which can be easily isolated and quantified whenever actual bioactives are unknown".

Characteristics of Good Marker

- Marker compounds refer to chemical constituents/active ingredients within a medicinal herb that can be used to verify its potency or identity.
- It should be sufficiently stable and commercially available.
- It should be unique to the given crude drug or herbal preparation.
- It should have established identity, chemical structure as well as present in sufficient quantity to perform validation methods.
- It should be accessible to quantify with the common analytical equipment (Table 4.2).

Table 4.2: Phytopharmaceuticals with their marker constituent

Phytopharmaceuticals with their marker constituents

Alkaloids are basically nitrogen bases (alkaline) and contain a secondary or tertiary amine function within a heterocyclic ring.

Plant name	Marker	Structure	Biological activity
Adhatoda vasica	Adhatodine	($C_{20}H_{21}N_3O_2$)	Not confirmed
	Vasicine	($C_{11}H_{12}N_2O$)	Bronchodilator
Atropa belladonna	Atropine	($C_{17}H_{23}NO_3$)	Mydriatic
Berberis aristata	Berberine	$C_{20}H_{18}NO_4$	Antiperodic

(Contd...)

Table 4.2: Phytopharmaceuticals with their marker constituent (*Contd.*)

Phytopharmaceuticals with their marker constituents

Alkaloids are basically nitrogen bases (alkaline) and contain a secondary or tertiary amine function within a heterocyclic ring.

Plant name	Marker	Structure	Biological activity
Strychnos nux-vomica	Brucine	($C_{23}H_{25}N_2O_4$)	Local anesthetic
	Strychnine	($C_{21}H_{22}O_2N_2$)	Convulsant
Camellia sinensis	Caffeine	($C_8H_{10}O_2N_4 \cdot H_{20}$)	CNS stimulant
Erythroxylon coca	Cocaine	($C_{17}H_{21}NO_4$)	Anesthetic

(*Contd.*)

Table 4.2: Phytopharmaceuticals with their marker constituent (*Contd.*)

Phytopharmaceuticals with their marker constituents

Alkaloids are basically nitrogen bases (alkaline) and contain a secondary or tertiary amine function within a heterocyclic ring.

Plant name	Marker	Structure	Biological activity
Papaver somniferum	Codeine	Codeine $C_{18}H_{21}NO_3$	Antitussive
	Morphine	Morphine $C_{17}H_{19}NO_3$	Narcotic analgesic
	Papaverine	Papaverine $C_{20}H_{21}NO_4$	Narcotic and antispasmodic
Hyoscyamus niger	Hyoscyamine	($C_{17}H_{23}NO_3$)	Antispasmodic

Table 4.2: Phytopharmaceuticals with their marker constituent *(Contd.)*

Phytopharmaceuticals with their marker constituents

Alkaloids are basically nitrogen bases (alkaline) and contain a secondary or tertiary amine function within a heterocyclic ring.

Plant name	Marker	Structure	Biological activity
Piper nigrum	Piperine	($C_{17}H_{19}NO_3$)	Antipyretic
Cinchona officinalis	Quinine	($C_{20}H_{24}N_2O_2$)	Antimalarial

A glycoside consists of two components, an aglycone (non-sugar) part and a sugar part (carbohydrate). The aglycone portion may be of several different types of secondary metabolite. Glycosides are water-soluble constituents, found in the cell sap. They are colorless, crystalline substances containing carbon, hydrogen and oxygen.

Cardiac glycosides *Digitalis purpureae*	Digitoxin	($C_{41}H_{64}O_{13}$)	Treatment of congestive cardiac failure

(Contd.)

Table 4.2: Phytopharmaceuticals with their marker constituent (Contd.)

Phytopharmaceuticals with their marker constituents

Alkaloids are basically nitrogen bases (alkaline) and contain a secondary or tertiary amine function within a heterocyclic ring.

Plant name	Marker	Structure	Biological activity
Anthracene glycosides *Aloe vera*	Aloin	($C_{21}H_{22}O_9$)	Purgative
Rheum emodi	Rhein	($C_{15}H_8O_6$)	Antioxidant, and Anti-infammatory activities allergy
Cassia angustifolia, Cassia acutifolia	Sennosides	($C_{42}H_{38}O_{20}$)	Purgative

(Contd.)

Table 4.2: Phytopharmaceuticals with their marker constituent (*Contd.*)

Phytopharmaceuticals with their marker constituents

Alkaloids are basically nitrogen bases (alkaline) and contain a secondary or tertiary amine function within a heterocyclic ring.

Plant name	Marker	Structure	Biological activity
Saponin glycosides *Glycyrhiza glabra*	Glychyrhizin		Antiviral
Bitter glycosides *Gymnema sylvestre*	Gymnemic acid	$C_{42}H_{62}O_{16}$	Antidiabetic
Ruta graveolans	Rutin	$C_{41}H_{64}O_{13}$ ($C_{27}H_{30}O_{16}$)	Anticoagulant

(*Contd.*)

Table 4.2: Phytopharmaceuticals with their marker constituent *(Contd.)*

Phytopharmaceuticals with their marker constituents

Alkaloids are basically nitrogen bases (alkaline) and contain a secondary or tertiary amine function within a heterocyclic ring.

Plant name	Marker	Structure	Biological activity

Resins are obtained by oxidization of volatile oils. Resins are brittle, non-volatile, solid substances. Resins are soluble in alkalies, alcohol and insoluble in water. They are obtained from plant exudates and are produced in special ducts. Oleoresins are natural products of resin mixed with volatile oils. Gum-resins are plant exudates and are mixtures of gum and resin and often volatile oils.

Plant name	Marker	Structure	Biological activity
Capsicum annum	Capsiacin	$C_{18}H_{27}NO_3$	Counterirritant
Zingiber officinale	Gingerol	$C_{15}H_{22}O_4$	Used in treatment of rheumatoid arthritis.
Podophyllum hexandrum	Podophyllin	$(C_{22}H_{22}O_8)$	Caustic.
Cinnamomum camphora	Camphor	$(C_{10}H_{16}O)$	Antipruritic and antiseptic.

(Contd.)

Table 4.2: Phytopharmaceuticals with their marker constituent (*Contd.*)

Phytopharmaceuticals with their marker constituents

Alkaloids are basically nitrogen bases (alkaline) and contain a secondary or tertiary amine function within a heterocyclic ring.

Plant name	Marker	Structure	Biological activity
Eugenia caryophyllus	Eugenol	$CH_3CH=CH_2$, OMe, OH ($C_{10}H_{12}O_2$)	Analgesic and antiseptic
Mentha spicata	Menthol	OH, isopropyl group, $C_{10}H_{20}O$	Antipruritic and antiseptic
Withania somnifera	Withaferin-A	($C_{28}H_{38}O_6$)	Anticancer

Tannins are phenolic compounds of high molecular weight. Tannins are soluble in water and alcohol and are found in root, bark, stem and outer layers of plant tissue. Tannins form complex with proteins, carbohydrates, gelatin and alkaloids.

Terminalia chebula	Ellagic acid	$C_{14}H_6O_8$	Antiproliferative and antioxidant

(*Contd.*)

Table 4.2: Phytopharmaceuticals with their marker constituent (*Contd.*)

Phytopharmaceuticals with their marker constituents

Alkaloids are basically nitrogen bases (alkaline) and contain a secondary or tertiary amine function within a heterocyclic ring.

Plant name	Marker	Structure	Biological activity
Quercus infectoria	Tannic acid	$C_{14}H_{10}O_9$	Anti-diarrhoeal agent and anti-tussives

Terpenes are flammable unsaturated hydrocarbons, existing in liquid form. They are found in essential oils, resins or oleoresins.

Plant name	Marker	Structure	Biological activity
Allium sativum	Allicin	$C_6H_{10}OS_2$	Hypolipidemic
Stevia species	Stevioside	$C_{38}H_{60}O_{18}$	Hypolipidemic

(*Contd.*)

Table 4.2: Phytopharmaceuticals with their marker constituent *(Contd.)*

Phytopharmaceuticals with their marker constituents

Alkaloids are basically nitrogen bases (alkaline) and contain a secondary or tertiary amine function within a heterocyclic ring.

Plant name	Marker	Structure	Biological activity
Taxus brevifolia.	Taxol	$C_{47}H_{51}NO_4$	Antitumor
Salvia officinalis	Ursolic acid	$(C_{18}H_{16}O_7)$	Antibacterial

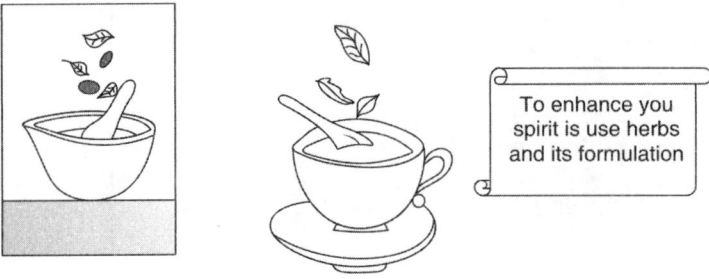

Use of phytopharmaceuticals

The detection and quantification of a marker can ensure genuineness of the crude drugs, but it does not guarantee the bioactivity or efficacy of the crude drugs. If the bioassay used is general and non-specific, then the isolated compounds can be labeled as "BIO-MARKER" for the crude drug. The development of a biomarker for this paradigm is not an easy task because of the complex interplay of many variables in this approach. But if the bioassay used is specific for a particular bioactivity, then the isolated compound can be called as the "BIO-ACTIVE MOLECULE" for that particular bioactivity.

Marker Analysis

Marker analysis is the uniform standardization tool to evaluate natural herbal products. It may help in different ways:
- To assess potency.
- Anticipate the active constituents.
- To ensure the quality and consistency of botanical raw materials and finished products.
- Validation of therapeutic doses by calculating the quantity of biological chemical entity required to produce specific pharmacological activity.
- Detecting the adulterants and monitoring decomposition.
- Essential in the stability study of herbals and deciding the shelf-life of a product.
- Post-market surveillance and pharmacovigilance studies to calculate quality, toxicity, stability and overdoses.

Marker compounds and chromatographic profiles may be used to evaluate the quality of products from herbal growers and suppliers, to standardise raw materials, and control formulation and tablet content uniformity. The marker analysis is carried out with the chromatographic testing of herbal medicine for identification and potency determination. The use of chromatographic fingerprinting for herbal drugs serves not only in identification but also assessment of the stability of the chemical constituents observed by chromatography. Thin layer chromatography (TLC) is most significant and commonly used method for analysis of marker compounds because it is simple, cost-effective, reproducible and visualizable. Further, fingerprinting of the chromatographic patterns and quantitative analysis of markers is possible using a densitometric scanner.

5
Drugs Derived from Natural Sources

5.1 CARBOHYDRATES

Carbohydrates are the most abundant class of organic compounds found in living organisms. They originate as products of photosynthesis, an endothermic reductive condensation of carbon dioxide requiring light energy and the pigment chlorophyll. They are hydrates of carbon $C_nH_{2n}O_n$. Chemically made up of skeletal C, H which is usually 2 × the number of C, highly variable number of O, occasional N and S. Carbohydrates are defined as polyhydroxyaldehyde or polyhydroxyketone, or substance that gives these compounds on hydrolysis.

$$nCO_2 + nH_2O + \text{energy} \rightarrow C_nH_{2n}O_n + nO_2$$

Table 5.1.1: Classes of carbohydrates

Classes	Example
Number of C	Triose, tetrose, pentose, hexose, heptulose
Number of saccharide units	Monosaccharides, disaccharides, oligosaccharides (2 to 10 units), polysaccharides
Position of carbonyl (C=O) group	Aldose, if terminally located Ketose, if centrally located
Reducing property	Reducing sugars (all monosaccharides), nonreducing sugars (sucrose)

Monosaccharides

Monosaccharides are sugars containing single units in total chain of 3–7 carbon atoms. They are simple sugar and serve as building blocks of larger molecules. A sugar containing:

- An aldehyde is known as aldose
- A ketone is known as ketose.

They all have the basic formula $(CH_2O)n$ and can be classified according to carbon atoms they contain:

2C = bioses sugars
3C = triose sugars, e.g. glyceraldehyde $C_3H_5O_2$
5C = pentose sugars, e.g. ribose $C_5H_{10}O_5$
6C = hexose sugars, e.g. glucose $C_6H_{12}O_6$

Disaccharides

When the alcohol component of a glycoside is provided by a hydroxyl function on another monosaccharide, the compound is called a **disaccharide**. Partial hydrolysis of starch and glycogen produces the disaccharide maltose.

Systematic nomenclatures for disaccharides are as follows:

Cellobiose	4-O-β-D-glucopyranosyl-D-glucose
Maltose	4-O-α-D-glucopyranosyl-D-glucose
Gentiobiose	6-O-β-D-glucopyranosyl-D-glucose
Trehalose	α-D-glucopyranosyl-α-D-glucopyranoside

Polysaccharides

Polysaccharides are large high-molecular weight molecules constructed by joining 10 or more monosaccharide units together by glycosidic bonds. Polysaccharides are

Table 5.1.2: Classification of carbohydrates

Category	Example	Site	STRUCTURES
Monosaccharides (made of 1 sugar molecule)	Glucose, galactose, fructose	Fruit, Fruit, nectar, Milk	α-Glucose, β-Glucose, Fructose
Disaccharide (made up of 2 monosaccharides joined together)	Maltose = α-glucose + α-glucose Sucrose = glucose + fructose Lactose = glucose + galactose	Germinating seeds Phloem tissue, fruit Milk	Maltose
Polysaccharide (made up of many monosaccharides joined together)	Starch = Polymer of glucose Glycogen = Polymer of α-glucose Cellulose = Polymer of β-glucose Chitin = Polymer of glucosamine	Chloroplast stroma Muscle cells Plant cell wall Exoskeleton of arthropods	Cellulose

polymers, i.e. they are made up of many repeating units. They are sometimes called **glycans**. The most important compounds in this class, cellulose, starch and glycogen are all polymers of glucose. As a polymer of glucose, cellulose has the formula $(C_6H_{10}O_5)_n$ where n ranges from 500 to 5,000, depending on the source of the polymer.

Homopolysaccharides: All the residues are the same monosaccharides.

Heteropolysaccharides: The residues are built from more than one type of monosaccharides.

Starch

Starch is the main storage polysaccharide in plants, made of two polymers of α-glucose—amylose and amylopectin. Both are insoluble in water, therefore, good storage compound, e.g. in stroma of chloroplast.

Amylose: A chain of glucose molecules joined by α-1, 4-glycosidic bonds which, by hydrogen bonding, forms a helix. It is this helix which holds and forms a complex with iodine. The helix forms a compact shape which allows tight packing and is, therefore, an excellent storage molecule (Fig. 5.1.1).

Amylopectin: Amylopectin has many protruding ends (glucose molecules) which can be hydrolysed rapidly allows rapid release of glucose to provide energy via respiration. Glucose molecules joined by β-1,4-glycosidic bonds but after every 25 glucose molecules adjacent chains are connected by α-1,6-glycosidic bonds, i.e. amylopectin is branched (Fig. 5.1.2).

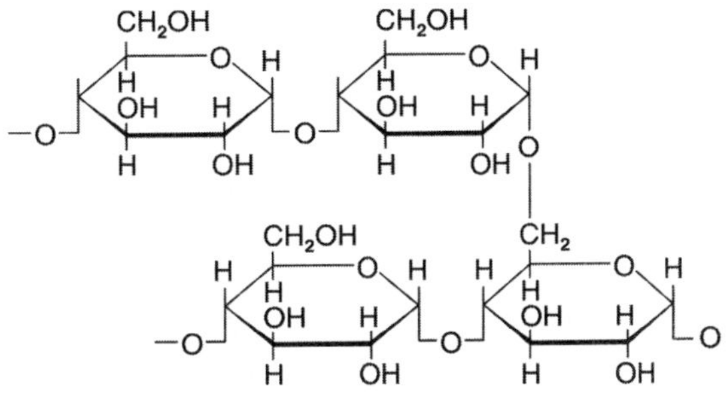

Fig. 5.1.2: Structure of amylopectin

Glycogen (Animal starch): Starch is the main storage polysaccharide of animal and fungal cells. Similar structure to amylopectin (in that it is a polymer of α-glucose) of starch but has many more branches and the branches are shorter. Glycogen is even more compact than amylopectin. The structure of glycogen allows faster hydrolysis than starch which is important as animals may need emergency glucose faster than plants.

Cellulose: It is the structural polysaccharide in plants. Long unbranched chains of glucose linked by β-1, 4-glycosidic bonds. The individual chains are then linked to each other by hydrogen bonds. These are formed into **strong** microfibrils. Hydrogen bonding prevents water entering the molecule. Cellulose is, therefore, resistant to enzyme hydrolysis which makes it an excellent **structural** polysaccharide. Cellulose cell walls provide protection to all plant cells (Fig. 5.1.3).

Chitin: It is a structural polysaccharide found in hard exoskeletons of all arthropods and in

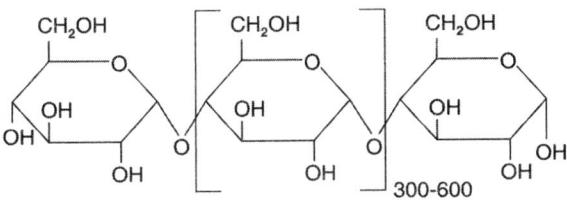

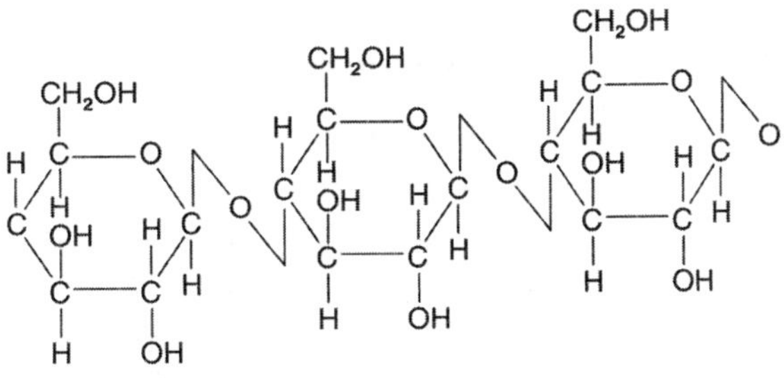

Fig. 5.1.1: Structure of amylose

Fig. 5.1.3: Structure of cellulose

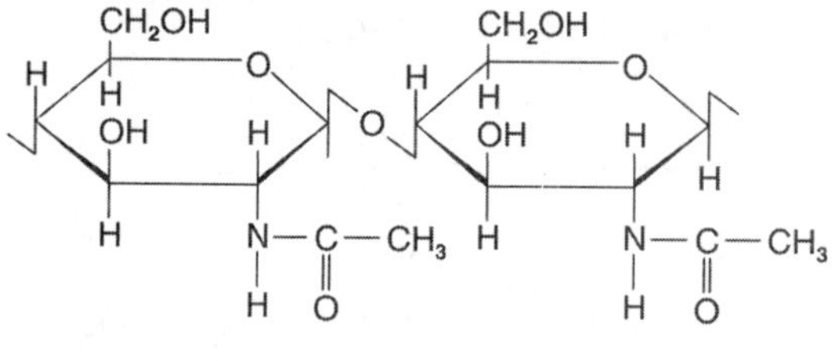

Fig. 5.1.4: Structure of chitin

hyphal walls of many fungi. Made of glucosamine units (glucose + amino acid) and is linked by β-1, 4-glycosidic bonds. The presence of the amino group causes even more hydrogen bonding between the chains than in cellulose. Chitin is, therefore, an extremely **resilient** and **tough** polysaccharide (Fig. 5.1.4).

Chemical Test of Carbohydrates

Test for starch: To the solution of carbohydrates, add 2–3 drops of iodine, blue/black precipitate (ppt) forms.

Test of reducing sugar: To the solution of carbohydrates, add equal quantity of Benedict's reagent, mix, heat to 70°C [(Do not boil because this would split a disaccharide, e.g. sucrose into reducing sugars glucose and fructose and may a false positive test)]. Solution turns from blue to pale green to yellow to orange to brick red ppt of copper (I) oxide, e.g. glucose, fructose and maltose.

Test of nonreducing sugar: To 2 ml test solution add 1ml dilute HCl, boil, cool and neutralize with excess NaOH. Repeat test for reducing sugar.

Functions of Carbohydrates

- Immediate respiratory substrates, e.g. glucose.
- Energy stores, e.g. glycogen in mammals, starch in plants.
- Structural components, e.g. cellulose in plant cell walls, chitin in arthropod exoskeleton.
- Pentose sugars—ribose and deoxyribose, are components of RNA and DNA, respectively.
- Metabolites, i.e. intermediates in biochemical pathways.
- Cell-to-cell attachment molecules, e.g. combined with proteins to form glycoproteins or lipids to form glycolipids on plasma membrane.
- Transport, e.g. sucrose in plant phloem tissue.

Bael (Fig. 5.1.5)

Synonyms: English—Wood apple, Bengal Quince, **Hindi** Bael, Sirphal.

Biological source: Bael consists of unripe or half ripe fruits or their slices or irregular pieces of *Aegle marmelos* Correab belonging to family Rutaceae.

Habitat: Woody tree, native to India, now naturalized in Sri Lanka, Pakistan, Bangladesh, Myanmar, Thailand and most of South Eastern Asian countries.

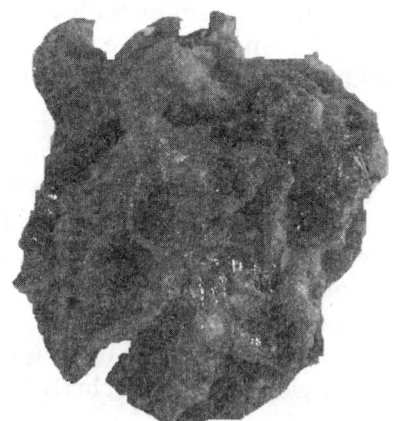

Fig. 5.1.5: Bael fruit
(*see also in colour Plate 1*)

Botany

- Kingdom   Plantae
- Order   Sapindales
- Family   Rutaceae

- Sub-family Aurantioideae
- Tribe Clauseneae
- Genus *Aegle*
- Species *marmelos*

Parts used: Fruit (both ripe and unripe), root-bark, leaves, rind of ripe fruits and flowers.

Organoleptic Characters

Color: Gray-green, yellow (ripe)
Odor: Aromatic
Taste: Mucilaginous
Shape: Sub-spherical berry
Size: 2 to 8 inches (5–20 cm) in diameter

Extra features: It consist of epicarp which is hard and woody in nature, mesocarp and endocarp embedded in the pulp are 10 to 15 seeds, flattened-oblong, about 3/8 inch (1 cm) long, bearing woolly hairs and each enclosed in a sac of adhesive, transparent mucilage that solidifies on drying.

Chemical constituents (Fig. 5.1.6): The main constituents are alkaloids, coumarin and steroids; detained from different parts of tree, such as leaves, fruit, wood, root and bark.

- Coumarin—marmelain, mormesin and mormin.
- Alkaloids—aegeline, aegelenine and mormelin.
- Polysaccharides—galactose, arabinose and L-rhamanose.

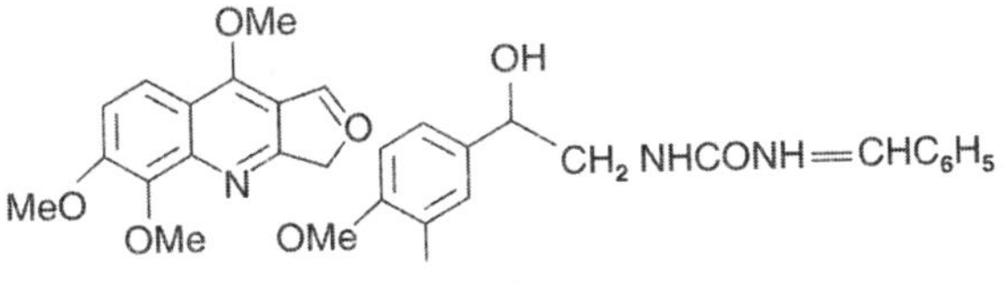

Fig. 5.1.6: Chemical constituents of Bael

Chemical Test

- Alcoholic extract when made alkaline, shows blue or green fluorescence in UV light.
- Take moistened dry powder in test tube. Cover the test tube with filter paper soaked with NaOH. Keep in water bath. After exposure of filter paper in UV light, it shows yellowish green fluorescence.
- Alcoholic/aqueous extract with 5% $FeCl_3$ gives deep blue black color and with lead acetate solution, it gives white ppt.

Uses: The fresh ripe fruits are taken for their mild laxative, tonic and digestive effects. Bael fruit is mildly astringent and used to cure dysentery, diarrhea, hepatitis, tuberculosis, dyspepsia and good for heart and brain.

Honey (Fig. 5.1.7)

Synonyms: hindi—Madhu, **English**—Purified honey.
Biological source: Honey is obtained from the sugary secretion deposited in honey comb by bees *Apis mellifera* and *Apis dorsata*; family—Apidae.
Habitat: West indies, California, Chile, Africa, Australia, New Zealand.

Organoleptic Characters

Color: Yellowish-brown liquid
Odor: Characteristic, pleasant
Taste: Sweet
Appearance: Syrupy thick, clear, viscid and translucent liquid when fresh.

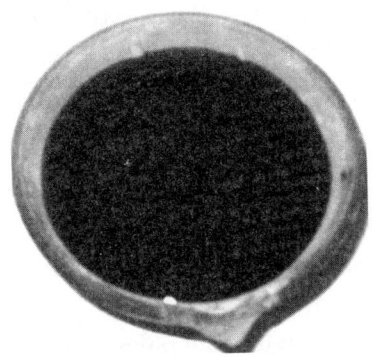

Fig. 5.1.7: Honey
(*see also in colour Plate 1*)

Weight per ml: 1.35 to 1.36

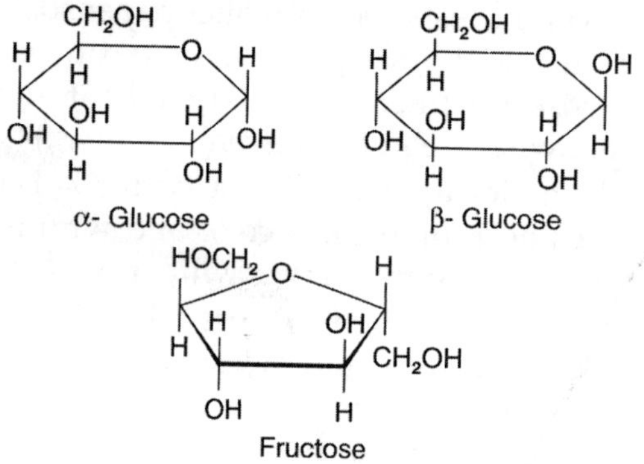

Fig. 5.1.8: Chemical constituents of honey

Solubility: Soluble in water, insoluble in alcohol and other organic solvents.

Rotation: Optically active with rotation between +0.6 and 0.3.

Chemical constituents (Fig. 5.1.8): Honey mainly consists of natural invert sugar, which is mixture of glucose (30–40%) and fructose (40–50%). It also contains sucrose, dextrin, formic acid, volatile oil and pollen grains in small amount together with vitamins, proteins

Table 5.1.3: Composition of honey

S. no	Constituents	Percentage
1.	Water	17–18%
2.	Levulose (fructose)	39%
3.	Dextrose (glucose)	34%
4.	Sucrose	1%
5.	Dextrin	0.5%
6.	Plant acids	0.5%
7.	Proteins	2%
8.	Salts	1%
9.	Undetermined residues	4%

and amino acids and traces of invertase and diastase enzymes (Table 5.1.3).

Chemical test

Honey solution is prepared by mixing one part of honey with five parts of water.
- *Reduction of Fehling's solution*: 1 ml of honey solution with 1 ml of Fehling's solution on heating, red color is produced due to reduction.
- Test for artificial invert sugar: 5 ml of honey solution + 2.5 ml of diethyl ether, shake and separate the ether layer, evaporate ether layer completely and to the residue add one drop of 1% w/v solution of resorcinol in concentrated HCl; pure honey should not give cherry red color. (*Note: Due* to prolonged heating and long storage, sometime pure honey also give cherry red color), Honey adulterated with artificial invert sugar due to presence of furfural gives cherry red color.
- Limit test: Limit test for chloride and sulfate is important as per pharmacopoeial standard.

Adulterants: Artificial invert sugar, commercial glucose, sucrose and polysaccharides.

Uses: It is used as a nutritive, as a demulcents in cough, cold and constipation, also as a sweetening agent, antiseptic and vehicle for ayurvedic preparations.

Ghatugum (Fig. 5.1.9)

Synonyms: English: Ghatti gum; **Hindi—**Bakla, **Gwalior—**Gond dhow; **Tamil—** Vakkali.

Biological source: Ghatti gum is obtained from *Anogeissus latifolia* Wallich, family Combretaceae. It is considered inferior to gum acacia. Its solution is dextrorotatory but it does not yield xylose on hydrolysis.

Habitat: Indigenous to India and Ceylon.

Botany

- Kingdom   Plantae
- Division   Magnoliophyta
- Class   Magnoliopsida
- Order   Myrtales
- Family   Combretaceae
- Genus   *Anogeissus*
- Species   *latifolia*

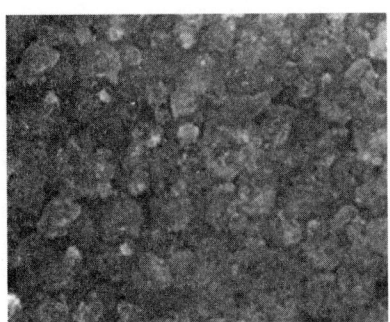

Fig. 5.1.9: Ghatugum
(see also in colour Plate 1)

Organoleptic Characters

Color: Best quality is colorless, inferior gum is yellow to brown in color
Odor: Odorless
Taste: Mucilaginous
Shape: Vermiform or round tears
Fracture: Uniform and glassy
Chemical constituents: Guar gum is an unbranched polysaccharide, galactomannan (Fig. 5.1.10), which consists of galactose attached to every other mannose unit. It consists of calcium and magnesium salt of a complex polysaccharide which contains L-arabinose, D-galactose, D-mannose, D-xylose and D-glucuronic acid. It also contains oxidase.

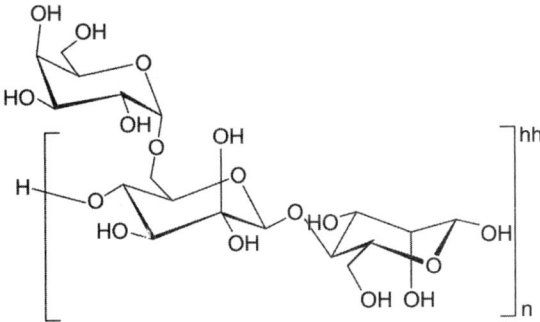

Fig. 5.1.10: Galactomannan

Chemical Test

- With 10% tannic acid, it gives white precipitate.
- Aqueous solution of gum gives slight precipitate with lead acetate.
- It forms colorless mucilage with water of much greater viscosity than that made with same proportion acacia.
- It does not form complete aqueous solutions but forms viscous dispersions in water at concentrations of 5.0%.

Uses: Gum is used in confectionery, used in scorpion sting and snakebite, emulsifier for oil and water emulsions, used as a waterproofing agent in liquid explosive, and to stabilize paraffin wax emulsions.

Agar (Fig. 5.1.11)

Synonyms: English–Agar-agar, vegetable gelatin, Japanese or Chinese Gelatin, Japanese Isinglass.

Biological source: It is the dried colloidal concentrate prepared from the decoction of red algae and from other species of the genus *Gelidium*, family Gelidaceae. Japanese agar is obtained from *Gelidium amansii*. It is also obtained from genus *Gracilaria*, family Gracilariaceae.

Habitat: Agar is produced on large scale in Japan, Korea, South Africa, USA, Spain, Mexico and New Zealand.

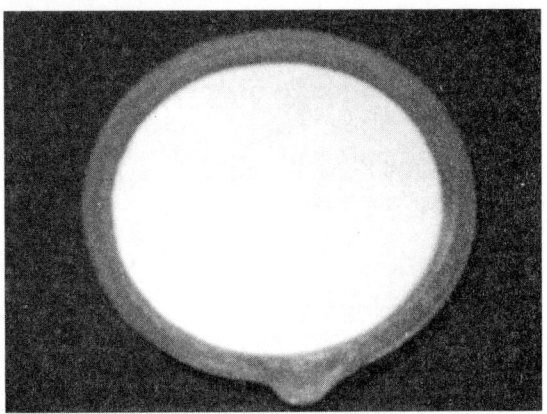

Fig. 5.1.11: Agar
(see also in colour Plate 1)

Botany

Kingdom	Archaeplastida
Division	Rhodophyta
Class	Rhodophyceae
Subclass	Rhodymeniophycidae
Order	Gelidiales
Family	Gelidiaceae
Genus	*Gelidium*

Morphological Characters

Form: It occurs in two forms: 1) Coarse powder or flakes; 2) bundles of translucent, and crumpled, strips, 2–5 mm wide.

Color: Colorless to pale yellow.

Fracture: Tough when damp and brittle when dry.

Odor: Not distinct

Taste: Mucilaginous

Solubility: Cold water—does not dissolve but swells to a gelatinous mass.

Boiling water—dissolves and 1% solution gives a stiff jelly on cooling.

Chemical constituents: Agar is a heteropolysaccharide which contains a calcium salt of sulfuric ester of carbohydrate complex. It consists of two principal constituents, agarose and agaropectin.
- Agarose (Fig. 5.1.12) is the neutral polymer of galactose disaccharides known as agarbiose and responsible for gel strength.
- Ageropectin is responsible for the viscosity of agar solution, is a sulfonated polysaccharide of galactose and uronic acid esterified with sulfuric acid.

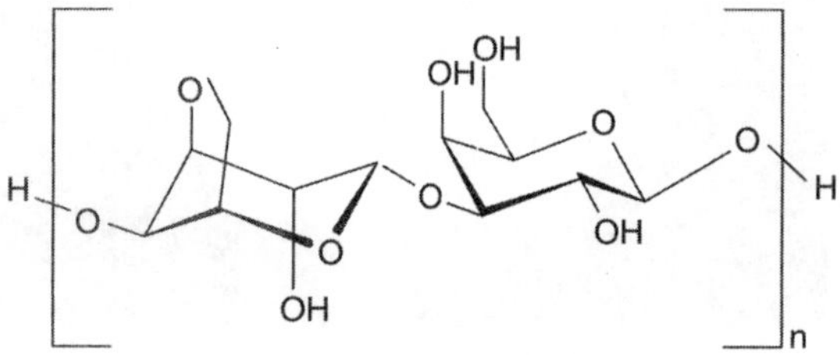

Fig. 5.1.12: Agarose

Chemical Test

- Agar with iodine solution gives crimson to brown color.
- Agar solution with ruthenium red gives pink color.
- Agar solution (hot) with $BaCl_2$ gives white precipitate.
- Agar with Fehling's solution (heat) gives red precipitate.
- Boil agar solution with water forms stiff jelly on cooling.
- Agar ash on slide with 2 drops of HCl when observed under microscope, sponge spicules of diatoms are seen.

Uses: Agar is widely used as a treatment for constipation, but is usually employed with Cascara. Its therapeutic value depends on the ability of the dry Agar to absorb and retain moisture. Its action is mechanical and analogous to that of the cellulose of vegetable foods, aiding the regularity of the bowel movements. It is sometimes used as an adulterant of jams and jellies. It is mainly used for preparation of nutrient media in bacteriological preparations.

Adulterants: The powdered drug is adulterated with starch. Mount the drug in chloral-iodine solution and observe the starch grains.

Acacia (Indian Gum—Fig. 5.1.13)

Synonyms: Gum acacia, Gum arabic.

Biological source: Acacia gum is a dried exudation from the stem and branches of *Acacia senegal*, family Leguminosae.

Habitat: Sudan, central and western African countries, such as Senegal, Nigeria and Senegambia

Botany

- Kingdom   Plantae
- Division   Magnoliophyta

- Class   Magnoliopsida
- Order   Fabales
- Family   Fabaceae
- Subfamily   Mimosoideae
- Genus   *Acacia*
- Species   *senegal*

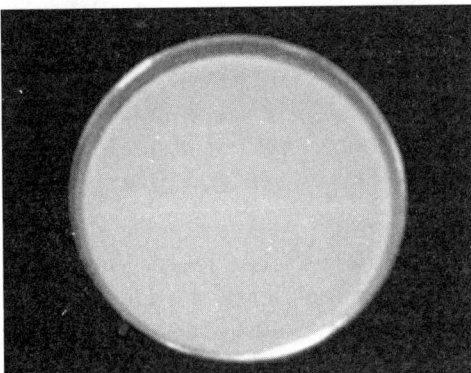

Fig. 5.1.13: Acacia gum
(*see also in colour Plate 1*)

Parts used: Gummy exudates from stems and branches.

Collection and Preparations

The gum harvest from the various species lasts about five weeks. About the middle of November, after the rainy season, it exudes spontaneously from the trunk and principal branches, but the flow is generally stimulated by incisions in the bark, a thin strip, 2 to 3 feet in length and 1 to 3 inches wide being torn off. In about fifteen days, it thickens in the furrow down which it runs, hardening on exposure to the air, usually in the form of round or oval tears, but sometimes in vermicular forms, white or red, according to whether the species is a white or red gum tree. About the middle of December, the Moors commence the harvesting. The masses of gum are collected, either while adhering to the bark, or after it falls to the ground, the entire product, often of various species, thus collected, is packed in baskets and very large sacks of tanned leather.

Characteristics

- Gum arabic is unique among the natural hydrocolloids because of its extremely high solubility in water. Gum arabic is insoluble in oils and in most organic solvents. It is soluble in aqueous ethanol up to a limit of about 60% ethanol. Limited solubility can also be obtained with glycerol and ethylene glycol.
- It can actually form a highly viscous, gel-like mass similar in character to a strong starch gel.
- High viscosities are not obtained with Gum arabic until concentrations of about 40–50% are obtained. This ability to form highly concentrated solutions is responsible for the excellent stabilizing and emulsifying properties of Gum arabic when incorporated with large amounts of insoluble matters.

Chemical constituents: Acacia gum consists almost entirely of a glucosidal acid of high molecular weight, i.e. arabic acid (Fig. 5.1.14), combined with potassium, magnesium, and calcium; by hydrolysis each molecule yields two molecules of the sugar arabinose and four of galactose. Gum acacia also contains an oxidase enzyme, and hence readily turns powdered guaiacum resin. It contains further a small percentage of nitrogen.

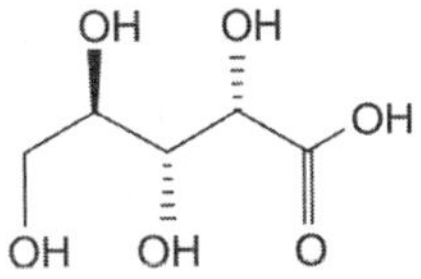

Fig. 5.1.14: Arabic acid

Chemical Test

- Acacia gum is insoluble in alcohol, but dissolves freely in water, forming a translucent, viscid, but not glairy or ropy liquid, that feebly reddens litmus paper.

- A 10% aqueous solution of good qualities is slightly levorotatory, and when boiled with an equal volume of Fehling's solution throws down a slight but distinct deposit of cuprous oxide.
- Solution of lead acetate produces no precipitate, but subacetate produces a copious white.
- A saturated solution of borax forms with a strong solution of gum a clear, translucent jelly.
- Inferior (brown) gum usually contains tannin which may be detected by solution of ferric chloride.

Uses: Acacia gum is used medicinally as a demulcent and as a means of suspending oils, resin, etc. in aqueous fluids. It is also used as binding agent in preparation of lozenges and compressed tablets.

Tragacanth (Fig. 5.1.15)

Synonyms: English – Gum Tragacanth, Gum Dragon

Biological source: Tragacanth is the gummy exudation obtained from the gummy exudation of *Astragalus gummifer*, family Leguminosae

Habitat: Asia Minor, Persia and Kurdistan

Botany

- Kingdom   Plantae
- Division   Magnoliophyta
- Class   Magnoliopsida
- Order   Fabales
- Family   Fabaceae
- Genus   *Astragalus*
- Species   *gummifer*

Parts used: Gummy exudation

Description: The plant is a small branching thorny shrub, the stem of which exudes a gum, vertical slits giving flat ribbon-shaped pieces and punctures giving tears; these have a horny appearance, are nearly colorless or faintly yellow, marked with numerous concentric ridges, the flakes break with a short fracture, are odorless and nearly tasteless; soaked in cold water, they swell and form a gelatinous mass 8 or 10% only dissolving.

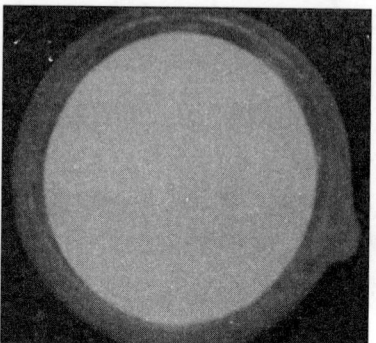

Fig. 5.1.15: Tragacanth gum (*see also in colour Plate 1*)

Chemical constituents: Gum tragacanth consists of a mixture of water-soluble polysaccharides which yield on hydrolysis. L-arabinose, D-xylose, D-galactose, D-galacturonic acid and water insoluble polysaccharides bassorin which consisting 60–70% of the gum as well as 1–3% starch, 1–4% cellulose; 3% ash, small amounts of invert sugar, 2–3% of a volatile acid (probably acetic acid), and about 15% water. Tragacanthic acid is composed of 40% D-galacturonic acid, 40% D-xylose, 10% L-fucose, 4% D-galactose, and three aldobiuronic acids. Arabinogalactan consists of 75% L-arabinose, 12% D-galactose, 3% D-galacturonic acid, and small amounts of L-rhamnose.

Characteristics

Color: White or pale yellowish white flakes
Odor: Odorless
Taste: Tasteless
Size: Flakes are 25 × 12 × 2 mm
Shape: Thin-flattened ribbon-like
Solubility: Partly soluble in water, swells, insoluble in alcohol.

Fracture: Short

Extra features: The gum is horny, translucent, transverse and longitudinal ridges.

Chemical Test

- Tragacanth gum when boiled with 10% aqueous ferric chloride solution, deep yellow precipitate is obtained.
- Tragacanth gum, if dissolved in precipitated copper oxide and conc. ammonium hydroxide, stingy precipitate is obtained.
- Gum in lead acetate gives white precipitate.
- Gum in Fehling's solution gives red precipitate.
- Gum in 5% caustic potash gives canary yellow color.

Uses: It is used as demulcent for the suspension of heavy, insoluble powders to impart consistence to lozenges, being superior to gum arabic, also in making emulsions, mucilage, etc. Mucilage of Tragacanth has been used as an application to burns.

Adulterants: The Indian gum, the product of *Coplospermum gossypium*, also acacia, dextrin wheat and corn starch.

Isapgol (Fig. 5.1.16)

Synonyms: Bengali—Isapgul; **Hindi**—Isapgol; **English**—Indian psyllium; **Mar**—Isapgola.

Biological source: It consist of dried seeds of *Plantago ovata* forsk, family Plantaginaceae.

Habitat: Mediterranean region and commercially grown in north western India.

Botany

- Kingdom   Plantae
- Division   Magnoliophyta
- Class   Magnolipisida
- Order   Lamiales

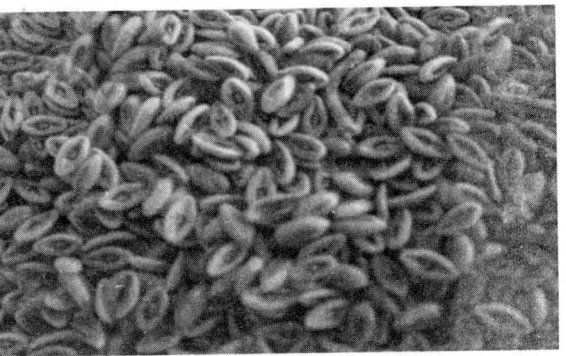

Fig. 5.1.16: Isapgol seeds
(*see also in colour Plate 2*)

- Family   Plantaginaceae
- Genus   *Plantago*
- Species   *ovate*

Parts used: Seeds, husk

Organoleptic Characters

Color: Light brown to moderate brown

Odor: Faint and characteristics

Taste: Bland, mucilaginous

Shake: Ovoid oblong, boat shaped.

Extra features: Seeds have convex and concave surfaces, convex surfaces has central glossy reddish brown elongated spots whereas concave surface is deeply groved with hilum.

Chemical constituents: Seed contains 30% mucilage, xylose, arabinose, galacturonic acid, galactose, albumin, tannin and acetylcholine. The seed pulp contains 14.7% linoleic acid and 5% stable oil.

Chemical Test: Test for Mucilage

- Seeds on slide with water show the zone of mucilage.
- Isapgol powder when treated with water forms jelly-like mass on keeping.
- Mucilage gives pink color with ruthenium red under microscope.

Standards

Total Ash: Not more than 4.0%
Particle size: Not more than 5.0%
Moisture (loss on drying): Not more than 12.0%
Acid insoluble ash: Not more than 1.0%
Foreign organic matter: Not more than 0.5%

Microscopy: Epidermal cell of testa is filled with mucilage which swells in contact with water. The cells are large, polyhedral, thin-walled, rounded in surface view. Small starch granules are simple or compound embedded in the mucilage. Inner layer of testa rather indistinct, thin-walled, cells containing brown pigment. Endosperm is composed of thick-walled cells with numerous piths and granular contents, embryo consisting of thin-walled polyhedral cells containing fixed oil and aleuronic grains.

Uses: The characteristics of psyllium seed husks make them useful for any treatment that requires improvement or maintenance of transit time in the gastrointestinal tract. Psyllium seed is considering as a good intestinal cleanser and stool softner. Psyllium seed is one of the most popular fibers and traditional herbal medicine. Psyllium seed husks are mainly used to treat constipation.

Adulterants: *Plantago lanceolata*

Starch (Fig. 5.1.17)

Synonyms: Amylum

Biological source: Starch or amylum is a polysaccharide carbohydrate produced by all green plants as an energy store and is a major food source for humans. Potato, rice, maize and wheat starch is obtained from *Solanum tuberosum* (Solanaceae), *Oryza sativa* (Gramineae), *Zea mays* (Gramineae), and *Triticum astivum* (Gramineae).

Habitat: Commercially, starch is produced in USA, India, China and Japan.

Organoleptic Characters

Color: Rice and maize: White; Potato: Slightly yellowish; Wheat: Cream
Odor: Odorless
Taste: Mucilaginous
Solubility: Insoluble in alcohol and cold water, but form colloidal solution with boiled water.
Specific gravity: 1.62–1.65
pH: Potato and maize–neutral–Rice–alkaline; Wheat–faint acidic.
Extra features: A typical feature of starch is that it becomes soluble in water when heated. The granules swell and burst, the semi-crystalline structure is lost and the smaller amylose molecules start leaching out of the granule. This process is called starch gelatinization.

Microscopical Characteristic

Potato starch (Fig. 5.1.18): Potato starch is mostly simple or compound. Subspherical grains are up to 35 μ in length and ovoid grains of 30 to 100 μ. They have usually a flattened ovoid shape and possess a small hilum that is often situated near the narrow extremity of the grain, whilst the broad end frequently

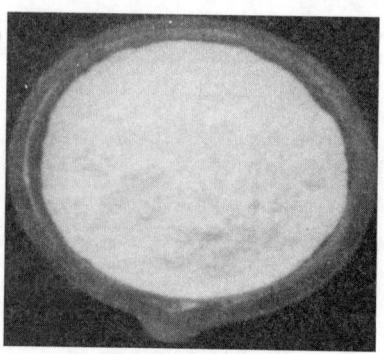

Fig. 5.1.17: Starch
(*see also in colour Plate 2*)

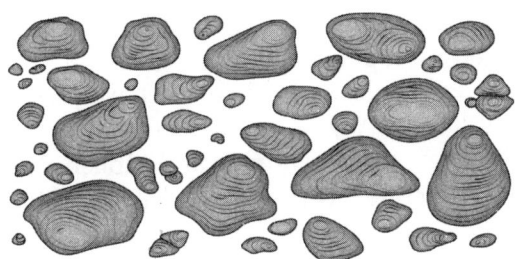

Fig. 5.1.18: Microscopy of potato starch

exhibits a sinuate outline; the concentric striae are well marked.

Rice starch (Fig. 5.1.19): The rice starch is simple and compound with polyhedral shape. No striations are visible but hilum can be distinguished by small central dot. The grains are up to 4 to 10 μ.

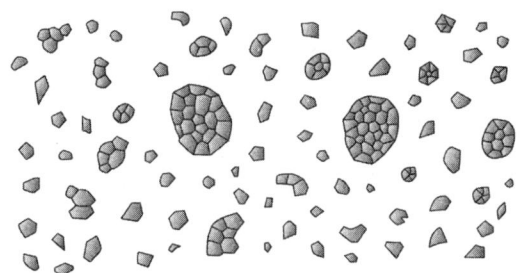

Fig. 5.1.19: Microscopy of rice starch

Maize starch (Fig. 5.1.20): Maize starch consists of grains that are nearly uniform in size and rather smaller than the large grains of wheat starch; (mostly 12 to 18 μ; they are polygonal

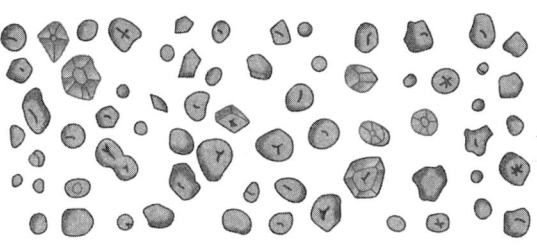

Fig. 5.1.20: Microscopy of maize starch

with blunt angles, or more or less rounded. In the center there is often a small cleft, or two or three radiating from a center (the hilum).

Wheat starch (Fig. 5.1.21): Wheat starch consists of large and small grains mixed together, with few intermediate in size; the former are lenticular in shape and sometimes marked with faint concentric rings. The hilum is central but not conspicuous. The larger of the large grains average about 30 to 38 μ in diameter, the smaller of the large grains 15 to 25 μ whilst the small grains average 6 to 7 μ.

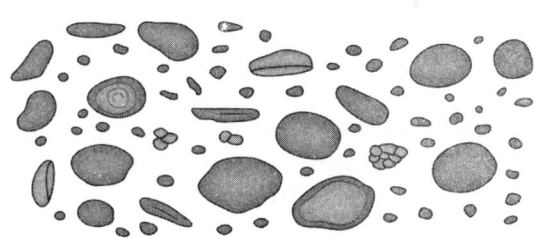

Fig. 5.1.21: Microscopy of wheat starch

Preparation of Starch

The cells are ruptured by grinding the softened grain to a pulp, and the gluten is removed by one of the following processes, viz.

a. A mixture of crushed grain and water is allowed to undergo putrefactive decomposition; the gluten is decomposed, lactic, acetic, and other acids being produced and removed by washing.
b. The crushed grain is mixed with a dilute solution of caustic soda by which the gluten is dissolved.
c. The grain is crushed and mixed with water to dough from which the starch grains are washed by kneading it in a stream of water, leaving a mass of gluten behind.

The starch is purified by washing, straining and allowing the milky liquid containing starch grains in suspension to clear, by which a more or less complete separation into pure starch and starch mixed with varying amounts of cell-debris is effected. It is finally dried, during which the moist mass gradually splits up into angular fragments. These are then ground to form starch powder.

Chemical Constituents

Starch consists of two types of molecules, amylose (normally 20–30%) and amylopectin (normally 70–80%). Both consist of polymers of α-D-glucose units. Amylose and amylopectin are inherently incompatible molecules; amylose having lower molecular weight with a relatively extended shape whereas amylopectin has huge but compact molecules. The presence of amylose tends to reduce the crystallinity of the amylopectin and influence the ease of water penetration into the granules. As they absorb water, they swell, lose crystallinity. The higher the amylose content, the lower is the swelling power and the smaller is the gel strength for the same starch.

Chemical test: Starch is a polysacharose of the formula $(C_6H_{10}O_5)n$. Boiled with water the grains swell, burst and partially dissolve, forming an opalescent solution which, sufficiently concentrated, gelatinises on cooling (starch paste).

Starch test: Add Iodine-KI reagent to a solution. A blue-black color results, if starch is present. If starch amylose is not present, then the color will stay orange or yellow. Starch amylopectin does not give the color, nor does cellulose, nor do disaccharides, such as sucrose in sugar.

It shows positive Fehling's and Molish test.

Uses: Starch is a versatile and cheap, and has many uses as thickener, water binder, emulsion stabilizer and gelling agent. Internally it is used as astringent, nutritive, demulcent, protective and absorbent. It is used as antidote in iodine poisoning. It is used as filler, binder and disintegrator in tablet. Starch is starting material for preparation of glucose, dextrose and dextrin.

Adulterants: Manihot esculenta (Euphorbiaceae).

5.2 GLYCOSIDES

Glycosides are the natural organic compounds, from plants or animal sources which on enzymatic or acid hydrolysis give one or more sugar moieties along with non-sugar moieties. These two different chemical compounds or compounds present in joined form in glycosides by a special linkage called glycosidal linkage. In which, the former is called glycone and the later aglycone or genin. Glycone is the sugar moiety and aglycone is the non-sugar moiety. In another words glycosides are the naturally occurring plant constituents which consists of a sugar portion attached by a special glycoside linkage to non sugar portion.

$$\text{Glycosides} \xrightarrow{\text{Acid/ enzymatic hydrolysis}} \text{Sugar component} + \text{Non-sugar component}$$
$$\text{(Glycone)} \quad \text{(Aglycone)}$$

$$R.OH + HO.X \underset{\text{Hydrolysis}}{\overset{\text{Condensation}}{\rightleftharpoons}} R.OX + H_2O$$

Example: Salicin is an example which represents formation of glycosides.

$$\underset{\text{Glucose}}{C_6H_{11}O_5OH} + \underset{\text{Salicyl alcohol}}{HOC_6H_4.CH_2OH} \rightleftharpoons \underset{\text{Salicin (glycosides)}}{C_6H_{11}O_5.C_6H_4.CH_2OH} + H_2O$$

Chemical Aspects

Chemically, the glycosides are considered as acetals in which the hydroxyl group of the sugar is condensed with a hydroxyl group of the non-sugar component and the secondary hydroxyl is condense within the sugar molecule itself to form an oxide ring so glycosides are also called sugar ether.

The usual linkage between sugar and aglycone is oxygen linkage which is between the reducing group of sugar and an alcoholic or phenolic group of aglycone and such glycosides are called O-glycosides. As sugar are found in two forms so, glycosides are of two types (α and β). Stereochemically, α and β stereoisomers are assigned. β glycosides are found in plants.

Glycosides can be hydrolyzed by enzyme, acid, alkali or sometimes only with moisture. The enzymes hydrolysed α-glycosides are invertase and maltase while myrosin, linarase, amygdalase, cellobiase and gentianase hydrolysed β glycosides. In simple form, the glycosides with these two isomers can be synthesized from union of methyl alcohol and glucose.

Aglycones

The aglycones or genin is that part of a glycoside molecule which is responsible for the pharmacological action of the drug of the glycosides. The aglycones belong to variety of different classes of definite chemical belong to compounds thus the glycosides can be grouped as cyanogenetic glycosides (amygdalin), glycosinolates (glucocapparin), lactone or coumarin (dasphnin, digitoxin), quinine glycosides (barbaloin), flavanoid (quercetin), steroidal alkaloid (salanine), saponin (glycyrrhizin).

Sugar

Mainly all kinds of sugars are present in the glycosides. They may be tetrose, pentose, hexoses or some special sugar, as in cardiac glycosides. When sugar moiety is glucose, fructose, rhamnoside, galactoside and riboside then glycosides are glycoside, fructoside, rhamnoside, galactoside and riboside, respectively.

Properties

Glycosides are colorless, crystalline or amorphous solid substances. Exceptional cases, like flavones glycosides are yellow-colored and anthracene glycosides are red or orange-colored. They are soluble in water and alcohol but insoluble in ether and chloroform. Glycosides are optically active and usually they are levorotatory means l-form. Glycosides are substances of profound physiological action or animal tissue and are many a times poisnous for human beings. They are generally the products of special metabolic process and their concentration in various morphological parts also varies considerably according to age and ecological factors of the plant. Those which are most significant therapeutic action are cardiac glycosides.

Classification

Glycosides are classified according to:
1. Nature of sugar
2. The chemical nature of aglycone
3. The therapeutic action
4. The glycosides linkage

Classification According to Nature of Sugar

Glycosides are classified according to nature of sugar and kind of sugar. Glycosides have glucose as a sole sugar. Examples, pentosides yield pentose. Sugar arabinose and rhamnosides yield the methyl-pentose and rhamnose. Some cardiac glycosides have special sugar component called deoxy or desoxy sugar found only in cardiac glycosides.

Classification According to Chemical Nature of Aglycone Group

The classification is based on the chemical nature of the aglycone group, such as steroid structure containing glycosides, etc. The main disadvantage of this classification is that it includes all kinds of plant constituents. Anthracene ring containing glycosides, flavone glycosides, cyanogenetic glycosides, alcohol, phenol, aldehyde group containing glycosides, etc.

Various aglycone groups are given in Table 5.2.1.

Table 5.2.1: Classification of glycosides with examples

Glycosides	Drugs
Cardiac or sterol	Digitoxin, gitoxin, digoxin from digitalis
Anthraquinone or anthracene	Sennosides from senna, cascarosides from cascara, barbolin from aloe
Saponin glycosides	Glycyrrhizin in glycyrrhiza, diosgenin from discorea
Cyanogenetic or cyanophoric glycosides	Amydalin—bitter almond Prussian—wild cherry bark
Isothiocyanate glycosides	Sinigrin—black mustard Sinalbin—white mustard
Flavanol glycosides	Rutin—ruta, Hesperidin-orange, kaempferol–senna
Alcohol glycosides	Salicin—salix
Aldehyde glycosides	Salinigrin—salix
Lactone or coumarin	Skimmin—staranise, aersculin—harsechest nut bean
Miscellaneous	Quassium–quassia, picrotoxin–anamista

Classification According to Therapeutic Action

This classification offers an excellent opportunity to group together glycosides which show characteristic or selective therapeutic action on a particular organ and/or against the particular aliment.

Examples:

1. *Digitalis glycosides:* Their action of heart/cardiac muscle called cardiac glycosides.
2. *Purgative glycosides:* Anthraquinone ring with which a definite structure activity relationship act as purgative principle.
3. *Bitter glycosides:* Glycosides of family Gentianaceae because of bitter taste are called bitter glycosides, which show their common use, understood by word bitter.

Classification based on Glycosides Linkage

This classification is based on the basis of the linkage which is formed between the aglycone and glycone part. The linkages are formed through oxygen, sulfur, nitrogen or carbon.

Extraction Procedure of Glucosidal Drugs

The extraction of glycosidal drug is performed by continuous hot percolation using soxhlet apparatus with alcohol as a solvent. But before it is required to inactivate the enzymes present in the glycosides for better yield. Thus methods for activation are:

- Fresh dry material is heated with boiling water or boiling alcohol for 10 to 20 min.
- Material is boiled with acetone, and treated with acid at cold temperature.

Stas-Otto Method

1. The fresh dry material is coarsely powdered and then enzymes are activated.
2. The extraction is carried out by percolation with mixture of methanol and water due to its solubility pattern.
3. The percolate is again treated with lead acetate to precipitate chlorophyll and tannins and marc is discarded.
4. Again filtrate and residue is obtained by filtration of sample, this filtrate is treated with H_2S gas to remove excess of lead acetate as lead sulfide.
5. Finally filtrate the solution and evaporate filtrate to get glycosidal residue.

Isolation Method for Glycosidal Drug

There are mainly three types of methods used for it:
1. By different solubility method
2. Fractional crystallization
3. By chromatography

By different solubility method: In this method, glycosidal extract is treated with many solvents, like mixture of water and methanol and thus glycosides are separate out.

Fractional crystallization: In this method, crystal of drug is prepared by isolation method and by crystal formation is separated out.

By chromatography: In chromatography, preparative type of TLC is formed in which the different color writing study is performed.

Identification Test for Glycosidal Drugs

For Normal Glycosides

a. *Xanthohydrol test:* The test solution is 0.125% of xanthohydrol in glacial acetic acid and 1% HCl is heated; red color is obtained.

b. *Antimony trichloride test:* Cardinolides are treated with antimony trichloride and trichloroacetic acid blue to violet color is obtained.

c. *Liberman test for steroidal glycosides:* Steroidal glycosides are treated with CCl_4, acetic anhydride and conc. H_2SO_4; violet blue color is obtained.

d. *Tollens test:* Test solution in pyridine is treated with silver paper, the solution liberates silver. The silver causes mirror on wall of test tube.

e. *Legal test:* Glycosides are treated with pyridine (for dissolution), 1 drop of 2% sodium nitroprusside and 1 drop of 20% NaOH deep red color is observed.

Applications

1. Cardiac stimulants (digitalis)
2. Purgative-laxative (aloe, rhubarb, seena, cascara)
3. Bitter tonics (picrorrhiza)
4. Expectorants (wild cherry)
5. Steriodal drug synthesis (dioscorea)

CARDIAC GLYCOSIDES

Many of the plants known to contain cardiac or cardiotonic glycosides have long been used as arrow poisons (e.g. *strophanthus*) or as heart drugs (e.g. *digitalis*). They are used to strengthen a weakened heart and allow it to function more efficiently, though the dosage must be controlled very carefully since the therapeutic dose is so close to the toxic dose. In plants, cardiac glycosides are confined to the angiosperms, but are found in both monocotyledons and dicotyledons.

The therapeutic action of cardioactive glycosides depends on the structure of the aglycone, and on the type and number of sugar units attached. Two types of aglycone are recognized, cardenolides, e.g. digitoxigenin from *Digitalis purpurea* and bufadienolides, e.g. hellebrigenin from *Helleborus niger*.

The cardenolides are more common, and the plant families the Apocynaceae (e.g. *Strophanthus*), Liliaceae (e.g. *Convallaria*), and Scrophulariaceae (e.g. *Digitalis*) yield medicinal agents. The rarer bufadienolides are found in some members of the Liliaceae (e.g. *Urginea*) and Ranunculaceae (e.g. *Helleborus*).

Biosynthesis

Formed through mevalonate and deoxyxylulose pathway

For cardiac glycosides:

a. *Raymond's test:* In this test, small amount of glycosides is dissolve in 1 ml of 50% ethanol then 0.1 ml of 1% solution of dinitrobenzene in ethanol is added with 2–3 drops of 20% NaOH; violet color appears which turn blue after sometime.

   Note: This color is due to the activation of methylene group of C-21 in the lactone ring of cardiac glycosides.

b. *Modified Raymond's test or Kidde's reagent test:* Glycosides treated with Kidde's reagent give blue violet color. This color disappears after sometime.

   Composition of Kidde's reagent: Mix equal quantity of 0.2% solution of 3,5 dinitrobenzoic acid in 50% methanol and 5.7% w/v of aq solution of KOH.

c. *Keller-Kiliani test:* In this test, 1 gm of powdered drug is extracted with 10 ml of 70% alcohol then filtered. 5 ml of filtrate is mixed with 10 ml of H_2O_2 and add 0.5 ml of strong lead acetate due to which precipitate formed and then filtered. Shake filtrate with 5 ml of $CHCl_3$ with 1 ml of 1 volume of 5% $FeSO_4$ and 99 volume of glacial acetic acid and then 1–2 drop of concentrated H_2SO_4 is added due to which blue color appears.

Note: Blue color is formed due to deoxy sugars.

Digitalis

Synonyms: English—Digitalis, Foxglove.

Biological source: Digitalis is dried leaves of *Digitalis purpurea* belonging to family Scrophulariaceae. Dried at not more than 60°C and moisture content not more than 5%.

Habitat: The common Foxglove of the woods (*Digitalis purpurea*; Fig. 5.2.1) is widely distributed throughout Europe and is common as a wild-flower in Great Britain, growing freely in woods and lanes, particularly in South Devon, ranging from Cornwall and Kent to Orkney, but not occurring in Shetland, or in some of the eastern counties of England.

Botany

- Kingdom   Plantae
- Division   Angiospermae
- Order   Lamiales
- Family   Plantaginaceae
- Genus   *Digitalis*
- Species   *purpurea*

Part used: Dried leaflets

Organoleptic Characters

Color : Greyish green (lower surface)
         Dark green (upper surface)
Odor : Characteristic
Taste : Bitter
Shape : Ovate-lanceolate
Size : 10 to 40 cm long, 3 to 10 cm wide

Chemical constituents: Digitalis contains four important glucosides of which three are cardiac stimulants. The most powerful is digitoxin (Fig. 5.2.2), an extremely poisonous and cumulative drug, insoluble in water. Digitalin, which is crystalline and also insoluble in water; digitalin, amorphous, but

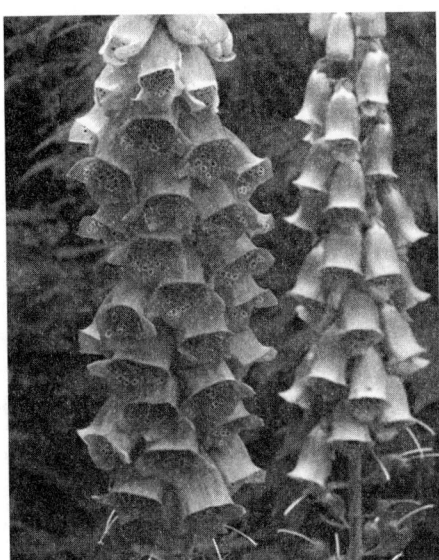

Fig. 5.2.1: Digitalis purpurea
(see also in colour Plate 2)

$CHCl_3$ with 1 ml of 1 volume of 5% $FeSO_4$ and 99 volume of glacial acetic acid and then 1–2 drop of concentrated H_2SO_4 is added due to which blue color appears.

Note: Blue color is formed due to deoxy sugars

Uses: Digitalis glycosides increase the force of contraction of heart without increasing the oxygen consumption and slow the heart rate when auricular fibrillation is present. To be used only under strict medical supervision. Digital in and digitoxin are powerful heart-muscle stimulants. Digitalis is useful as an antidote to aconite poisoning, nitrite poisoning and in agaricin poisoning.

Adulterants: Verbascum thapsus leaves primula vulgaris.

readily soluble in water, rendering it, therefore, capable of being administered subcutaneously, in doses so minute as rarely to exceed of a grain. Digitonin, which is a cardiac depressant, containing none of the physiological actions peculiar to digitalis. Other constituents are volatile oil, fatty matter, starch, gum, sugar, etc.

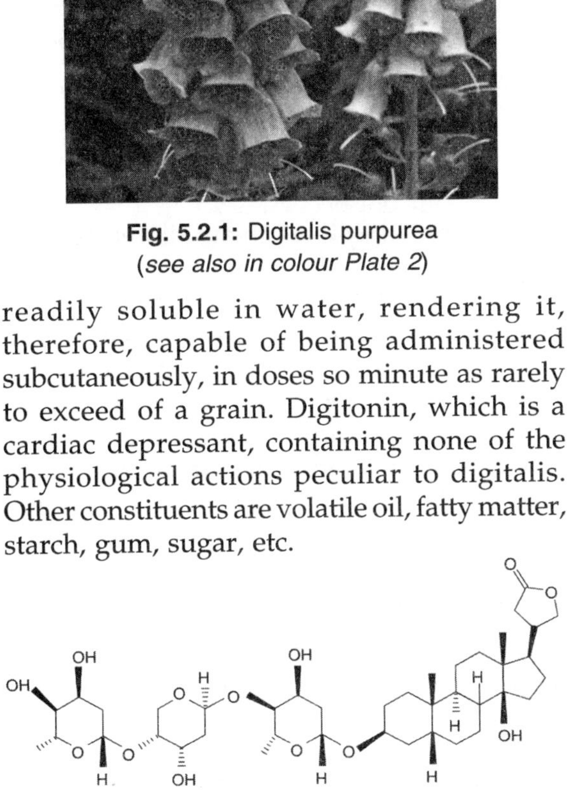

Fig. 5.2.2: Digitoxin

Chemical test

Keller-Kiliani test: In this test, 1 gm of powdered drug is extracted with 10 ml of 70% alcohol then filtered. 5 ml of filtrate is mixed with 10 ml of H_2O_2 and add 0.5 ml of strong lead acetate due to which precipitate formed and then filtered. Shake filtrate with 5 ml of

Squill

Synonyms: English—White squill, squill bulb (European squill); **Hindi**—Chhoti jungli, **Bengali**—Suphadiekhus; *Tamil*—Shirunari.

Biological source: Squill consists of dried slices of the bulb of *Urginea indica* (Indian squill) and *Urginea maritima* (European squill) belonging to family Liliaceae.

Habitat: European squill is found in dry, sandy places, especially the seacoast in most of the Mediterranean districts, and is found in Portugal, Morocco, Algeria, Corsica, southern France, whereas Indian squill is found throughout India including Konkan and Saurashtra.

Botany

- Kingdom   Plantae
- Order   Asparagales
- Family   Hyacinthaceae
- Genus   *Scilla*
- Species   *indica, maritime*

Part used: Bulb cut into slices, dried and powdered.

Organoleptic characters: Organoleptic characters of squill are given in Table 5.2.2.

Table 5.2.2: Organoleptic characters of squill

Macroscopic characters	Indian squill	European squill
Color	Yellowish white	Pale yellow
Odor	Slight	Slight
Taste	Bitter and acrid	Bitter, mucilaginous and acrid
Shape	Curved and sickle-shaped	Curved strips
Size	1 to 5 cm long 5 to 10 mm broad	5 to 6 cm long 3 to 8 mm broad

Chemical constituents: Scilla contains cardiac glycosides scillaren A (Fig. 5.2.3) and B and enzyme scillarenase. Three bitter glucosidal substances namely scillitoxin, scillipicrin and scillin were isolated. The first two are amorphous and act upon the heart, the former being the more active; scillin is crystalline and causes numbness and vomiting. Other constituents are mucilaginous and saccharine matter, including a peculiar mucilaginous carbohydrate named sinistrin, an inulin-like substance, which yields laevulose on being boiled with dilute acid present in Indian squill.

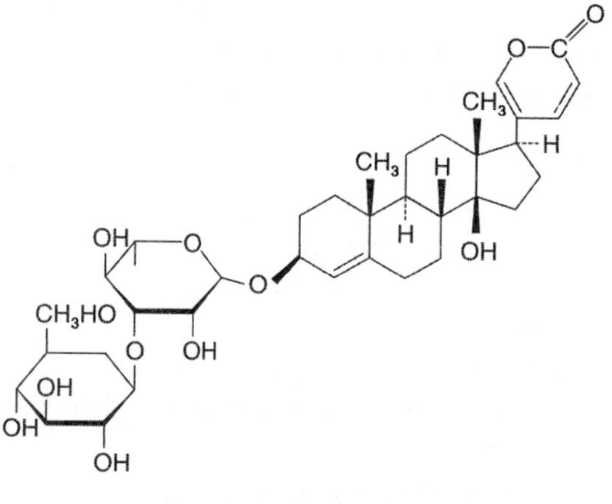

Fig. 5.2.3: Scillaren A

Chemical Test

1. For cardiac glycosides:
   Keller-Kiliani test: In this test, 1 gm of powdered drug is extracted with 10 ml of 70% alcohol then filtered. 5 ml of filtrate is mixed with 10 ml of H_2O_2 and add 0.5 ml of strong lead acetate due to which precipitate formed and then filtered. Shake filtrate with 5 ml of $CHCl_3$ with 1ml of 1 volume of 5% $FeSO_4$ and 99 volume of glacial acetic acid and then 1–2 drop of concentrated H_2SO_4 is added due to which blue color appears.

   Note: Blue color is formed due to deoxy sugars.

2. Mucilage stains reddish purple with iodine water. This test distinguishes between European scilla and Indian scilla.

Uses: Stimulating, Expectorant, diuretic, cardiac tonic, acting in a similar manner to digitalis, slowing and strengthening the pulse, though more irritating to the gastrointestinal mucous membrane. On account of its irritant qualities, it is not administered in diseases of an acute inflammatory nature. It has also been given as an emetic in whooping-cough and croup, usually combined with ipecacuanha, but as an emetic is considered very uncertain in its action.

ANTHRACENE GLYCOSIDES OR ANTHRAQUINONE GLYCOSIDES

They are found abundantly in dicot plant families: Ericaceae, Euphorbiaceae, Leguminoseae, and Rubiaceae. These glycosides contain an aglycone group that is a derivative of anthraquinone like anthraquinone anthrone, anthranol, dianthranol, oxanthrone and dianthrone.

For Anthraquinone Glycosides

a. *Borntrager test:* Powder drug is treated with dil H_2SO_4 and boiled for 5–10 minutes and filtered. The filtrate is shaked with organic solvent (benzene/chloroform). The organic layer is separated and treated with ammonia solution. The ammonical layer appears pink.

b. *Modified anthraquinone test:* Powder drug is treated with dil HCl and 5 ml of 5% $FeCl_3$ cooled and shake with organic solvent, the organic layer is treated with ammonia pink; red color is obtained.

Note: Addition of $FeCl_3$ is due to break of C-C linkage of glycosides which is stronger than C = O linkage.

Senna Pod (Fig. 5.2.4)

Synonyms: Hindi—Hindisana; **Bengali**—Sonamukhi; **Tamil**—Nila Vakai.

Biological source: Senna pods are dried ripe fruits of *Cassia angustifolia* (Tinnevelly senna pods) and *Cassia acutifolia* (Alexandrian senna pods) belonging to family Leguminosae.

Habitat: Cultivated in dry lands of southern and western India, and indigenous to Arabia.

Botany

- Kingdom — Plantae
- Division — Angiospermae
- Order — Fabales
- Family — Fabaceae
- Genus — *Senna*
- Species — *angustifolia, acutifolia*

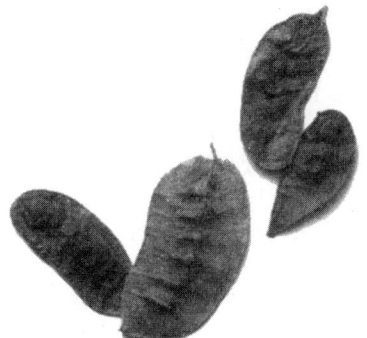

Fig. 5.2.4: Senna pod
(see also in colour Plate 2)

Table 5.2.3: Organoleptic characters of senna

Macroscopic characters	Alexandrian senna	Tinnevelley senna
Color	Green on surface	Brownish green veins
Odor	Faint	Faint
Taste	Slightly bitter	Slightly bitter
Shape	Broadly oblong	Oblong and slightly curved
Size	5 cm long, 2 to 2.5 cm broad	5 cm long, 1.5 to 2 cm broad

Part used: Dried leaflets (Folium sennae), Pods (Fructus sennae).

Organoleptic characters: Organoleptic characters of senna pod are given in Table 5.2.3.

Chemical constituents: Tinnevelly senna pods contain approximately 3% dianthrone glycosides (sennosides A-D) whereas Alexandrian senna pods contain approximately 4–5%; anthraquinones including aloe-emodin and rhein 8-glucoside; mucilage; tannins; flavonoids especially kaempferol; and resinous substances. Senna pods contain higher levels of glucosennosides and smaller amounts of anthraquinone glycosides compared with the leaves (Fig. 5.2.5).

R=COOH: Sennoside A trans
R=CH$_2$OH: Sennoside C trans
R=COOH: Sennoside B meso
R=CH$_2$OH: Sennoside D meso

Fig. 5.2.5: Sennosides

Chemical Test

- Borntrager test is positive due to presence of anthraquinone glycosides. Boil plant material with dilute H_2SO_4, filter and shake with organic solvent (ether or benzene). Separate the organic layer and add ammonia, ammonical layer turns pink or red.
- Treat ether extract of hydrolysed acid solution of senna with methanolic magnesium acetate solution. Alexandrian senna gives pink color in daylight and pale green-orange color in filtered UV light while Tinnevelly senna gives orange color in daylight and yellow-green color in filtered UV light.

Standards

- Foreign matter: NMT 1%
- Loss on drying: NMT 12%
- Total ash: NMT 9.0%
- Acid insoluble ash: NMT 2.0%

Uses: It is used as, anti-diarrheal, anti-inflammatory, in cellular regeneration, cleansing, constipation, detoxifying, hemorrhoids, laxative, pre and postoperative cleansing.

Senna Leaf (Fig. 5.2.6)

Synonyms: Alexandrian Senna, Senna-ki-patti, Nubian Senna, Cassia Senna.
Biological source: It consists of dried leaves of *Cassia angustifolia* (Tinnevelly senna) and of *Cassia acutifolia* (Alexandrian senna) belonging to family Leguminosae.
Habitat: Egypt, Nubia, Arabia, Sennar.

Botany

- Kingdom   Plantae
- Division   Angiospermae
- Order   Fabales
- Family   Fabaceae
- Genus   *Senna*
- Species   *C. angustifolia, C. acutifolia*

Parts used: Dried leaflets, pods.

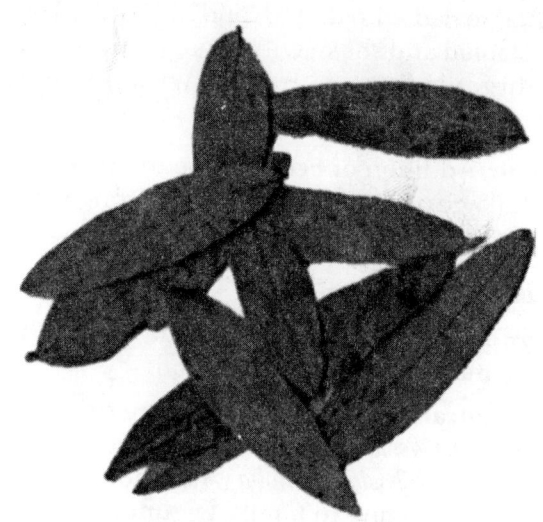

Fig. 5.2.6: Senna leaves
(*see also in colour Plate 2*)

Organoleptic Characters

Color: Yellowish green
Odor: Slight
Taste: Bitter and mucilaginous
Extra features: Isobilateral leaf with trichomes on both sides. The leaf has asymmetrical base with lanceolate shape.

Microscopy of Senna Leaf (Fig. 5.2.7)

Type: The leaf is isobilateral.
Epidermis: Upper and lower epidermises are similar in appearance; they are composed of cells with thin, straight or slightly sinuous walls, polygonal in outline except in the regions over the veins where they are more elongated and may show faint cuticular striations.
Stomata: Numerous paracytic stomata are present.

Trichomes: The covering trichomes which are found scattered as well as attached to fragments of the epidermis; they are unicellular, conical, with thick and distinctly warted walls.

Calcium oxalate crystals: The calcium oxalate crystals are very abundant, occur as prisms in the cells of the parenchymatous sheath surrounding the groups of fibers, and also as cluster crystals of moderate size in the cells of the spongy mesophyll.

Fibers: The fibers, occur in groups; they are thick-walled, lignified with few pits and are surrounded by a calcium oxalate prism sheat

Others: The fragments of the lamina in sectional view showing the palisade under both epidermises. The palisade cells under the upper epidermis are much elongated and more or less straight-walled whereas those under the lower epidermis are shorter and have distinctly sinuous walls. The rounded spongy mesophyll cells between the two layers of palisade frequently contain cluster crystals of calcium oxalate.

Staining Reagents

Phloroglucinol: HCl- 1:1 (Lignified tissues are seen red/pink)

Ruthenium red: Mucilaginous cell of epidermis seen red/pink.

Acetic acid: Crystals are insoluble.

Sudan red III: Cutin/cuticles are seen pink.

Chemical constituents: Senna leaf contains: approximately 3% dianthrone glycosides (sennosides A, A1, B, C, D, E, F and G); and small amounts of anthraquinones including aloe-emodin and rhein 8-glucoside; approximately 10% mucilage; tannins; and flavonoids. The medical action of senna can be attributed mainly to anthraquinone glycosides especially sennosides A and B.

Chemical test: Both Borntrager test and modified Borntager test are positive due to presence of anthraquinone glycosides.

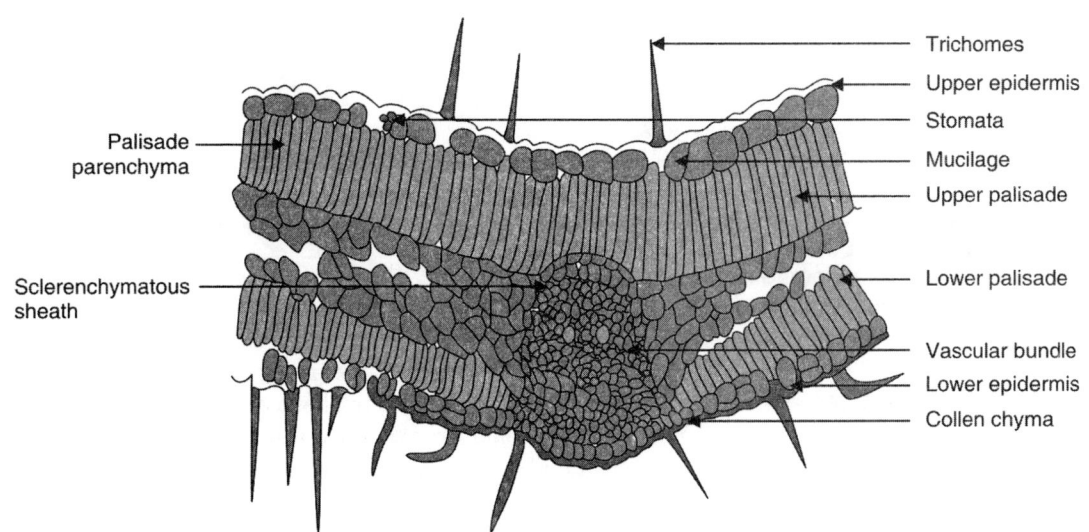

Fig. 5.2.7: Microscopy of senna leaf

Standards

- Foreign matter: NMT 1%
- Loss on drying: NMT 12%
- Total ash: NMT 9.0%
- Acid insoluble ash: NMT 2.0%

Uses: Senna leaves pods are used as laxative, purgative, antipyretic and cathartic it promotes the excretion of toxins and alleviate constipation by increasing the amount of water and electrolytes in the intestine.

Adulterants: Arabian or Bombay senna, Mecca senna.

Aloe (Fig. 5.2.8)

Synonyms: Sanskrit—Ghrita kumari; **English**—Indian aloe; **Hindi**—Ghik anvar kumari; **Gujrati**—Kunvar.

Biological source: It consists of dried juice collected by incision of bases of leaves of various species of aloe, *viz. Aloe perryi, Aloe vera, Aloe ferox*, family Liliaceae.

Habitat: Aloes are indigenous to east and south Africa, but have been introduced into the West Indies (where they are extensively cultivated) and into tropical countries, and will even flourish in the countries bordering on the Mediterranean.

Botany

- Kingdom   Plantae
- Order   Asparagales
- Family   Asphodelaceae
- Genus   *Aloe*
- Species   *A. perryi, A. vera, A. ferox*

Parts used: Leaves and dried gel.

Organoleptic characters: Organoleptic characters of different species of aloe are given in Table 5.2.4.

Chemical constituents (Fig. 5.2.9): The most important constituents of Aloes are the two aloins, barbaloin and isobarbaloin, which constitute the so-called crystalline aloin,

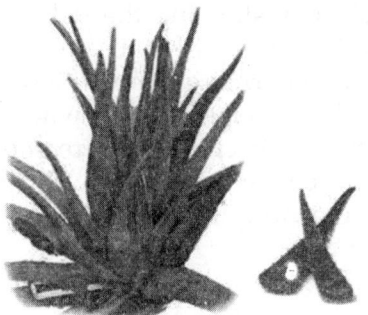

Fig. 5.2.8: Aloe leaves
(*see also in colour Plate 2*)

Table 5.2.4: Organoleptic characters of different species of aloe

Characters	Curacao	Socotrine	Zanzibar	Cape
Form	Opaque and translucent	Opaque	Opaque	Transparent and glossy
Color	Reddish brown	Dark brown	Liver color	Dark brown to greenish brown
Fracture	Smooth	Porous	Fairly smooth and porous	Smooth, even and glossy
Odor	Strong and unpleasant	Slight and disagreeable	Pleasant	Unpleasant
Taste	Disagreeable Bitter	Disagreeable Bitter	Disagreeable Bitter	Disagreeable Bitter

present in the drug at from 10 to 30%. Other constituents are amorphous aloin, resin and aloe-emodin. Aloe contains two classes of aloins: (1) nataloins, which yield picric and oxalic acids with nitric acid, and do not give a red coloration with nitric acid; and (2) barbaloins, which yield aloetic acid ($C_7H_2N_3O_5$), chrysammic acid ($C_7H_2N_2O_6$), picric and oxalic acids with nitric acid, being reddened by the acid. Aloes also contain a trace of volatile oil, to which its odor is due.

Chemical test: Boil plant material with 5 ml dilute HCl and 5 ml $FeCl_3$, filter and shake with organic solvent (ether or benzene). Separate the organic layer and add dilute ammonia, ammonical layer turns pink or red.

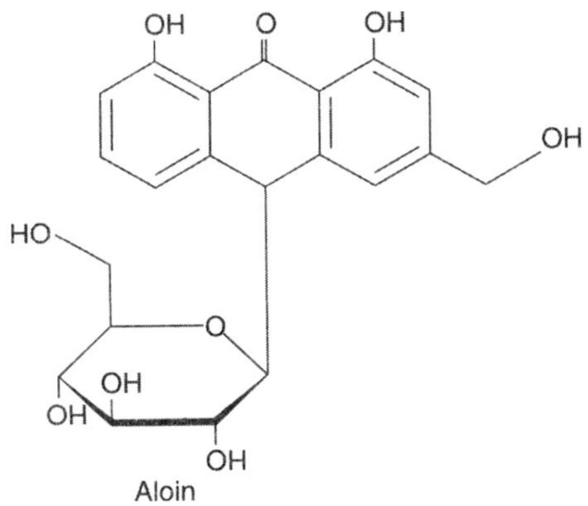

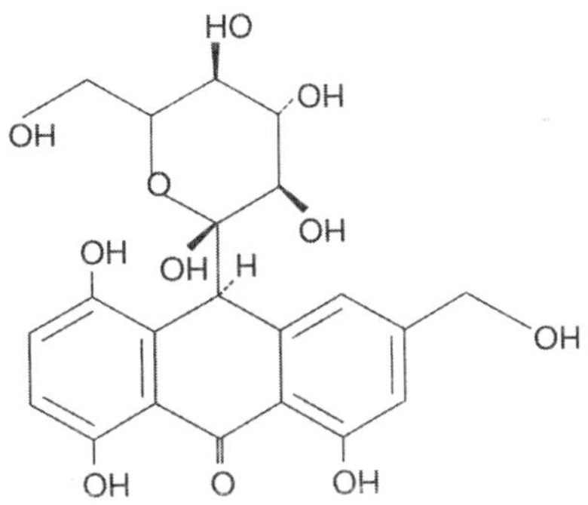

Isobarbaloin

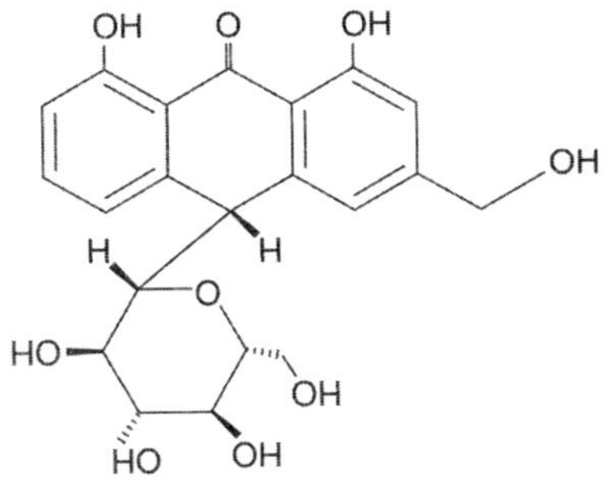

Fig. 5.2.9: Chemical constitents of Aloe

Uses: Aloe has been used for its healing properties, and both oral intake and topical dressings include blisters, insect bites, rashes, sores, herpes, urticaria, athlete's foot, fungus, vaginal infections, conjunctivitis, sties, allergic reactions, and dry skin. Other topical uses include acne, sunburn, frostbite (it appears to prevent decreased blood flow), shingles, screening out X-ray radiation, psoriasis, preventing scarring, rosacea, warts, wrinkles from aging, and eczema. It is also used as purgative.

Adulterants: Natal aloes, Mocha aloes, black catechu and pieces of iron and stones.

Aloin

Barbaloin

Rhubarb (Fig. 5.2.10)

Synonyms: Sanskrit—Amlavetusa; **English**—Himalayan rhubarb; **Hindi**—Revand Chini; **Bengali**—Rheuchini; **Tamil**—Variyattu

Biological source: It consists of dried rhizomes of *Rheum emodi*, family Polygonaceae.

Habitat: It is found in Astore, Nagar, Nalter, Ishkomen, mostly rocky and sandy places where moisture remains for long time.

Botany

- Kingdom   Plantae
- Family   Polygonaceae

- Genus   *Rheum*
- Species   *emodi*

Parts used: Rhizome, roots

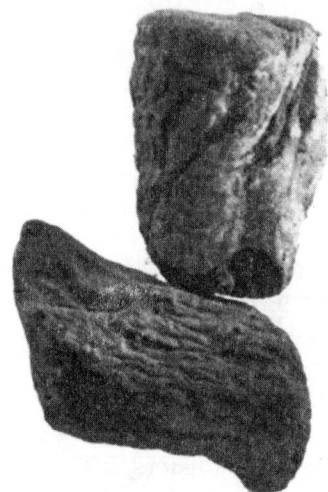

Fig. 5.2.10: Rhubarb
(*see also in colour Plate 2*)

Organoleptic Characters

Color: Yellowish brown

Odor: Fragnant

Taste: Bitter and astringent

Shape: Somewhat cylindrical, barrel-shaped/conical

Size: 2–20 cm in length, 1.5–8 cm in dia

Extra features: Outer surface is irregular and wrinkled, transverse wrinkles and annulations are present.

Microscopy of Rhizome of Rhubarb
(Fig. 5.2.11)

Parenchyma: The parenchyma cells are thin-walled, elongated cells tapering at the ends. These cells are filled with starch in longitudinal view.

Medullary rays: It is composed of cells with slightly thickened walls and both the walls and the cell contents are deep brownish-yellow.

Ground tissue: It is composed of cells varying from rounded to oval to rectangular in outline, they are filled with starch granules or with large cluster crystals of calcium oxalate.

Calcium oxalate: The cluster crystals of calcium oxalate found scattered and in some of the parenchymatous cells.

Starch granules: The starch granules are simple, spherical and compound with distinct, central hilum in the form of a cleft or radiating split.

Vessels: The *vessels* are large, reticulately thickened and do not give a reaction for lignin, occur singly or in small groups and are frequently found in fragments.

Chemical constituents: It consists of anthraquinone derivatives, such as chrysophanic acid, emodin, aloe-emodin, rhein and physician, with their O-glycosides, such as glucorhein, chrysophanein, glucoemodin; sennosides A-E, reidin C and others. It also contains d-catechin and epicatechin gallate, with various cinnamoyl and coumaroyl golloyl glucosides and fructoses. Stilbene derivatives, related stilbene glycosides present in other types drug also have volatile oil, containing diisobutyl phthalate, cinnamic and ferulic acids; rutin, fatty acids, calcium oxalate, etc.

$R = CH_3$ (Chrysophanol)
$R = CH_2OH$ (Aloeemodin)
$R = COOH$ (Rhein)

Chemical Test

- It gives red coloration with 5.0% NaOH
- It gives pink color with ammonia.
- It gives Borntrager test positive.
- Under ultraviolet radiation, *Rheum emodi* gives brown color and *Rheum rhaponticum* gives violet color.

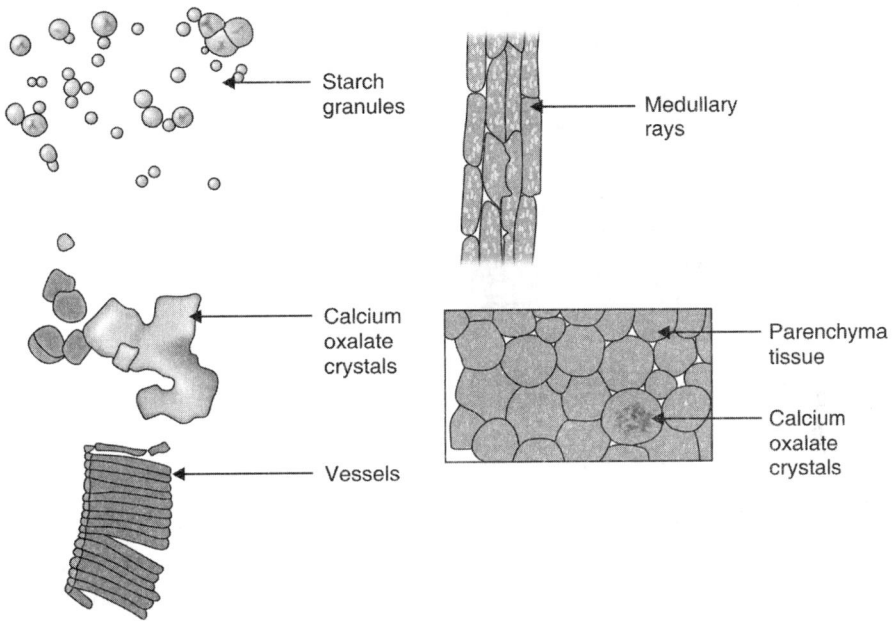

Fig. 5.2.11: Microscopy of rhizome of rhubarb

Standards

Total ash:	NMT 7.0%
Acid insoluble ash:	NMT 4.0%
Alcohol-soluble extractive:	NMT 19.0%
Water-soluble extractive:	NMT 12.0%

Uses: The roots are astringent, tonic and purgative. The tuber is pungent, bitter, alexiteric, emmenagogue, chronic bronchitis asthma, sore eyes and bruises. **Locally,** roots are used to chronic constipation. The tuber is used in biliousness, sore eyes and fever. It is also used as blood purifier.

Adulterants: *Rheum rhaponticum* is an adulterant of the official drug.

Cascara Bark (Fig. 5.2.12)

Synonyms: English—Buckthorn

Biological source: It is obtained from dried bark of *Rhamnus purshiana* belonging to family Rhamnaceae.

Habitat: Native to Europe; introduced in Kashmir, Himachal Pradesh, Bhutan and the Nilgiris.

Botany

- Kingdom   Plantae
- Family   Rhamnaceae
- Genus   *Rhamnus*
- Species   *purshiana*

Part used: Bark

Organoleptic Characters

Color: Pale black to brown in color

Shape: Quilled, channeled or flat pieces

Size: 20 cm long, 1 to 4 mm thick.

Fracture: Short and granular

Chemical constituents (Figs 5.2.13 and 5.2.14): The bark contains up to 8–10% of a complex mixture of anthraquinone glycosides of which 60–70% are cascarosides A, B, C and

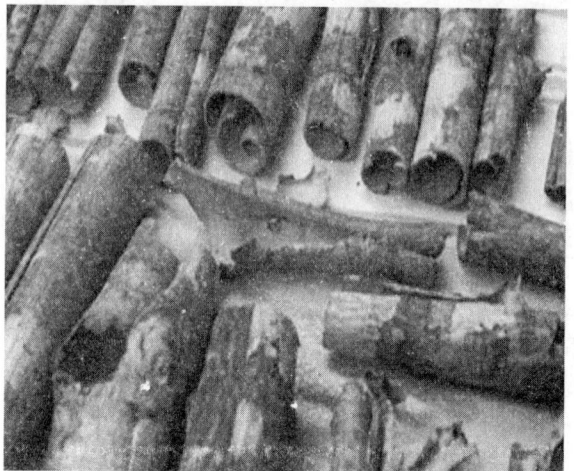

Fig. 5.2.12: Cascara bark
(see also in colour Plate 2)

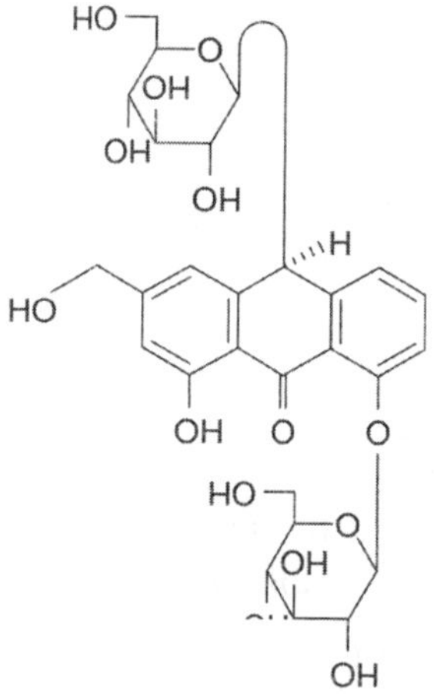

	X	Y	R^3	R^6	R^8
Aloin A	Glc	H	OH	H	H
Aloin B	H	Glc	OH	H	H
Cascaroside A	Glc	H	OH	H	Glc
Cascaroside B	H	Glc	OH	H	Glc
Cascaroside C	Glc	H	H	H	Glc
Cascaroside D	H	Glc	H	H	Glc
Cascaroside E	Glc	H	H	OH	Glc
Cascaroside F	H	Glc	H	OH	Glc
Chrysaloin A	Glc	H	H	H	H
Chrysaloin B	H	Glc	H	H	H

Fig. 5.2.13: Cascarosides A

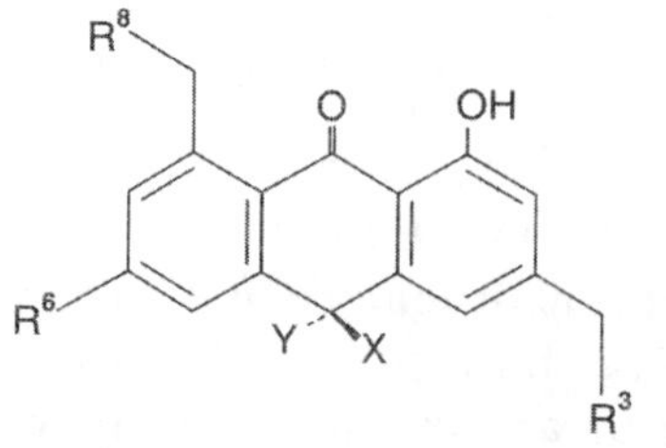

Fig. 5.2.14: Chemical constituents of cascara bark

D, other glycosides in minor concentrations include chrysanol, frangulin, barbaloin, glycosides based on aloe-emodin, emodin, chrysophanol and emodinoxanthrone, dianthrones, and free aglycones. The bark contains barbaloin and O-glycosides of emodin (e.g. frangulin), emosin oxanthrone and palmidin A, B, and C (also found in Rhubarb root). The bark also contains linoleic acid, myristic acid and syringic acid. It also contains resins, tannins and lipids. Cascarosides A and B are aloin O- and C-glycosides and cascarosides C and D are deoxyaloin O- and C-glycosides.

Chemical test: With 5% KOH, it shows red color.

Uses: Stool-softener, bitter stomachic, stimulant, laxative, pancreatic stimulant, and tonic.

Adulterants: Frangula bark

SAPONIN GLYCOSIDES

Steroidal saponins widely distributed in nature. They possesses some common characteristics:

a. They produce foam in aqueous solution
b. They cause hemolysis of RBC.

Aglycone of the saponin glycosides are known as sapogenins. They are found in many monocotyledon families, especially the Dioscoreaceae (e.g. *Dioscorea*) and the Liliaceae (e.g. *Smilax, Trillium*), e.g. dioscin (*Dioscorea*). Acid hydrolysis of dioscin liberates the aglycone diosgenin.

Biosynthesis: Formed through mevalonate and deoxyxylulose pathway

Test for saponin: About 2 g of the powdered sample was boiled in 20 ml of distilled water in a water bath and filtered. 10 ml of the filtrate was mixed with 5 ml of distilled water and shaken vigorously for a stable persistent froth. The frothing was mixed with 3 drops of olive oil and shaken vigorously, then observed for the formation of emulsion.

Dioscorea (Fig. 5.2.15)

Synonyms: English—Wild yam; greater yam, rheumation root.

Biological source: It is obtained from root and rhizomes of various Discorea species, viz *D. atropurpurea* Roxb, *D. globosa* Roxb, *D. purpurea* Roxb and *D. deltoidea* belonging to family Dioscoreaceae.

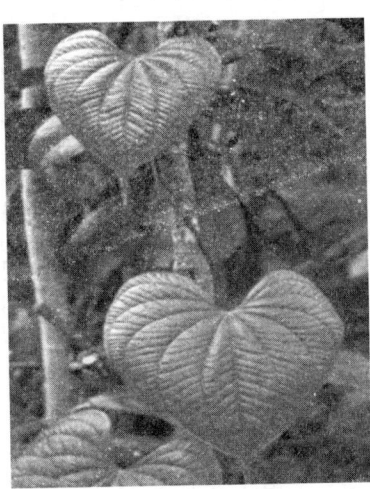

Fig. 5.2.15: Dioscorea
(*see also in colour Plate 3*)

Habitat: Native to east Asia; cultivated in Assam, Vadodara, Tamil Nadu, Bengal and Madhya Pradesh.

Botany

- Kingdom   Plantae
- Family   *Dioscoreaceae*
- Genus   *Diosorea*
- Species   *deltoidea*

Parts used: Root and rhizomes.

Organoleptic Characters

Color: Sightly brown

Taste: Acrid

Odor: None

Shape: Long, branched, crooked and woody

Extra features: The therapeutical value is lost after the first year, so that it should be freshly gathered and carefully dried each year.

Chemical constituents: The main bioactive components of wild yam are the saponin, diosgenin, and the alkaloids, dioscorin (Fig. 5.2.16) and dioscorine. It also contains anthocyanins, cyanidin and peonidin-3-gentiobioside acylated with sinapic acid. Rhizomes contain enzyme sapogenase, whereas tuber contains glycosides and phenolic compounds.

Uses: Wild yams are used as cholagogue, antispasmodic, anti-inflammatory, antirheumatic, diuretic. Also used for painful periods,

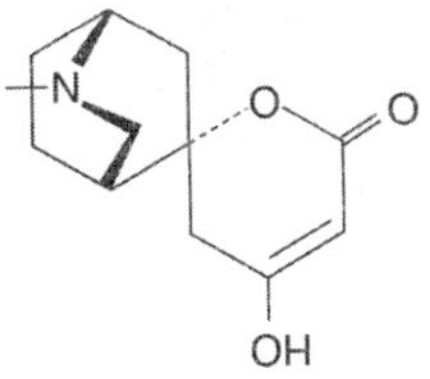

Fig. 5.2.16: Dioscorin

cramps and muscle tension. It is used in first commercial production of oral contraceptives, topical hormones, systemic corticosteroids, androgens, estrogens, progestogens and other sex hormones.

Shatavari (Fig. 5.2.17)

Synonyms: English—Satavari; **Hindi**—Shakakul; **Gujrati**—Satavar.

Biological source: Satavari consists of dried roots of *Asparagus racemosus*, belonging to family Liliaceae.

Habitat: Shatavari is a perennial much branched climbing herb found all over India, especially in tropical and sub-tropical parts and in Himalayan region up to 1400 m elevation.

Botany

- Kingdom   Plantae
- Order   Asparagales
- Family   Asparagaceae
- Genus   *Asparagus*
- Species   *racemosus*

Parts used: Fleshy roots and leaves.

Organoleptic Characters

Color: Leaves are green, roots are white to buff color sometimes pale brownish.

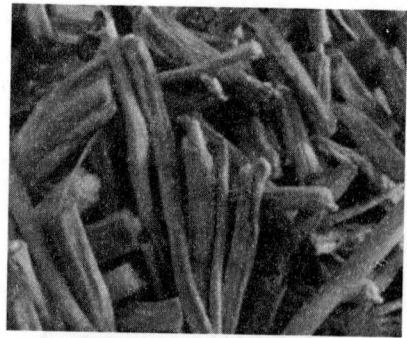

Fig. 5.2.17: Shatavari
(see also in colour Plate 3)

Odor: Odorless
Taste: Bitter
Shape: Roots are fascicled at the stem base, smooth tapering at both ends.
Size: Tuberous succulent roots are 30 cm to a metre or more in length.
Extra features: Entire roots are tapering on both ends, drug swells when soaked in water and becomes soft and flaccid.

Chemical constituents: Root contains 4 steroidal saponin shatavarins I-IV, water soluble constituents 52.1/2%, moisture 1%, glucose 7% and ash from dried root 4% (Fig. 5.2.18).

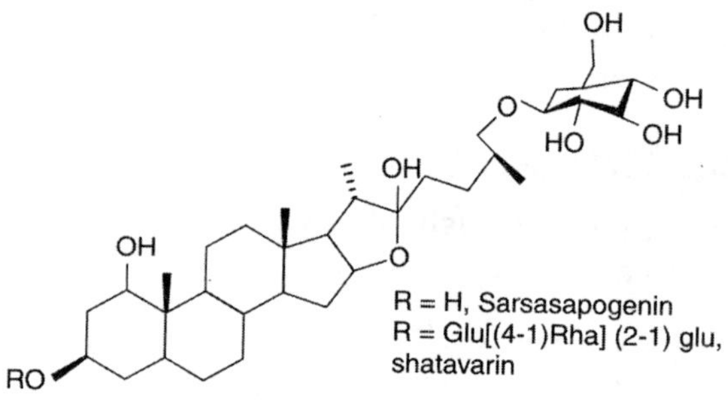

R = H, Sarsasapogenin
R = Glu[(4-1)Rha] (2-1) glu, shatavarin

Fig. 5.2.18: Chemical constituents of shatavari

Chemical test: Shake drug with water, persistent foam is observed.

Uses: The root of *Asparagus racemosus* (Shatavari) is a nutritive, aphrodisiac, astringent, used in treatment of general debility, male infertility (due to low sperm count), loss of libido, epilepsy (fits), mental debility and in many male diseases. It is also used in female ailments, such as menopausal syndrome, anemia, lower quantity of breast milk secretion, and for both mental and physical ailments.

Ginseng (Fig. 5.2.19)

Synonyms: English—Ginseng

Biological source: Ginseng consists of dried roots of *Panax ginseng* (Asian ginseng) or *Panax quinquefolius* (American ginseng), belonging to family Araliaceae.

Plate 1

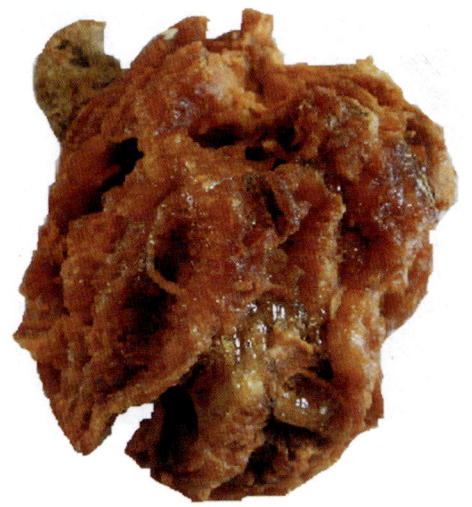

Fig. 5.1.5: Bael fruit

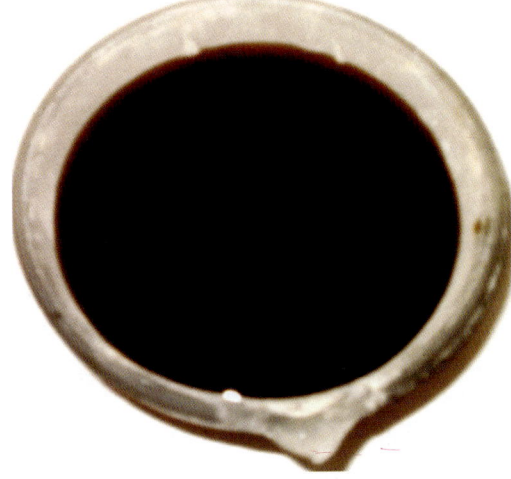

Fig. 5.1.7: Honey

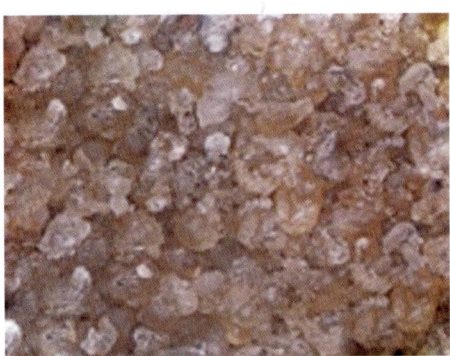

Fig. 5.1.9: Ghatugum

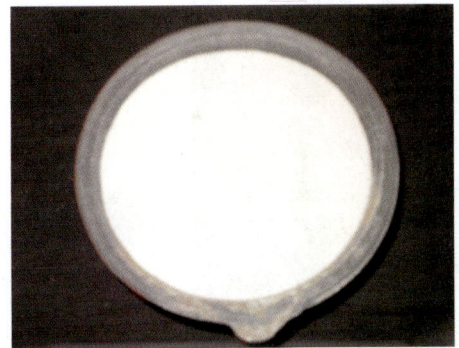

Fig. 5.1.11: Agar

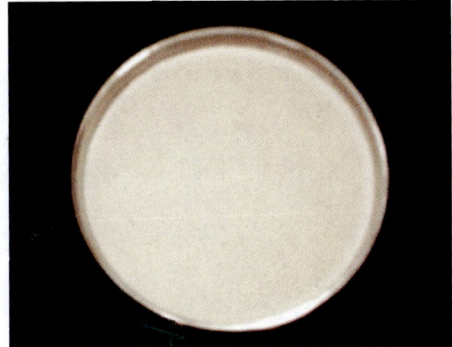

Fig. 5.1.13: Acacia gum

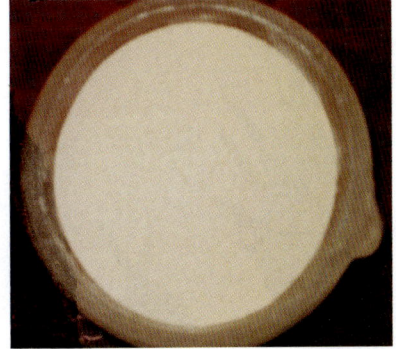

Fig. 5.1.15: Tragacanth gum

Plate 2

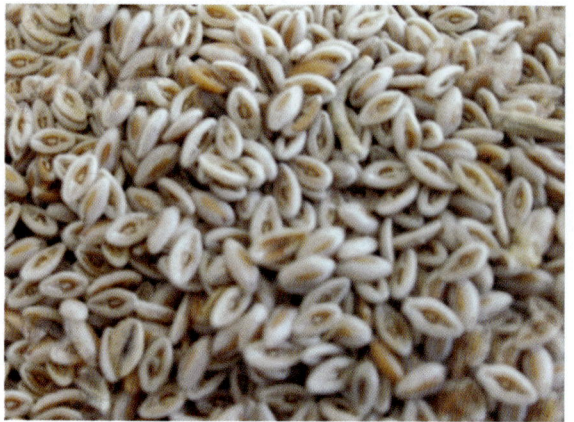

Fig. 5.1.16: Isapgol seeds

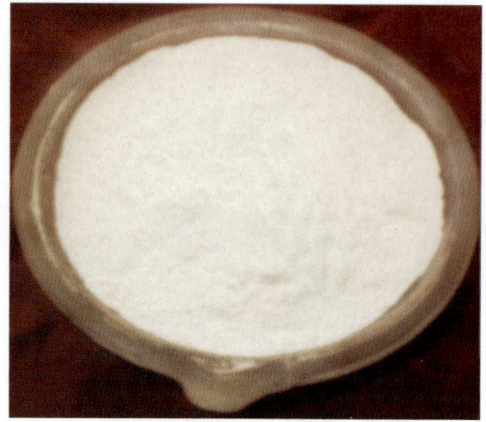

Fig. 5.1.17: Starch

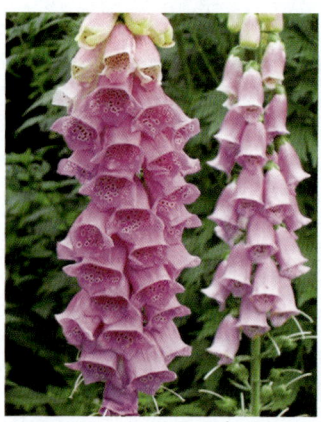

Fig. 5.2.1: Digitalis purpurea

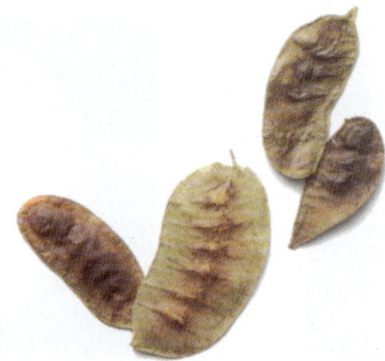

Fig. 5.2.4: Senna pod

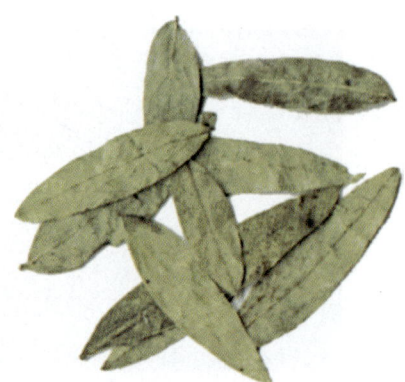

Fig. 5.2.6: Senna leaves

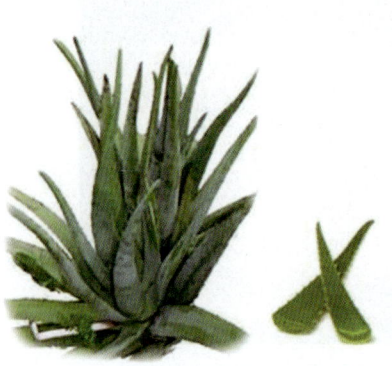

Fig. 5.2.8: Aloe leaves

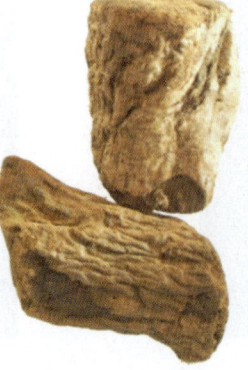

Fig. 5.2.10: Rhubarb

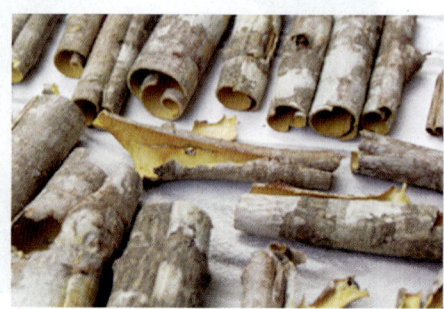

Fig. 5.2.12: Cascara bark

Plate 3

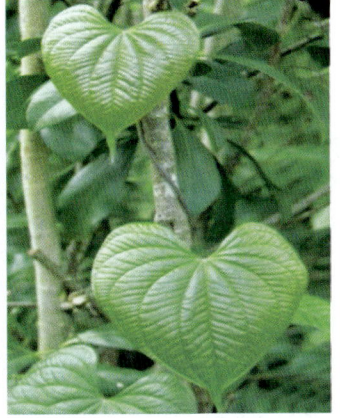

Fig. 5.2.15: Dioscorea

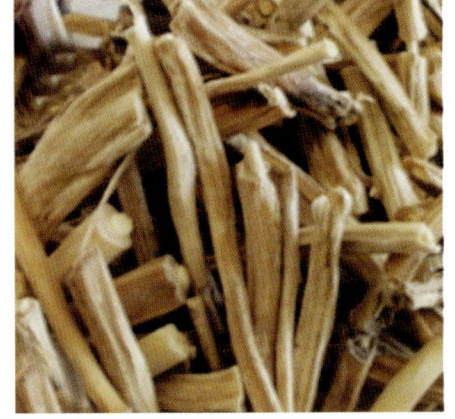

Fig. 5.2.17: Shatavari

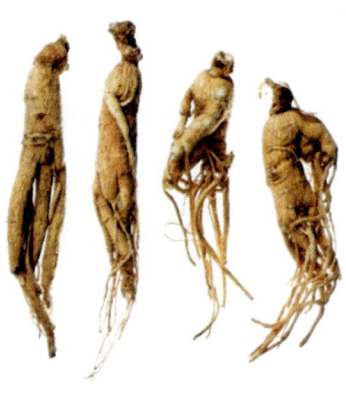

Fig. 5.2.19: Ginseng roots

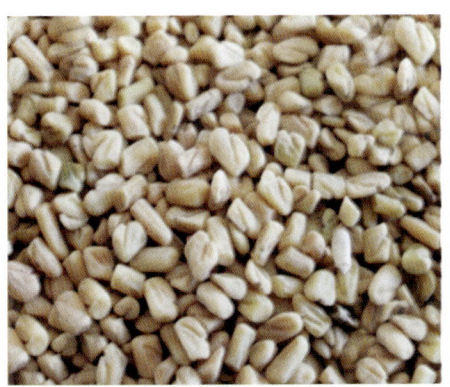

Fig. 5.2.21: Fenugreek

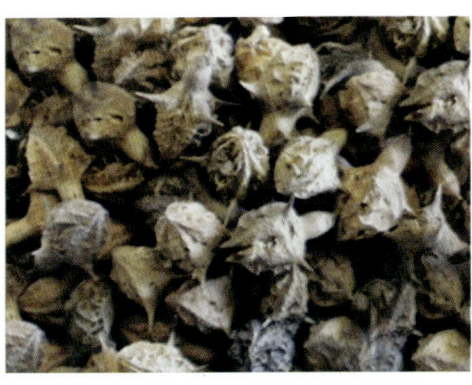

Fig. 5.2.23: Large gokhru

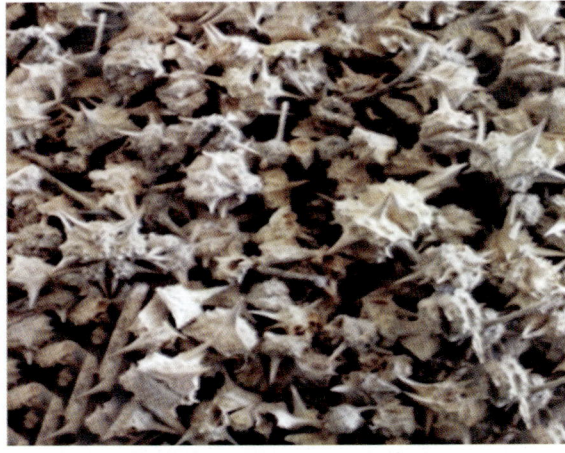

Fig. 5.2.24: Small gokhru

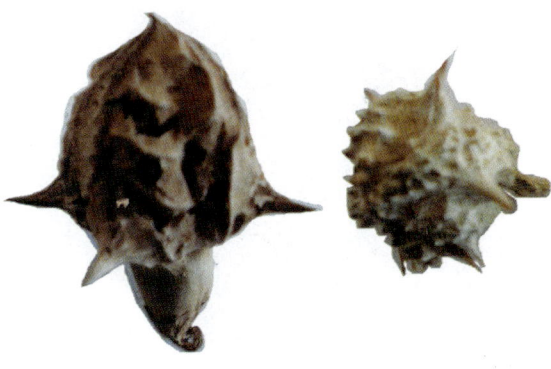

Fig. 5.2.25: Comparison of large and small gokhru

Plate 4

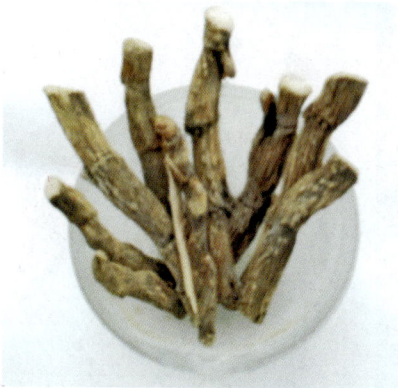

Fig. 5.2.27: Liquorice root

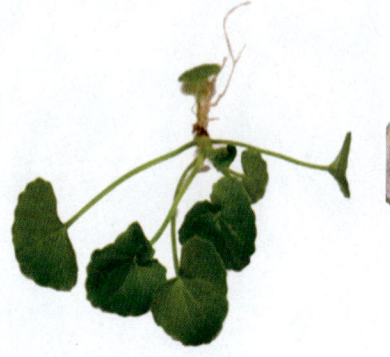

Fig. 5.2.30: Brahmi

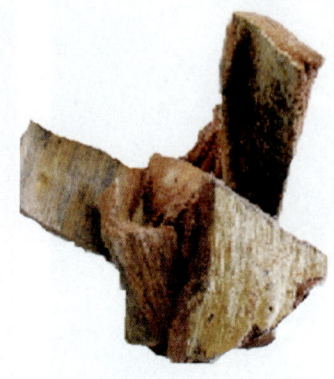

Fig. 5.2.32: Arjuna bark

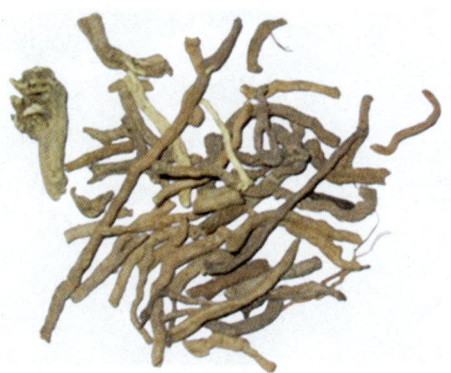

Fig. 5.2.34: Senega root

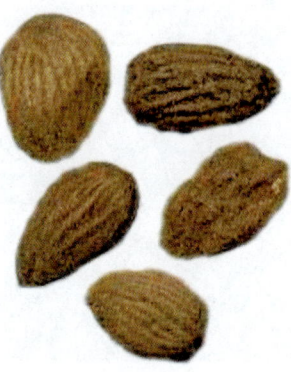

Fig. 5.2.36: Bitter almond

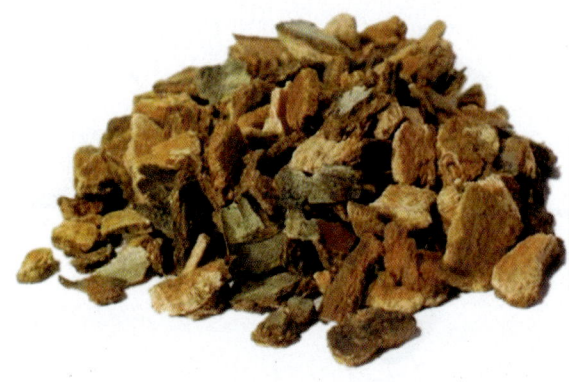

Fig. 5.2.38: Wild cherry bark

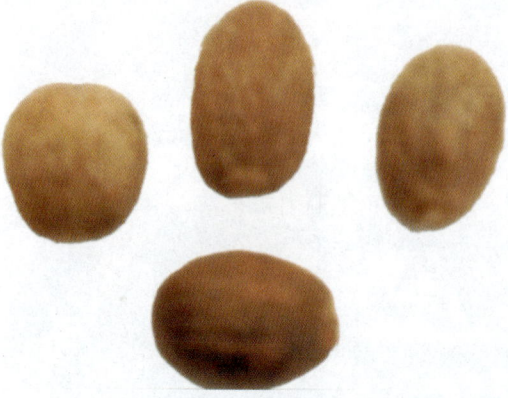

Fig. 5.3.1: Nutmeg

Plate 5

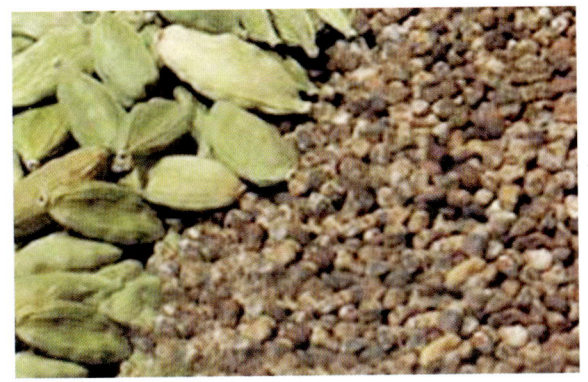

Fig. 5.3.3: Cardamom fruits and seeds

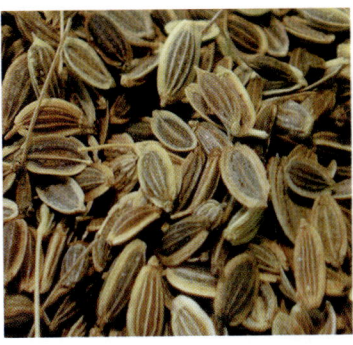

Fig. 5.3.5: Dill

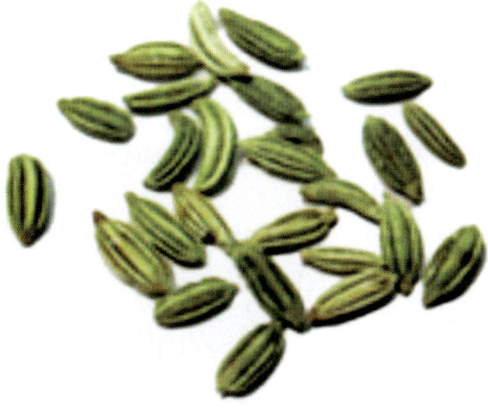

Fig. 5.3.8: Fennel

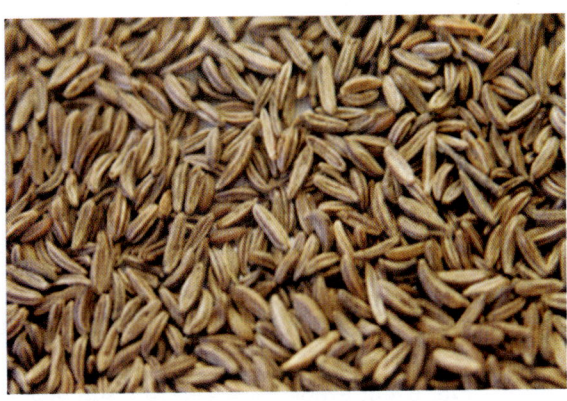

Fig. 5.3.11: Caraway

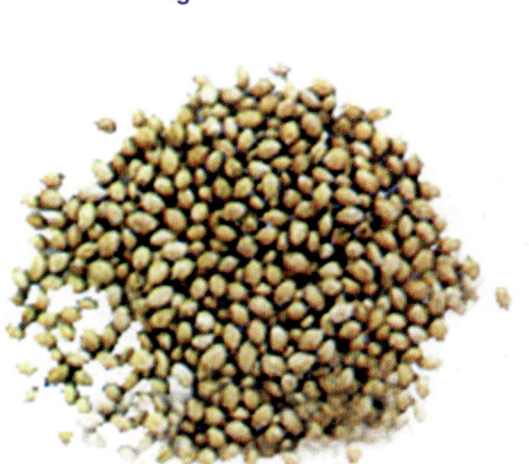

Fig. 5.3.14: Coriander

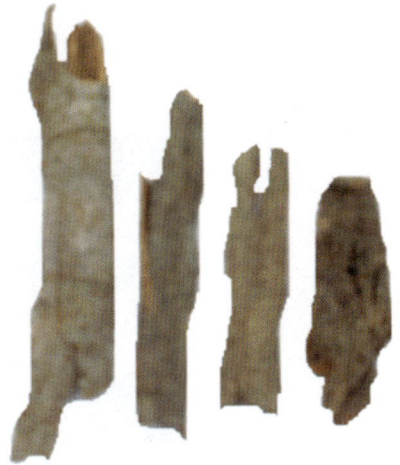

Fig. 5.3.17: Cinnamon bark

Plate 6

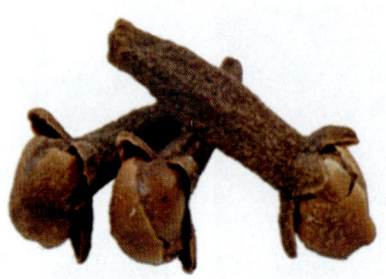 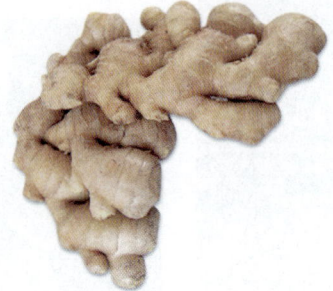 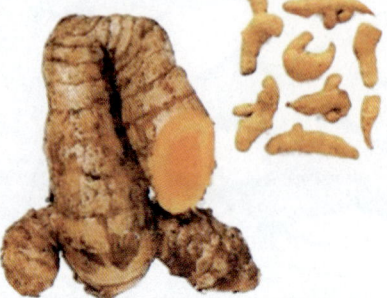

Fig. 5.3.21: Clove bud **Fig. 5.3.24:** Ginger **Fig. 5.3.27:** Turmeric

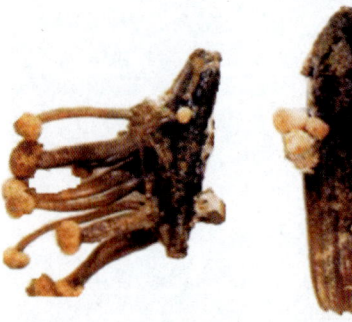 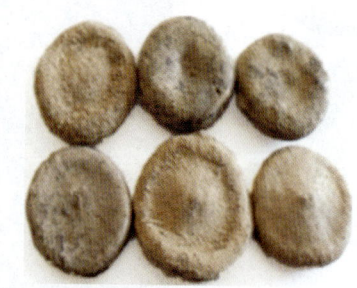 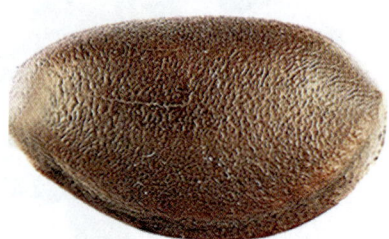

Fig. 5.4.4: Ergot **Fig. 5.4.7:** Nux vomica **Fig. 5.4.10:** Calabar bean

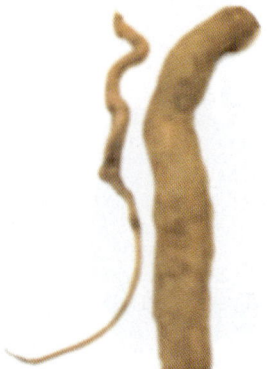 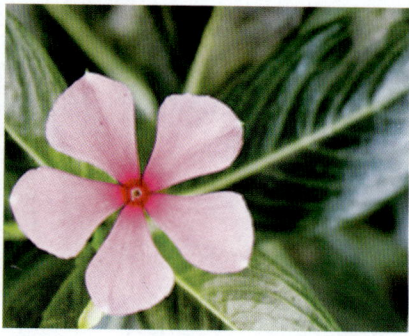 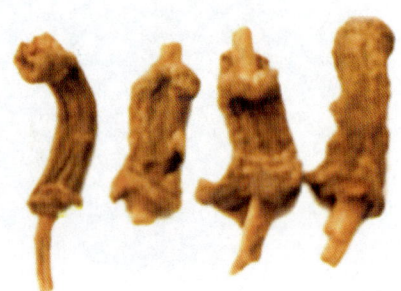

Fig. 5.4.12: Rauwolfia **Fig. 5.4.15:** Vinca **Fig. 5.4.25:** Ipecacuanha

Plate 7

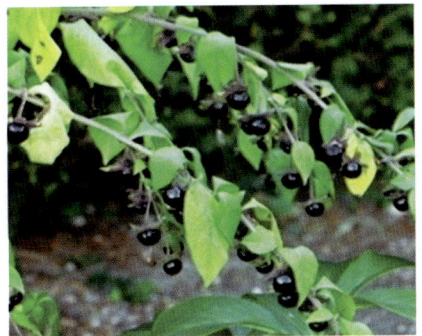

Fig. 5.4.28: Belladonna

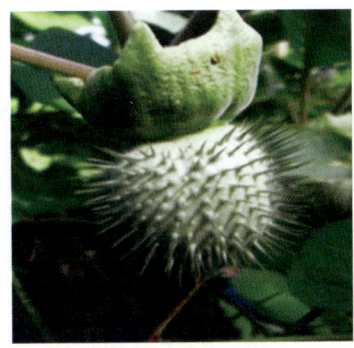

Fig. 5.4.31: Datura

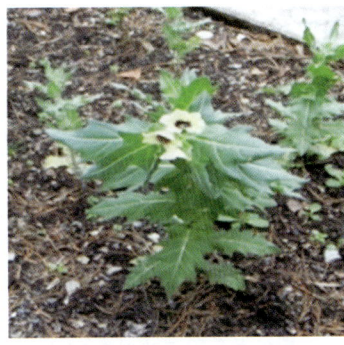

Fig. 5.4.34: Hyoscyamus

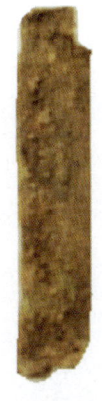

Fig. 5.4.37: Cinchona bark

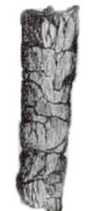 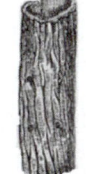 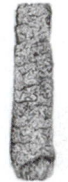 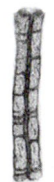

C.calisaya   C.succirubra   C.officinalis   C.ledgeriana

Fig. 5.4.38: Types of Cinchona

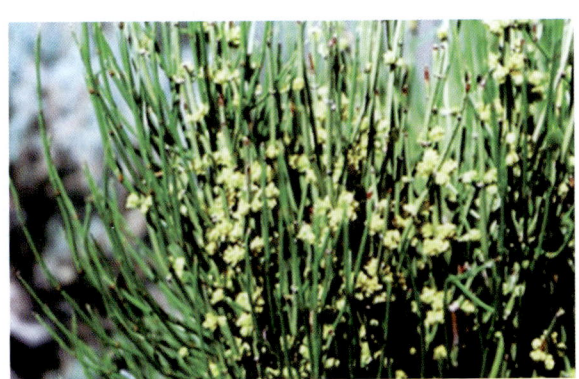

Fig. 5.4.41: Ephedra

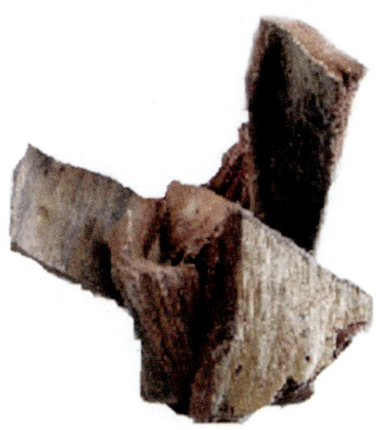

Fig. 5.5.1: Arjuna bark

Plate 8

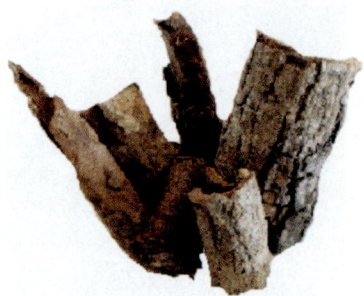

Fig. 5.5.3: Ashoka bark

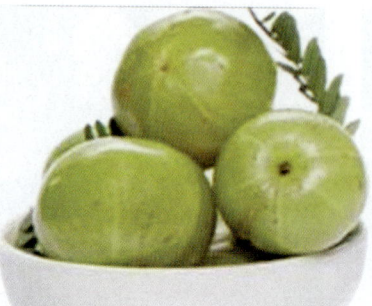

Fig. 5.5.5: Amla fruit

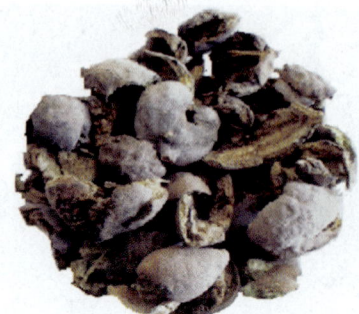

Fig. 5.5.7: Bahera fruits

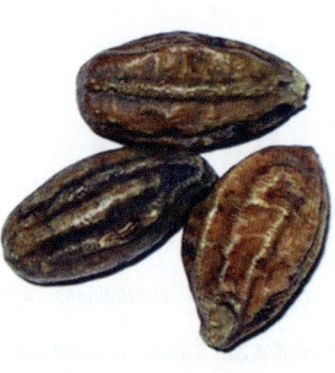

Fig. 5.5.9: Myrobalan fruits

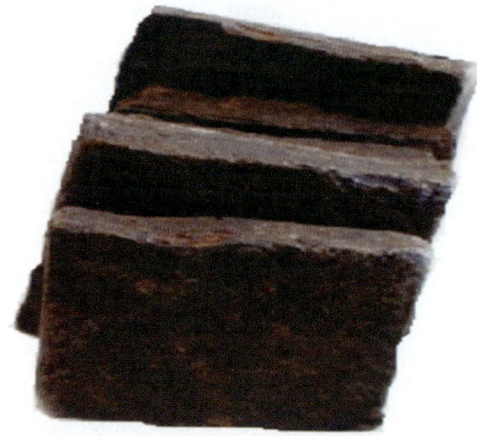

Fig. 5.5.11: Catechu

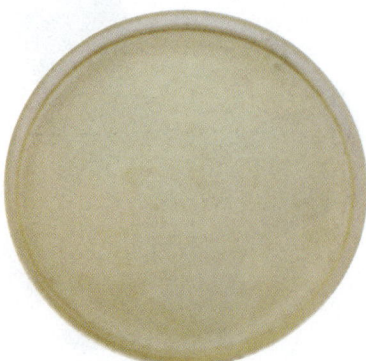

Fig. 5.6.1: Castor oil

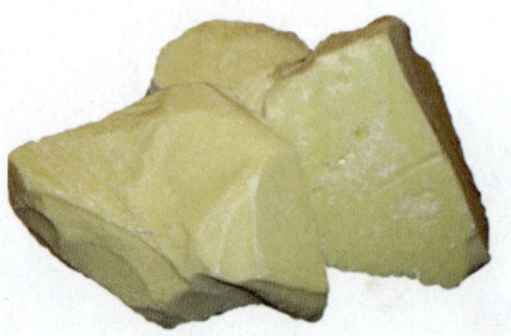

Fig. 5.6.7: Cocoa butter

Habitat: Ginseng is now found throughout the world.

Botany

- Kingdom   Plantae
- Family   Araliaceae
- Genus   *Panax*
- Species   *ginseng, quinquefolius*

Part used: Roots

Organoleptic Characters

Asian ginseng: It is an herbaceous perennial plant from 30 to 80 cm high with divided palmate leaves and clusters of red berries in the autumn.

American ginseng: The herbaceous perennial plant grows to a height of twelve to twenty four inches and has three compound leaves, with five toothed leaflets, that are joined at the top of an erect stem. Greenish-white flowers bloom in late spring or early summer. Green berries follow and ripen to red by late summer.

Chemical constituents: The main bioactive components of ginseng are a diverse group of steroidal saponins called as ginsenosides or panaxosides (Fig. 5.2.20). The other constituents are ginseng oils and phytosterol, carbohydrates and sugars, organic acids, nitrogenous substances amino acids and peptides, vitamin minerals and enzymes.

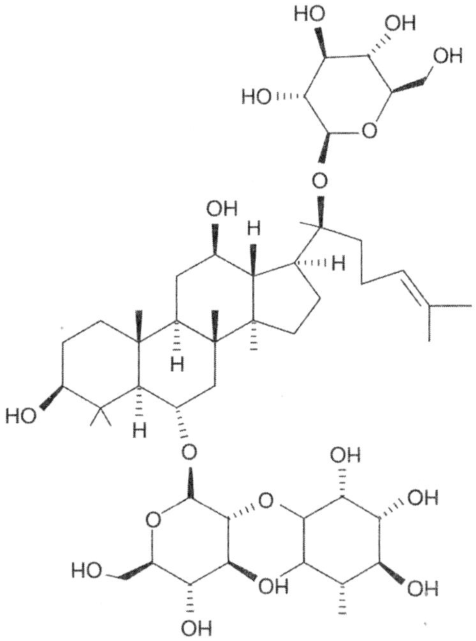

Ginsenosides

Fig. 5.2.20: Chemical constituent of ginseng

Uses: Ginseng is used to relieve stress, increase energy, and improve mental acuity. It has been used to increase physical endurance and lessen fatigue, to improve the ability to cope with stress, and to improve concentration. It is also used for anemia, diabetes, gastritis, neurasthenia, erectile dysfunction, impotence and male fertility, fever, hangover, and asthma. Panax ginseng is also used for bleeding disorders, loss of appetite, vomiting, colitis, dysentery, cancer, insomnia, neuralgia, rheumatism, dizziness, headache, convulsions, disorders of pregnancy and childbirth.

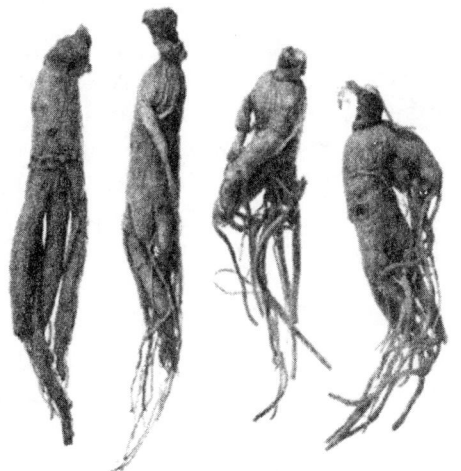

Fig. 5.2.19: Ginseng roots
(*see also in colour Plate 3*)

Methi Seeds (Fig. 5.2.21)

Synonyms: Sanskrit—Medhika; **English**—Fenugreek; **Gujrati**—Methi, **Telgu**—Mentulu.

Biological source: It is obtained from seeds of *Trigonella foenum-graecum* belonging to family Fabaceae.

Habitat: Indigenous to the countries on the eastern shores of the Mediterranean. It is cultivated in India, Africa, Egypt, Morocco, and occasionally in England.

Botany

- Kingdom   Plantae
- Division   Magnoliophyta
- Order   Fabales
- Family   Fabaceae
- Genus   *Trigonella*
- Species   *foenum-graecum*

Parts used: Seeds, pods and leaves

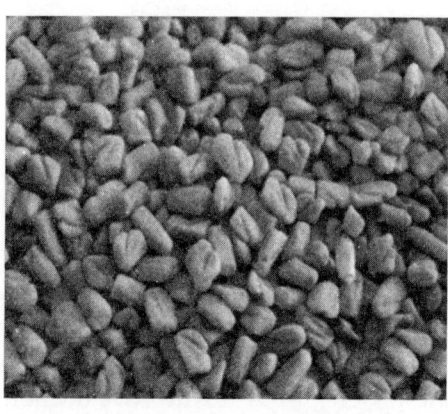

Fig. 5.2.21: Fenugreek
(*see also in colour Plate 3*)

Organoleptic Characters

Color: Yellow hard seeds
Odor: Strong and characteristic
Taste: Strong
Shape: Irregularly rhomboidal, flattened

Chemical constituents (Fig. 5.2.22): It contains 28% mucilage, 5% stronger-smelling bitter fixed oil, 22% proteins. It also contains two alkaloids, trigonelline and choline, and a yellow coloring substance. It is rich in phosphates, lecithin and nucleoalbumin, considerable quantities of iron in an organic form.

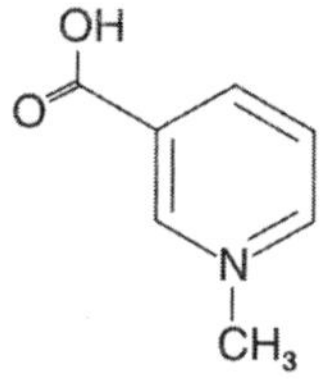

Trigonelline

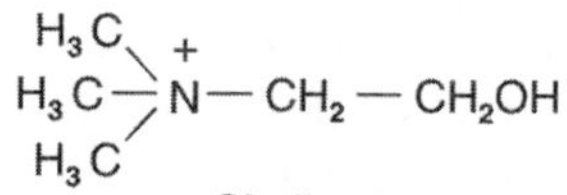

Choline

Fig. 5.2.22: Chemical constituent of fenugreek

Chemical test: The chemical test of alkaloids, glycosides and steroids can be performed.

Uses: Externally, it is used as a poultice for abscesses, boils, carbuncles, etc. It can be employed as a substitute for cod-liver oil in scrofula, rickets, anemia, debility following infectious diseases. The ground seeds are used also to give a maple-flavoring to confectionery and nearly all cattle like the flavor of fenugreek in their forage. The powder is also employed as a spice in curry.

Gokhru (Figs 5.2.23 to 5.2.25)

Synonyms: Large gokhru Hindi—Farib duti; **Bengali**—Bara gokhru; **Gujrati**—Kadva gokhru.

Small Gokhru Sanskrit—Ikshugandha; **English**—Small gokhru; **Hindi**—Chota gokhru; **Bengali**—Gokhuri.

Biological source: Large gokhru consists of dried ripe fruits of *Pedalium murex* belonging to family pedaliaceae. Small gokhru consists of dried ripe fruits of *Tribulus terrestris* belonging to family Zygophyllaceae.

Habitat: Throughout India, Gujrat, Srilanka, Africa, etc.

Organoleptic characters: Organoleptic characters of large and small gokhru are given in Table 5.2.5.

Botany

- Kingdom   Plantae
- Family   Pedaliaceae, Zygophyllaceae
- Genus   *Pedalium, Tribulus*
- Species   *murex, terrestris*

Part used: Whole plant, fruits and seeds.

Table 5.2.5: Organoleptic characters of large and small gokhru

Parameters	Large gokhru	Small gokhru
Color	Brown	Yellowish white
Shape	Pyramid, ovoid shape tapering at base	Globose
Surface	Each fruit has four spines and does not show separate cocci	Spiny having five woody cocci and coccus which contain several seeds

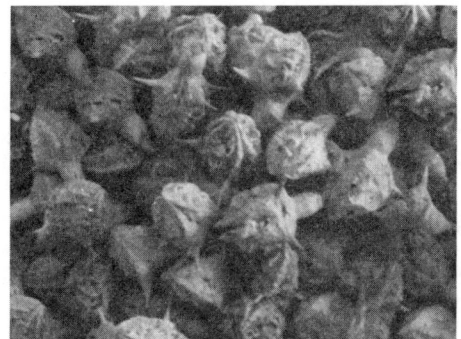

Fig. 5.2.23: Large gokhru
(*see also in colour Plate 3*)

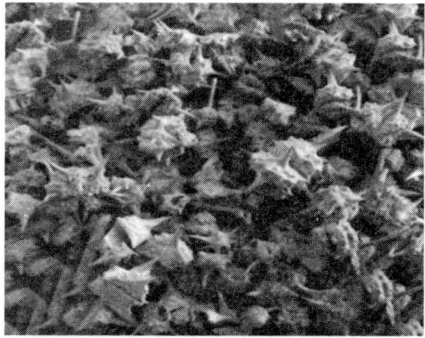

Fig. 5.2.24: Small gokhru
(*see also in colour Plate 3*)

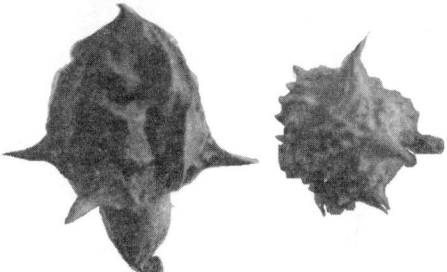

Fig. 5.2.25: Comparison of large and small gokhru
(*see also in colour Plate 3*)

Chemical constituents (Fig. 5.2.26): It consists of saponins which on hydrolysis yield diosgenin, ruscogenin and gitogenin. It also contains three flavone glycosides, traces of alkaloids, fixed oil and potassium nitrate.

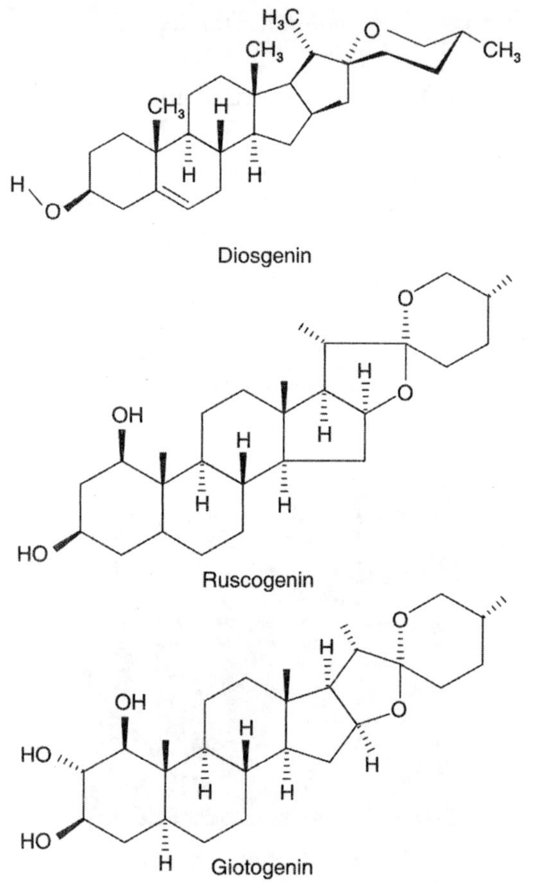

Fig. 5.2.26: Chemical constituents of gokhru

Uses: Bara gokhru: Seeds are demulcant, diuretic, tonic, muscilaginous, aphrodisiac, gonorrhea, and incontinence.

Chotta gokhru: The roots and fruits are sweet, cooling, emollient, appetizer, alternate, laxative, cardiotonic, styptic, lithontriptic and tonic. They are useful in strangury, dysuria, vitiated conditions of *vat* and *pitta*, renal and vesical calculi, anorexia, dyspepsia, helminthiasis, cough, asthma. The seeds are astringent, strengthening and are useful in epistaxis, hemorrhages and ulcerative stomatitis. The ash of the whole plant is good for external application in rheum arthritis.

Glycyrrhiza (Fig. 5.2.27)

Synonyms: Sanskrit—Yashti-madhu; **English**—Sweetwood; liquorice; **Hindi**— Mithilakdi, Mulathee.

Biological source: It consists of dried, peeled or unpeeled roots and stolons of *Glycyrrhiza glabra*, belonging to family Leguminosae.

Habitat: Natives of South-east Europe and South-west Asia.

Botany

- Kingdom   Plantae
- Division   Magnoliophyta
- Class   Magnoliopsida
- Order   Fabales
- Family   Fabaceae
- Genus   *Glycyrrhiza*
- Species   *glabra*

Part used: Roots

Organoleptic Characters

Color: Unpeeled–Yellowish brown to dark brown; Peeled—Pale yellow.

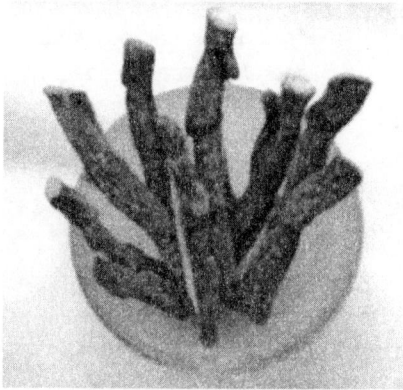

Fig. 5.2.27: Liquorice root
(*see also in colour Plate 4*)

Odor: Faint and characteristic
Taste: Sweet, free from bitterness
Fracture: Fibrous
Extra features: Peeled drug is fibrous and angular in shape.

Microcopy of Liquorice Root (Fig. 5.2.28)

Cork: Fairly abundant, polygonal fragments of orange-brown cork composed of thin-walled cells.

Starch: The abundant starch granules, most of which are simple; they are rather small, spherical to ovoid and slightly flattened; a slit-shaped hilum is visible in some of the larger granules.

Fibers: The very abundant fibers which occur in groups surrounded by a calcium oxalate prism sheath.

Vessels: The vessels are found singly or in small groups. Some of the individual vessels are very large and are frequently found fragmented. The larger vessels are usually accompanied by lignified xylem parenchyma composed of moderately thin-walled cells, square to elongate rectangular in outline with variably pitted walls.

Calcium oxalate: The prisms of calcium oxalate are fairly uniform in size and occur in the cells forming the crystal sheath surrounding the fibers.

Parenchyma cells: The abundant thin-walled parenchyma from the cortex, medullary rays and pith. The cells vary from rounded to rectangular in outline and are usually filled with starch granules.

Sieve tissue: Occasional groups of sieve tissue, composed of very thin-walled cells with faint sieve areas, may be found associated with the medullary rays. A small amount of collenchyma is also present.

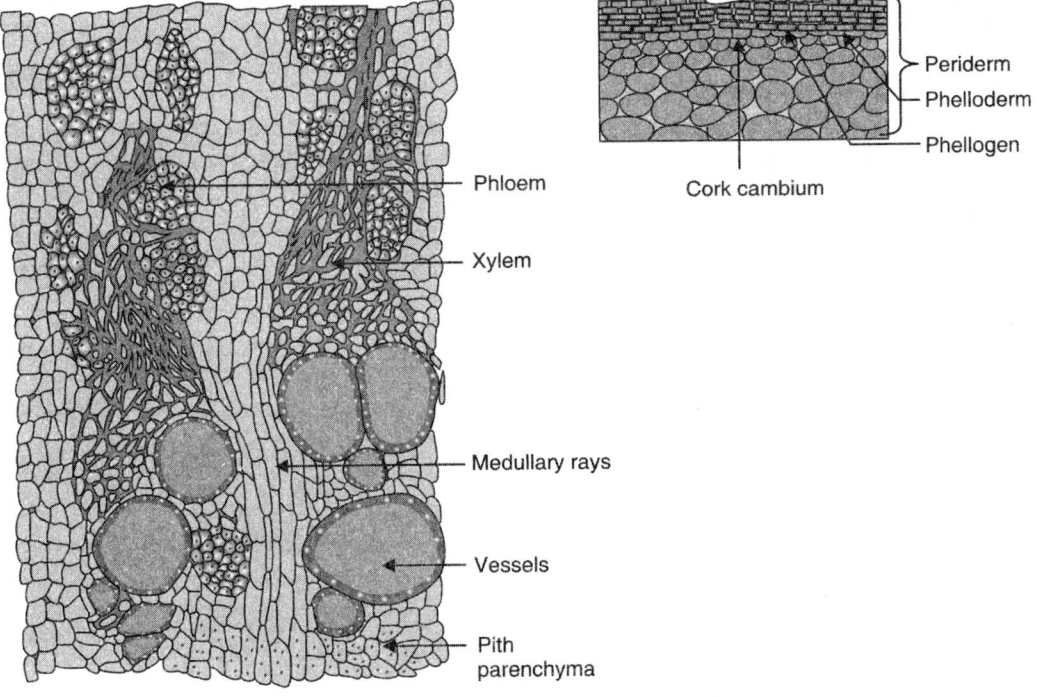

Fig. 5.2.28: Transverse section of liquorice root

Staining Reagents

Phloroglucinol: HCl-1:1 (Lignified tissues are seen red/pink.)

Acetic acid: Crystals are insoluble.

Iodine solution: Starch (blue).

Sulfuric acid: Calcium oxalate crystals are seen.

Chemical constituents: The chief constituent of liquorice root, which gives it sweet taste, is glycyrrhizin (6 to 8%), obtainable in the form of a sweet, white crystalline powder, consisting of the calcium and potassium salts of glycyrrhizic acid (Fig. 5.2.29). The drug also contains sugar, starch (29%), gum, protein, fat (0.8%), resin, asparagin (2 to 4 per cent), a trace of tannin in the outer bark of the root, yellow coloring matter, and 0.03% of volatile oil.

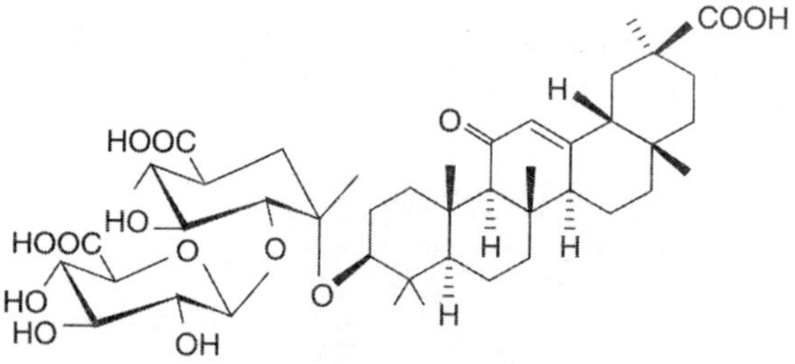

Fig. 5.2.29: Glycyrrhizin (glycyrrhizic acid)

Chemical Test

Test for phenolics: Aqueous extract treated with $FeCl_3$ gives dark coloration.

Test for flavonoids: Aqueous extract treated with mineral acid (HCl/H_2SO_4) gives reddish orange coloration which disappears after addition of alkali and reappears again.

Test for saponin: Powder treated with water gives persistent foam.

Standards

- *Foreign matter:* Powdered glycyrrhiza shows no stone cells.
- *Loss on drying:* NMT 12%
- *Total ash:* NMT 7.0%
- *Acid insoluble ash:* NMT 2.0%

Uses: Powdered liquorice root is an effective expectorant, especially in ayurvedic medicine where it is also used in toothpowders and is known as Jastimadhu. Additionally, liquorice may be useful in conventional and naturopathic medicine for both mouth ulcers and peptic ulcers.

Adulterants: Indian liquorice (*Abrus pracatorious*)

Brahmi (Fig. 5.2.30)

Synonyms: English—Water Hyssop; **Tamil**—Nirbrahmi; **Gujarati**—Jalanevari.

Biological source: It is obtained from the herb of *Bacopa monnieri*, belonging to family Scrophulariaceae.

Habitat: Brahmi is a perennial creeping herb with small white flowers. Its leaves are bright green and look almost like a succulent. It grows in damp, marshy areas, in both fresh and brackish water. It is commonly found throughout southeast Asia, but has since migrated with great success to Florida and several other southern states in the US. Because of its easy adaptability, it is a favorite foliage for aquariums both big and small.

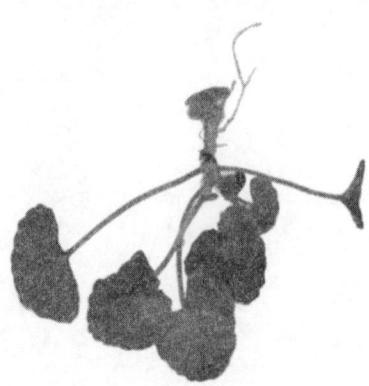

Fig. 5.2.30: Brahmi
(*see also in colour Plate 4*)

Botany

- Kingdom — Plantae
- Family — Scrophulariaceae.
- Genus — *Bacopa*
- Species — *monnieri*

Part used: Whole plant

Organoleptic Characters

Leaves: The succulent leaves are sessile, opposite, decussate, obovate-oblanceolate in shape, 1.0–2.5 cm × 0.4–1.0 cm in size.

Flowers: The flowers are small and white, with four or five petals.

Stem: 10 to 30 cm long rooting at nodes, branches numerous ascending.

Chemical constituents (Fig. 5.2.31): The active principle is alkaloids brahmine (0.1–0.2%) and hersaponin in leaves. It also contain bacoside A and bacoside B, betulic acid, β sitosterol and stigmasterol.

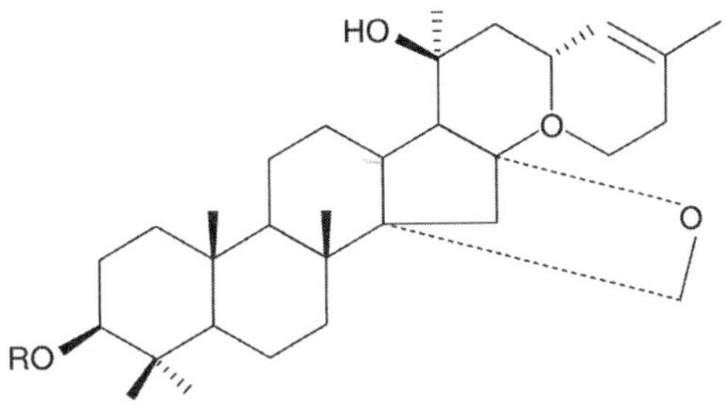

Bacoside A: R = Ara (3-1) Ara
Bacoside B: R = Rlu (2-1) Araj (3-1) Glu

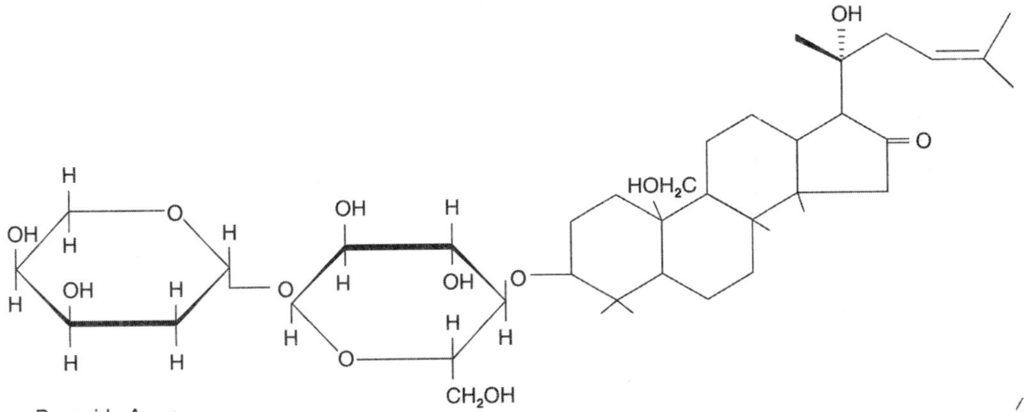

Bacoside A

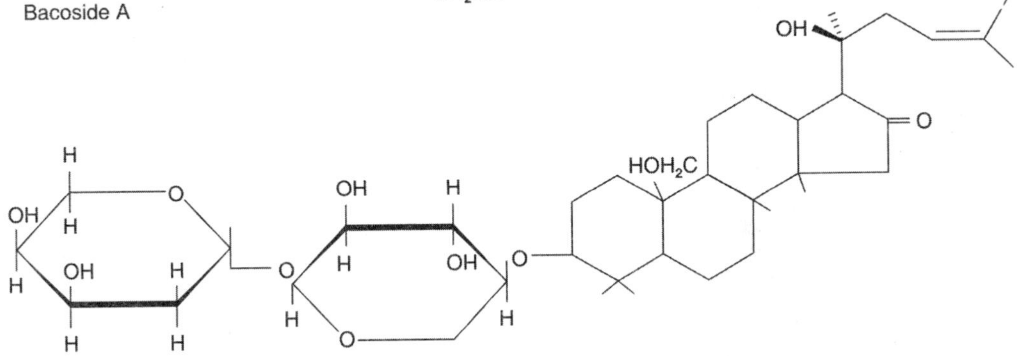

Bacoside B

Fig. 5.2.31: Chemical constituents of Brahmi

Uses: Brahmi has antioxidant properties. It has been reported to reduce oxidation of fats in the bloodstream, which is a risk factor for cardiovascular diseases. It has been used for treatment of epilepsy, memory capacity, increase concentration, and reduce stress-induced anxiety. It is listed as a nootropic, a drug that enhances cognitive ability.

In Ayurveda: It is bitter, pungent, heating, emetic, laxative and useful in bad ulcers, tumors, ascites, enlargement of spleen, indigestion, inflammations, leprosy, anemia, biliousness, etc.

In Unani system of medicine: It is bitter, aphrodisiac, good in scabies, leucoderma, syphilis, etc. It is promising blood purifier and useful in diarrhea and fevers.

Arjuna Bark (Fig. 5.2.32)

Synonyms: Sanskrit—Arjuna; **English**—Arjuna myrobalan; **Hindi**—Arjun, Kahu; Guj; Sajadan.

Biological source: Arjuna is dried bark of *Terminalia arjuna*, belonging to family Combretaceae.

Origin: *Terminalia arjuna* is common throughout India especially in the sub-Himalayan tracts and eastern India.

Botany

- Kingdom   Plantae
- Division   Magnoliophyta
- Class   Magnoliopsida
- Order   Myrtales
- Family   Combretaceae
- Genus   *Terminalia*
- Species   *arjuna*

Organoleptic Characters

Color: Externally, it is pink or flesh-colored with mealy coating and internal surface is reddish brown.

Odor: None

Taste: Gritty and astringent

Fracture: Fibrous

Size: Varying size with 5 to 10 mm thickness

Extra features: 40 meters high deciduous tree. Leaves are simple, 4–6″ long oppositely arranged, rectangular or oval. At the base of the lamina, two glands are present. Flower: Green and star-like spikes, calyx smooth. Fruit: Truncate.

Chemical constituents (Fig. 5.2.33): The bark contains specific medicinal active constituents namely triterpene glycosides, like arjunetosides I, II, III, IV, arjunine and arjunetin. It is also rich in saponins, natural anti-oxidants (flavonoids—arjunone, arjunolone, leteilin) gallic acid, ellagic acid, oligomeric proanthocyanidins, phytosterols, rich in minerals like calcium, magnesium, zinc and copper.

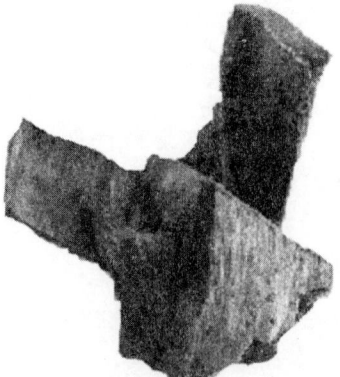

Fig. 5.2.32: Arjuna bark
(*see also in colour Plate 4*)

(a) Arjunolic acid

Senega (Fig. 5.2.34)

Synonyms: Senega root, Senega snake root, Radix senegae, Rattlesnake root.

Biological source: Senega consists of dried roots and root stocks of *Polygala senega* linn and *Polygala chinensis*, belonging to family Polygalaceae.

Habitat: North western USA, India (Indian senega)

Botany

- Kingdom — Plantae
- Family — Polygalaceae.
- Genus — *Polygala*
- Species — *senega*

Parts used: Roots and root stocks

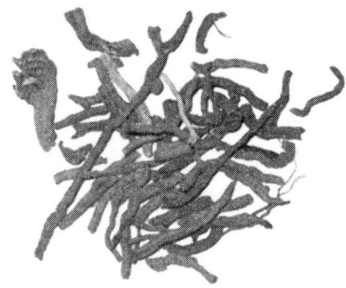

Fig. 5.2.34: Senega root (*see also in colour Plate 4*)

Organoleptic Characters

Color: Grayish brown to yellowish brown

Odor: Characteristic, resembling methyl salicylate

Taste: First sweet than bitter, acrid and irritating

Shape: Longitudinal stratified

Size: Length 5 to 20 cm, diameter 2 to 12 cm

Chemical constituents (Fig. 5.2.35): Triterpenoid saponins, senegin, polygalic acid, sapogenin, phenolic acids, methyl salicylate and polygalitol.

(b) Arjunic acid

(c) Arjungenin

Fig. 5.2.33: Chemical constituents of Arjuna bark

Chemical Test

Fluorescence analysis: The fluorescence analysis is carried out with 10% extract of ether and petroleum ether in UV chamber (Table 5.2.6).

Table 5.2.6: Comparative chemical test of *Terminalia* species

Chemicals	T. arjuna	T. tomentosa
Ether	Pinkish white	Pale blue
Petroleum Ether	Bright pinkish Red	Pale white Blue

Uses: The bark is astringent, sweet, acrid, cooling, aphrodisiac, cardiotonic, urinary astringent, expectorant, alexiteric and is useful in fractures, ulcers, cirrhosis of the liver, hyperhidrosis, otalgia and hypertension.

Adulterants: *Terminalia tomentosa* (dried bark). It is distinguished by Arjuna bark by fluorescence test.

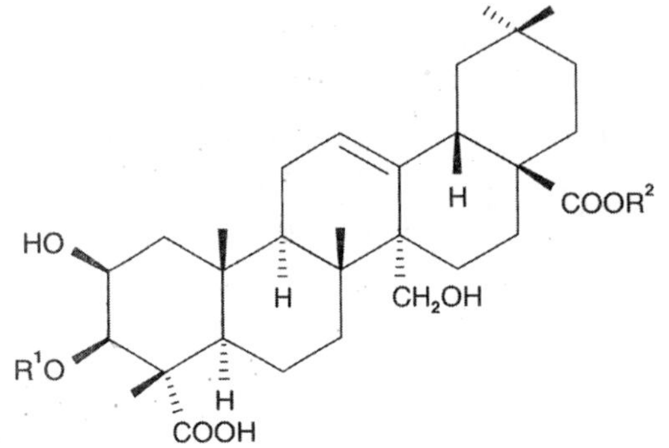

Fig. 5.2.35: Chemical constituents of senega

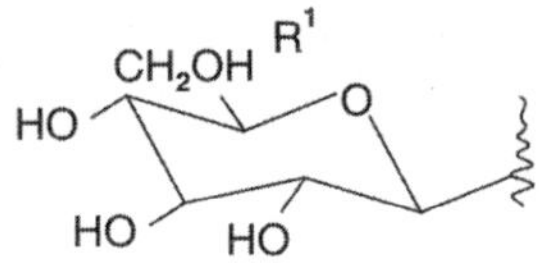

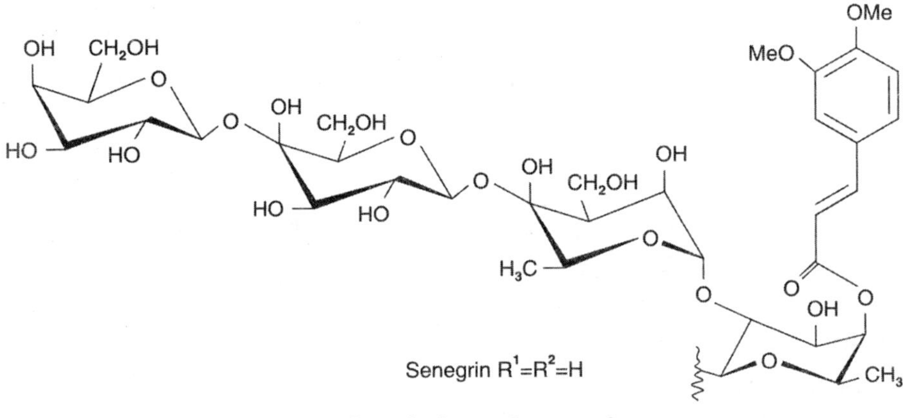

Chemical test: Shake drug with water, persistent foaming is seen.

Uses: It is used in bronchitis, asthma, tracheitis, emphysema and inflammation of the respiratory tract. Also used for the treatment of rheumatism, colds, inflammation, and bleeding wounds. It stimulates bronchial mucous gland secretion.

Adulterants: White senega, Indian senega and *Polygala tenuifolia*.

CYANOGENIC GLYCOSIDES

Cyanogenic glycosides are a group of mainly plant-derived materials, which liberate hydrocyanic acid (HCN) on hydrolysis, and are thus of concern as natural toxicants. The group is identified by **amygdalin,** a constituent in the kernels of bitter almonds (*Prunus amygdalus*; Rosaceae) and other *Prunus* species, such as apricots, peaches, cherries, and plums. When plant tissue containing a cyanogenic glycoside is crushed, glycosidase enzymes, usually located in different cells, are brought into contact with the glycoside and begin to hydrolyse it. Thus, amygdalin is hydrolysed sequentially by α-glucosidase-type enzymes to **prunasin** and then **mandelonitrile**. Cyanogenetic glycoside contains nitrogen, but the sugar moiety is attached to oxygen. The enzyme emulsin found in almond consists of two enzymes—amygdalase and prunase.

The main amino acids utilized in the biosynthesis of cyanogenic glycosides are phenylalanine (e.g. prunasin, sambunigrin, and amygdalin), tyrosine [e.g. **dhurrin** from sorghum (*Sorghum bicolor*; Graminae/Poaceae)], valine [e.g. linamarin from flax (*Linum usitatissimum*; Linaceae], isoleucine (e.g. from flax), and leucine [e.g. **hetero-dendrin** from *Acacia* species (Leguminosae/Fabaceae].

Chemical Test: Sodium Picrate Test

A strip of filter paper is dipped in 10% aqueous solution of picric acid. It is drained and redipped in 10% sodium carbonate solution and drained again. To powdered drug in a flask, water is added to moisten it. Sodium picrate is kept on the mouth of the flask. Hydrocyanic acid vapours turn the paper brick red or maroon-colored.

Biosynthesis: Through shikimic acid and phenylalanine pathway.

Bitter Almond (Fig. 5.2.36)

Biological source: Bitter almond is dried ripe seeds of *Prunus amygdalis var amara* belonging to family rosaceae.

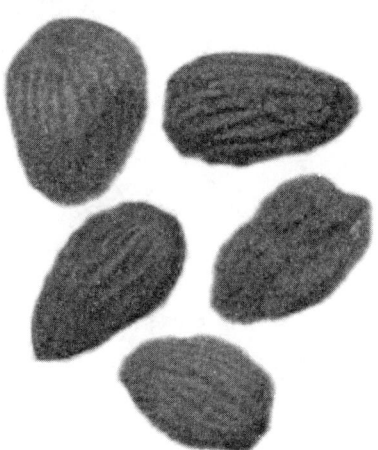

Fig. 5.2.36: Bitter almond
(*see also in colour Plate 4*)

Habitat: The almond tree is a native of the warmer parts of western Asia and of north Africa, but it has been extensively distributed over the warm temperate region of the Old World, and is cultivated in all the countries bordering on the Mediterranean.

Botany

- Kingdom   Plantae
- Family   Rosaceae
- Genus   *Prunus*
- Species   *amygdalis*

Part used: Seeds

Chemical constituents: The bitter almond seed contains a ferment emulsin, which in presence of water acts on the soluble glucoside amygdalin (Fig. 5.2.37) yielding glucose, prussic acid and the essential oil of bitter almonds, or benzaldehyde, which is not used in medicine. Bitter almonds yield from 6 to 8% of prussic acid.

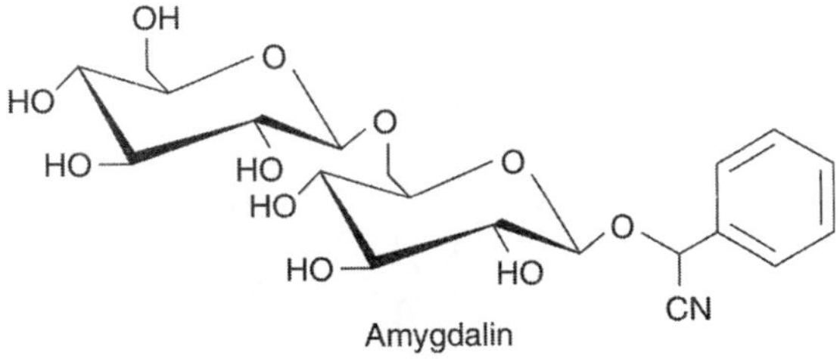

Fig. 5.2.37: Chemical constituent of bitter almond

Uses: This essential volatile oil of bitter almonds, is used in confectionery and as a culinary flavoring, but on account of its poisonous nature, great care ought to be exercised in its use. Bitter almonds and their poisonous properties used in intermittent fevers, as a vermifuge, as an aperient and diuretic, and as a cure for hydrophobia. Simple water, strongly impregnated by distillation with the volatile oil, will cause giddiness, headache and dimness of sight, and has been found also poisonous to animals, and there are instances of cordial spirits flavored by them being poisonous to man.

Wild Cherry Bark (Fig. 5.2.38)

Synonyms: English—Virginian prune; black cherry.

Biological source: It is obtained from dried bark of *Prunus serotina* belonging to family Rosaceae.

Habitat: North America generally, especially in northern and central states.

Botany

- Kingdom   Plantae
- Family   Rosaceae
- Genus   *Prunus*
- Species   *serotina*

Parts used: Bark of root, trunk and branches

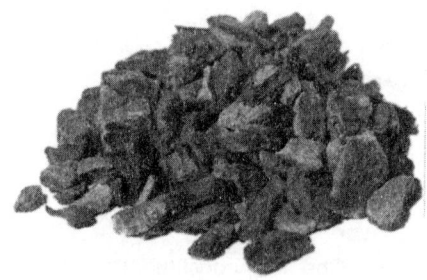

Fig. 5.2.38: Wild cherry bark
(*see also in colour Plate 4*)

Organoleptic Characters

This tree grows from 50 to 80 feet high, and 2 to 4 feet in diameter. The bark is black and rough and separates naturally from the trunk.

Leaves deciduous, 3 to 5 inches long, about 2 inches wide, on petioles which have two pairs of reddish glands, they are obovate, acuminate, with incurved short teeth, thickish and smooth and glossy on upper surface.

Flowers bloom in May, and are white, in erect long terminal racemes, with occasional solitary flowers in the axils of the leaves.

Fruit about the size of a pea, purply-black, globular drupe, edible with bitterish taste, is ripe in August and September.

Root-bark must be freshly collected each season as its properties deteriorate greatly, if kept longer than a year. It has a short friable fracture and in commerce it is found in varying lengths and widths (1 to 8 inches), slightly curved, outer bark removed, a reddish-fawn color. These fragments easily powder. It has the odor of almonds, which almost disappears on drying, but is renewed by maceration. Its taste is aromatic, prussic, and bitter. It imparts its virtues to water or alcohol, boiling impairs its medicinal properties.

Chemical constituents: Starch, resin, tannin, gallic acid, fatty matter, lignin, red coloring matter, salts of calcium, potassium, and iron, also a volatile oil associated with hydrocyanic acid by distillation of water from the bark. It also contains prunasin (a cyanogenic glycoside; Fig. 5.2.39), emulsin, eudesmic acid, p-coumaric acid, scopoletin, tannins, sugars, etc.

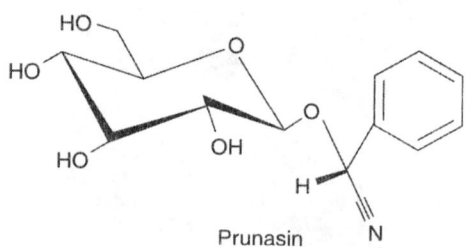

Fig. 5.2.39: Prunasin

Uses: Astringent tonic, pectoral, sedative and flavouring agents. It has been used in the treatment of bronchitis of various types. It is valuable in whooping-cough, and dyspepsia.

FLAVANOID GLYCOSIDES

Flavanoid glycosides are mostly occurring as o-glycosides or c-glycosides containing in the cell sap of higher plants belonging to the families, like Compositeae, Leguminoseae, Rutaceae and Umbelliferae.

Different types of flavanoid glycosides are:
1. Flavone glycosides, e.g. apiin and diosmin
2. Flavonol glycosides, e.g. rutin and quercetin
3. Flavanone glycosides, e.g. hesperidin and Liquiritin
4. Chalcone glycosides, e.g. carthamin
5. Isoflavanoid glycosides, e.g. tephrosin and prunetrin
6. Anthrocyanidin glycosides, e.g. cyanidin and malvidin

Flavonoids are particularly beneficial, acting as antioxidants and giving protection against cardiovascular disease, certain forms of cancer, and it is claimed age-related degeneration of cell components. Their polyphenolic nature enables them to scavenge injurious free radicals, such as superoxide and hydroxyl radicals. **Quercetin** is almost present in substantial amounts in plant tissues, and is a powerful antioxidant, chelating metals, scavenging free radicals, and preventing oxidation of low density lipoprotein.

Flavonoids in red wine (**quercetin, kaempferol**, and anthocyanidins) and in tea (**catechins** and catechin gallate esters) are also demonstrated to be effective antioxidants. Flavonoids contribute to plant colors, yellows from chalcones and flavonols, and reds, blues, and violets from anthocyanidins. Even the colorless materials, e.g. flavones, absorb strongly in the UV and are detectable by insects, probably aiding flower pollination.

Chalcones act as precursors for a vast range of **flavonoid** derivatives found throughout the plant kingdom. Flavanones can then give rise to many variants on this basic skeleton, e.g. **flavones, flavonols, anthocyanidins**, and **catechins**.

Chemical Tests

1. It exhibits a brown fluorescence under UV light.
2. It gives yellow precipitate with basic lead acetate solution.
3. It gives greenish brown precipitate with ferric chloride.
4. It produces a silver mirror with ammoniacal silver nitrate solution.

Biosynthesis: Through acetate pathway and shikimic acid pathway.

Rutin (Fig. 5.2.40)

Synonyms: Rutoside, quercetin-3-rutinoside and sophorin

Biological source: Rutin is a citrus flavonoid glycoside found in the fruits and fruit rinds (especially *citrus* fruits—orange, grapefruit, lemon, lime) and berries, such as mulberry and cranberries. Its name comes from the name of *Ruta graveolens*, a plant that also contains rutin. It is sometimes referred to as vitamin P.

Rutin is a yellow crystalline flavonol glycoside ($C_{27}H_{30}O_{16}$) that occurs in various plants (rue, tobacco, buckwheat, etc.). Upon hydrolysis (a chemical reaction that uses water to breakdown a compound), rutin yields quercetin and rutinose. Rutin is used in many countries as a vasoprotectant and is an ingredient in numerous multivitamin preparations and herbal remedies. The rutosides are naturally occurring flavonoids that have effects on capillary permeability and edema (swelling) and have been used for the treatment of disorders of the venous and microcirculatory systems.

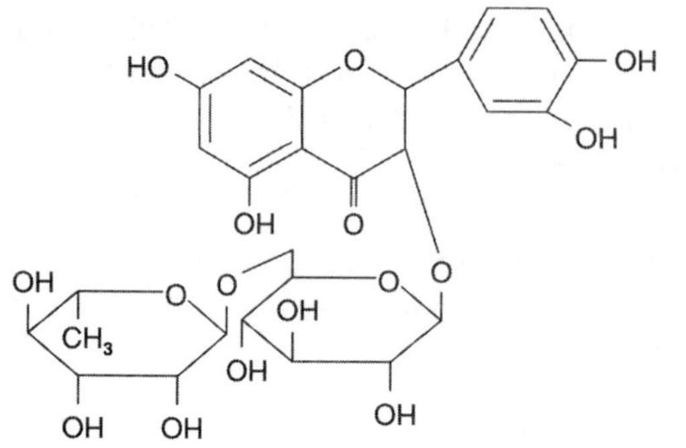

MW: 610, 53, Formula: $C_2H_{30}O_{16}$

Fig. 5.2.40: Rutin

Biological source: Hesperidin is a flavanone glycoside (flavonoid) ($C_{28}H_{34}O_{15}$) found abundantly in citrus fruits. Its aglycone form is called hesperetin. Hesperidin is the predominant flavonoid in lemons and oranges. The peel and membranous parts of these fruits have the highest hesperidin concentrations. Sweet oranges (citrus sinensis) and tangelos are the richest dietary sources of hesperidin. Hesperidin is classified as a citrus bioflavonoid. Hesperidin, rutin and other flavonoids thought to reduce capillary permeability and to have anti-inflammatory action were collectively known as vitamin P.

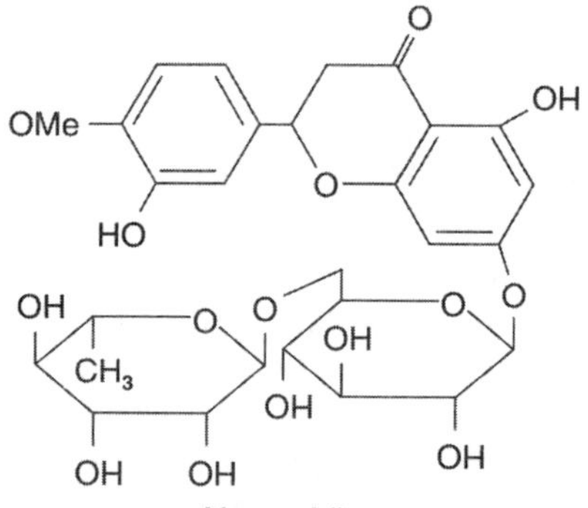

Uses

- Rutin inhibits platelet aggregation, as well as capillary permeability making the blood thinner and improving circulation. Rutin has anti-inflammatory activity.
- Rutin inhibits aldose reductase activity. Aldose reductase is an enzyme normally present in the eye and elsewhere in the body. It helps change glucose (sugar-glucose) into a sugar alcohol called sorbitol.
- Rutin also strengthens the capillaries, and, therefore, can reduce the symptoms of hemophilia.
- Rutin, as ferulic acid, can reduce the cytotoxicity of oxidized LDL cholesterol and lower the risk of heart disease.
- Rutin is also an antioxidant, along with quercetin, acacetin, morin, hispidulin, hesperidin, and naringin, it was found to be the strongest. Hydroxyethylrutosides, synthetic hydroxyethyl acetylations of rutin are used in the treatment of chronic venous insufficiency.

Hesperidin (Fig. 5.2.41)

Synonyms: Hesperetin 7-rhamnoglucoside, hesperetin-7-rutinoside

MW: 610, Formula: $C_{28}H_{34}O_{15}$

Fig. 5.2.41: Hesperidin

Uses: Hesperidin has antioxidant, anti-inflammatory, hypolipidemic, vasoprotective and anticarcinogenic and cholesterol lowering actions. Hesperdin can inhibit following enzymes: phospholipase A2, lipoxygenase, HMG-CoA reductase and cyclo-oxygenase. Hesperidin improves the health of capillaries by reducing the capillary permeability. Hesperidin is used to reduce hay fever and other allergic conditions by inhibiting the release of histamine from mast cells. The possible anti-cancer activity of hesperidin could be explained by the inhibition of polyamine synthesis.

ISOTHIOCYANATE GLYCOSIDES

Isothiocyanate glycosides contain sulfur and present in many cruciferous plants. On hydrolysis, they produce isothiocyanate aglycones. Sinigrin from black mustard and sinalbin from white mustard are isothiocyanate glycosides. Sinigrin on hydrolysis in the presence of enzyme myrosin, yields allyl isothiocyanate, glucose and potassium acid sulfate. These glycosides are irritant and employed as counterirritant in neuralgia and rheumatism.

Chemical Test

1. The powdered black mustard seeds on treatment with sodium hydroxide yields bright yellow coloration.
2. The hydrolysed products of sinalbin (white mustard) are crystalline and give rise a bright yellow coloration in alkaline medium.

PHENOLIC GLYCOSIDES

Simple phenolic glycosides have their aglycone portion loaded with phenolic moieties, alcoholic moieties or carboxylic acid functions. Commonly found phenolic glycosides are salicin, populin, arbutin, gaultherin, etc.

Biosynthesis: Through shikimic acid pathway.

Chemical Tests

1. It gives a bright yellow coloration with conc. sulfuric acid that fades out on addition of water.
2. It yields blue coloration with ferric chloride solution.

5.3 TERPENOIDS, VOLATILE OILS AND RESINS

TERPENOIDS

Terpenes are unique, widespread and chemically diverse groups of hydrocarbon-based natural products whose structure may be derived from combinations of several 5-carbon base (C5) units called isoprene, giving rise to structures which may be divided into isopentane (2-methylbutane) units. The terpenes are of a biogenetic origin, in which isopentenyl pyrophosphate and dimethylallyl pyrophosphate combine to yield geranyl pyrophosphate, leading to monoterpenes. Similarly, sesquiterpenes and triterpenes are formed from two equivalents of farnesyl pyrophosphate. A terpene containing oxygen is called a terpenoids.

Terpenes are thus classified by the number of 5-carbon units they contain (Table 5.3.1):

1. Hemiterpene C_5
2. Monoterpene C_{10}
3. Sesquiterpene C_{15}
4. Diterpene C_{20}
5. Sesterterpene C_{25} (very rare)
6. Triterpene C_{30}
7. Tetraterpenes C_{40}

The function of terpenes in plants is as follows, they are generally considered to be both ecological and physiological:

- They inhibit the growth of competing plants (allelopathy).
- They show insecticidal activity as well as found to attract insect pollinators.
- The plant hormone, abscisic acid, is one of the sesquiterpenes.
- Gibberellic acid is a type of terpene, and is major plant hormones.

Table 5.3.1: Types of terpenes

The monoterpenes are formed from the coupling of two isoprene units (c10). They are the most representative molecules constituting 90% of the essential oils and allow a great variety of structures. They consist of several functions:

1.	Carbures	Acyclic: Myrcene, ocimene, etc. Monocyclic: Terpinenes, p-cimene, phellandrenes, etc. Bicyclic: Pinenes, -3-carene, camphene, sabinene, etc.
2.	Alcohols	Acyclic: Geraniol, linalol, citronellol, lavandulol, nerol, etc. Monocyclic: Menthol, a-terpineol, carveol Bicyclic: Borneol, fenchol, chrysanthenol, thuyan-3- ol, etc.
3.	Aldehydes	Acyclic: Geranial, neral, citronellal, etc.
4.	Ketone	Acyclic: tegetone, etc. Monocyclic: Menthones, carvone, pulegone, piperitone, etc. Bicyclic: Camphor, fenchone, thuyone, ombellulone, pinocamphone, pinocarvone, etc.
5.	Esters	Acyclic: Linalyl acetate or propionate, citronellyl acetate, etc. Monocyclic: Menthyl or a-terpinyl acetate, etc. Bicyclic: Isobornyl acetate, etc.
6.	Ethers	1,8-cineole, menthofurane, etc. Peroxydes: Ascaridole, etc.
7.	Phenols	Thymol, carvacrol, etc.

Examples of plants containing monoterpeniods are (+)-α-pinene from *Pinus palustris*, (−)-β-pinene from *Pinus caribaea*, (−) linalol from coriander, (+)-linalol from some camphor trees, (±)-citronellol is widespread, the form (+) is characteristic of *Eucalyptus citriodora*

The sesquiterpenes are formed from the assembly of three isoprene units (c15). The extension of the chain increases the number of cyclisations which allows a great variety of structures. The structure and function of the sesquiterpenes are similar to those of the monoterpenes:

1.	Carbures	Azulene, β-bisabolene, cadinenes, β-caryophyllene, logifolene, curcumenes, elemenes, farnesenes, zingiberene, etc.
2.	Alcohols	Bisabol, cedrol, β-nerolidol, farnesol, carotol, β-santalol, patchoulol, viridiflorol, etc.
3.	Ketones	Germacrone, nootkatone, cis-longipinan-2,7-dione, β-vetinone, turmerones, etc.
4.	Epoxide	Caryophyllene oxide, humulene epoxides, etc.

Examples of plants containing these compounds are angelica, bergamot, caraway, celery, citronella, coriander, eucalyptus, geranium, juniper, lavandin, lavander, lemon, lemongrass, mandarin, mint, orange, peppermint, petitgrain, pine, rosemary, sage, thyme.

Aromatic compounds are derived from phenylpropane, the aromatic compounds occur less frequently than the terpenes.

1.	Aldehyde	Cinnamaldehyde
2.	Alcohol	Cinnamic alcohol
3.	Phenols	Chavicol, eugenol
4.	Methoxy dioxy compounds	Apiole, myristicine, safrole

The principal plant sources for these compounds are anise, cinnamon, clove, fennel, nutmeg, parsley, sassafras, star anise, tarragon, and some botanical families (Apiaceae, Lamiaceae, Myrtaceae, Rutaceae).

VOLATILE OILS

Volatile oils are volatile, natural, complex compounds characterized by a strong odor and are formed by aromatic plants as secondary metabolites. They can be synthesized by all plant organs, i.e. buds, flowers, leaves, stems, twigs, seeds, fruits, roots, wood or bark, and are stored in secretory cells, cavities, canals, epidermic cells or glandular trichomes. They are liquid, volatile, rarely colored, lipid soluble and soluble in organic solvents with a generally lower density than that of water. They are usually obtained by steam or hydro-distillation, known for their antiseptic, i.e. bactericidal, virucidal and fungicidal, and medicinal properties and their fragrance. They are used in embalment, preservation of foods and as antimicrobial, analgesic, sedative, anti-inflammatory, spasmolytic and locally anesthesic remedies. Due to their bactericidal and fungicidal properties, pharmaceutical and food uses are more and more widespread as alternatives to synthetic chemical products to protect the ecological equilibrium. Volatile oils are very complex natural mixtures which can contain about 20–60 components at quite different concentrations, also known as essential oils (Table 5.3.2).

Physical Properties of Volatile Oil

- Volatile essential oils are volatile and become liquid at room temperature.
- When distilled they are at first colorless or slightly yellowish.
- They are soluble in alcohol and in the usual organic solvents, such as ether or chloroform.
- They are less dense than water (sassafras essence and clove essence being exceptions).
- They are nearly always rotational and have a high refractory index.
- They are lipo-soluble and not very soluble in water, but can be dragged using steam.

Table 5.3.2: Plant essential oil with chemical constituents

S. no.	Plant essential oil	Chemical constituents
1.	Origanum compactum	Carvacrol (30%) and thymol (27%)
2.	Coriandrum sativum	Linalol (68%)
3.	Artemisia herba-alba	α- and β-thuyone (57%) and camphor (24%)
4.	Cinnamomum camphora	1,8-cineole (50%)
5.	Anethum graveolens (leaf)	α-Phellandrene (36%) and limonene (31%)
6.	Anethum graveolens (seed)	Carvone (58%) and limonene (37%)
7.	Mentha piperita	Menthol (59%) and menthone (19%)

Classifying Essential Oils

Essential oils may be classified using different criteria: consistency, origin, and chemical nature of the main components.

a. Consistency

Depending on their consistency, essential oils are classified as:

Essences, balsams, resins.

1. Fluid **essences** are liquids which are volatile at room temperature.
2. **Balsams** are natural extracts obtained from a bush or tree. They usually have a high benzoic and cynamic acid content with their corresponding esters. They are thicker, not very volatile, and less likely to react by polymerising. Examples of balsams are copaiba balsam, Peruvian balsam, banguy balsam, tolu balsam, liquid amber.

Within the resin group we find a number of possible combinations and mixes:

3. i. **Resins:** These are amorphous solid or semisolid products of a complex chemical nature. They are physiological or physiopathological in origin. Colophony, for example, is obtained by separating trementine an oleoresin. It contains abietic acid and derivates.

   ii. **Oleoresins:** The term oleoresin is also used to refer to vegetable extracts obtained using solvents. Because of their advantages, (viz. stability, microbiotic and chemical uniformity, and easy to add), they have the aroma of the plant in concentrated form and are highly viscous liquids or semi-solid substances. These are homogeneous mixes of resins and essential oils. Trementine, for example, is obtained by making incisions in the trunk of different pine species. It contains resin (colophony) and essential oil (trementine essence) which are separated by steam drag distillation, e.g. black pepper, paprika oleoresin, cloves.

   iii. **Gum-resins:** These are natural plant or tree extracts. They are a mix of gums and resins.

b. Origin

Depending on their origin, essential oils are classified as: Natural, artificial, synthetic.

Natural oils are obtained straight from the plant and are not modified physically or chemically afterwards. However, they are expensive because of their limited yield.

Artificial oils are obtained using processes of enriching the essence with one or several of its components. For example, essences of rose, geranium, and jasmine are enriched with linalool, and aniseed essence with athenol.

Synthetic oils are usually produced by combining their chemically synthesized components. These are the cheapest and are thus much more commonly used as fragrance and taste enhancers (vanilla, lemon and strawberry essences).

c. Chemical Nature

The total essential oil content of a plant is generally low (less than 1%), highly concentrated form which is used in industrial processes. Most of these are highly complex chemical compounds. The proportion of these substances varies depending on the oil, season, time of day, growing conditions, and genetics.

The term **chemotype** refers to the variation in chemical composition of an essential oil, even of the same species. A chemo-type is a distinct chemical entity, different from secondary metabolites. Certain small variations in the environment, geographical location, genes, which have little or no effect on a morphological level can, however, produce big changes in chemical phenotypes. Thyme (*Thymus vulgaris*) is a typical example. It has 6 different chemo-types depending on which is the main component of its essence (timol, carvacrol, linalool, geraniol, tuyanol-4, or terpineol). For example, *Thymus vulgaris* linalool, *Thymus vulgaris* timol.

Extraction

There are several methods for extracting essential oils. These may include use of liquid carbon dioxide or microwaves, and mainly low or high pressure distillation employing boiling water or hot steam. The chemical profile of the essential oil products differs not only in the number of molecules but also in the stereochemical types of molecules extracted. The type of extraction is chosen according to the purpose of the use. The extraction product can vary in quality, quantity and in composition according to climate, soil composition,

Table 5.3.3: Classification of terpenoids

Classification	Functional (suffix)	Important group	Examples constituents	Properties
Terpenoids Hydrocarbons (—ene)	—C=C—	Cadinene, camphene, pinene, lemonene	Turpentine, junipes, cade	Stimulant, Antiviral, Antitumoral
Alcohol (—OH)	C—OH	Linalol, menthol, santalol, geraniol	Coriander, peppermint, sandal wood	Antimicrobial, antiseptic, spasmodic
Aldehyde (—al)	CHO	Cinnamaldehyde, citral, citonellal	Cinnamon, clove, lemon peel	Spasmodic, sedative, antiviral
Esters (—ate)	$R_1-C(=O)-O-R_2$	Linalyl acetate, bornyl acetate	Ceaultheria, lavender, rosemary	Spasmodic, antifungal, sedative
Ketones (—one)	$R_1-C(=O)-R_2$	Carvone, camphor, menthone	Caraway, dill, camphor	Mucolitic, neurotoxic, regenator cellular
Ethers	—C—O—C—	Chavical methyl ether cineol, mepisticin, ascaridol	Arise, eucalyptus, nutmeg	Expectorant and stimulant
Peroxides Non-terpenoids	—O—O—	Ascaridole	Chenopodium	Insect repellant, increase digestion
Phenol (—ol)	Ar—OH	Eugenol, thymol, carvacrol	Clove, cinnamon leaf, thyme	Antimicrobial, stimulant, irritant
Phenolic ether	Ring—O—C	Safrol, anetol, miristicine	Sassafras, anise seed	Flavoring agent, carminative, expectorant
Glycoside derived	Sugar and non sugar group	Methyl salicylate allyl isothiocynate benzaldehyde	Wintergreen, mustard, bitter almond	Flavoring agent

plant organ, age and vegetative cycle stage. So, in order to obtain essential oils of constant composition, they have to be extracted under the same conditions from the same organ of the plant which has been growing on the same soil, under the same climate and has been picked in the same season. There are four ways of extraction of volatile oils:

1. Expression
2. Steam distillation
3. Extraction by volatile solvents
4. Adsorption in purified fat (effleurage)
5. Extraction with supercritical gases

1. Expression

The plant material is crushed and the juice is screened to remove the large particles. The rind is macerated, and the contents of the ruptured secretory cavities are recovered.

Classic process: An abrasive action is applied on the surface of the fruit in a flow of water. The solid waste is eliminated, and the essential oil separated from the aqueous phase by centrifugation.

Other process: Machines break the cavities by depression, and collect the essential oil directly. It prevents the degradation linked to the action of water.

The screened juice is centrifuged at a high speed when nearly half of the essential oils is extracted. The other half of the oil is generally not extracted and such residue is used for isolation of the inferior quality of oil by distillation.

Example: Citrus, lemon and grass oils.

2. Steam Distillation

i. **Simple steam distillation:** This is most widely used method, the plant material is macerated and then steam distilled. Heterogeneous vapours are condensed on a cold surface. Essential oil separates based on difference in density and immiscibility. However, the method should be used with a great care, since some essential oils are decomposed during distillation and some (esters) are hydrolysed to non- or less-fragment compounds.

ii. **Saturated steam:** When plant does not come into contact with the water, steam is injected through the plant material placed on perforated trays. It is possible to operate under moderate pressure.

Advantages: Limits the alteration of the constituents of the oil, it shortens the duration of the treatment, it conserves energy and it can also be conducted on online in automated set ups.

iii. **Hydrodiffusion:** In this method, pulses of steam are sent through the plant material at very low pressure from top to bottom.

Advantage: Normally produces a product of high quality and it saves time as well as energy.

iv. **Steam distillation by microwaves under vacuum:** In this procedure, the fresh plant (require no water) is heated selectively by microwave radiation in a chamber inside which the pressure is reduced sequentially.

Advantage: This method is fast, consumes little energy and yields a product which is most often of a higher quality than the traditional steam distillation product.

3. Extraction by Means of Volatile Solvents

Some volatile essential oils are sensitive to heat and hence decomposed during distillation, in such cases, the plant material is directly treated with light petrol at 50°C and the solvent is then removed by distillation under reduced pressure.

4. Enfluerage

The fat taken in glass plates is warmed to about 50°C, then its surface is covered with the petals and it is allowed to be kept as such for several days until the fat is saturated with the essential oils for which the old petals may be replaced by the fresh ones. The petals are then removed and the fat is digested with ethyl alcohol when the essential oils present in fat are dissolved in ethyl alcohol. And if some fat is also dissolved during digestion, it is removed by cooling to about 20°C. The extract having ethyl alcohol and essential oils is distilled under reduced pressure to remove the solvent. But recently, the activated coconut charcoal is used in place of fat owing to the greater stability and more surface as compared to fat.

5. Extraction by Supercritical Gasses

For perfume uses, extraction with lipophilic solvents and sometimes with supercritical extraction is favored because beyond its critical point, a fluid can have the density of a liquid and the viscosity of a gas, therefore, diffuses well through solids, resulting in a good solvent. CO_2 is the main gas used due to its advantages that are chemically inert, non-flammable, non-toxic, selective, inexpensive, readily available and easy to completely eliminate.

Disadvantages: Technical constraints and high cost of initial investment.

Advantages: It obtains extracts which are very close in composition to the natural product and it is possible to adjust the selectivity and viscosity, etc. by fine tuning the temperature and pressure.

Example: Ginger, paprika, celery (spice extracts), black tea, oak wood smoke.

Separation

i. Chemical Methods

1. Volatile oil treated with NaCl in chloroform. The product separated is and decomposed and collected.
2. Terpenoid alcohol and volatile oil are separated with reaction with phthalic anhydride to form diesters.
3. Terpenoid aldehyde and ketone are separated by reaction with carbonyl reagent, $NaHCO_3$ and 2–4 drops of di-nitrophenyl hydrazine and Grignard reagent.

i. Physical Distillation

1. Fractional distillation
2. Chromatography

1. **Fractional distillation:** During such type of distillation, monoterpenoid hydrocarbon and tryoxygenated derivatives and residue contain sesquiterpenes are unextracted.

2. **Chromatography:** Adsorption chromatography is generally used by using silica gel and alumina used as isolation technique. Most of the commercialized essential oils are chemotyped by gas chromatography and mass spectrometry analysis.

Identification Tests of Volatile Oils

1. Volatile oil treated with Sudan red–III reagent produces red color.
2. Volatile oil treated with tincture of alkana shows red color.
3. Volatile oil treated with cosmic acid does not show stain.
4. Volatile oil at filter paper does not show stain.

Nutmeg (Fig. 5.3.1)

Synonyms: Sanskrit—Jati palam; **English**—Nutmeg; **Bengali**—Jayiphal; **Telgu**—Jajikaya.

Biological source: It is obtained from dried kernel of seeds of *Myristica fragrans* belonging to family Myristicaceae.

Habitat: Banda Islands, Malayan Archipelago, Molucca Islands, and cultivated in Kerala and Tamil Nadu.

Botany

- Kingdom   Plantae
- Order   Magnoliales
- Family   Myristicaceae
- Genus   *Myristica*
- Species   *fragrans*

Parts used: Dried kernel of the seed.

Organoleptic Characters

Color: Externally: Greenish brown
Odor: Strongly aromatic
Taste: Pungent and aromatic
Shape: Ellipsoidal
Size: 20 to 30 mm in length, 20 mm broad.

Chemical constituents: Nutmeg contains lignin, stearin (Fig. 5.3.2), volatile oil, starch, gum and 0.08 of an acid substance. The volatile oil contains 4–8% myristicin, elimicin and safrole.

Chemical Test

- Thin section of drug is treated with Sudan red III solution, red-colored globules are seen under microscope.
- Thin section of drug is treated with few drops of tincture alkana, red color is seen.

Uses: Powdered nutmeg is rarely given alone, though it enters into the composition of a number of medicines. The expressed oil is sometimes used externally as a gentle stimulant. It is used as a local stimulant to the gastrointestinal tract.

Adulterants: Bombay nutmeg, Papua nutmeg.

Cardamom Fruits and Seeds (Fig. 5.3.3)

Synonyms: Sanskrit—Ela, Truti, Kapita; **English**—Cardamom; **Bengali**—Chota Elachi; **Hindi**—Chhoti Elachi.

Biological source: It is obtained from dried ripe seeds and fruits of *Elettaria cardamomum* belonging to Family. Zingiberaceae.

Habitat: Southern India.

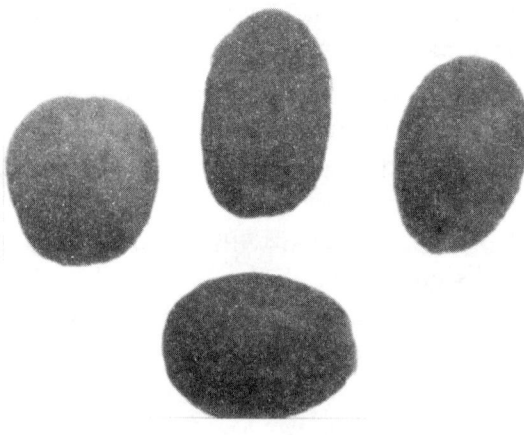

Fig. 5.3.1: Nutmeg
(*see also in colour Plate 4*)

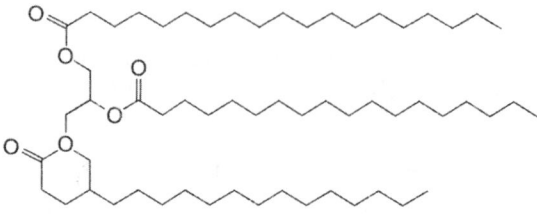

Fig. 5.3.2: Stearin

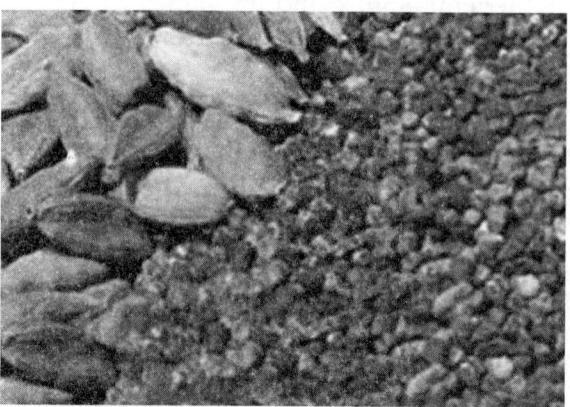

Fig. 5.3.3: Cardamom fruits and seeds
(*see also in colour Plate 5*)

Botany

- Kingdom   Plantae
- Order   Zingiberales
- Family   Zingiberaceae
- Genus   *Elettaria*
- Species   *cardamomum*

Parts used: Dried ripe seeds, oil from fruits.

Organoleptic characters: Organoleptic characters of cardamoms are given in Table 3.5.4.

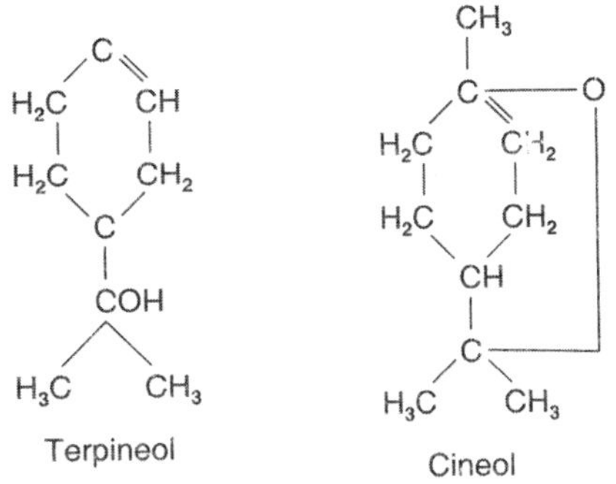

Fig. 5.3.4: Chemical constituents of cordamom

Table 5.3.4: Organoleptic characters of cardamom

Macroscopic characters	Cardamom seeds	Cardamom fruits
Color	Dark reddish brown	Pale buff
Odor	Characteristic	Characteristic
Taste	Strongly aromatic	Strongly aromatic
Shape	Irregularly angular	Ovoid and oblong
Size	Up to 4 mm	1 to 2 cm long

Extra features: Seeds: The seeds consist of Periderm: Large and it contains starch; Endosperm: Small translucent contains aleurone grains and Embryo: Small and contains aleurone grain.

Fruits: Fruit consists of apex which is beaked and rounded base with stalk.

Chemical constituents (Fig. 5.3.4): The seeds contain volatile oil, fixed oil, salt of potassium, a coloring principle, starch, nitrogenous mucilage, ligneous fiber, an acrid resin, and ash. The volatile oil contains terpenes, terpineol and cineol. It is colorless when fresh, but becomes thicker, more yellow, and less aromatic. It is very soluble in alcohol and readily soluble in four volumes of 70%. alcohol, forming a clear solution.

Chemical Test

- Thin section of drug is treated with sudan red III solution, red-colored globules are seen under microscope.
- Thin section of drug is treated with a few drops of tincture alkana, red color is seen.

Standards

Acid value: 1 to 4

Ester value: 90 to 150

Refractive index: 1.4620 to 1.4675

Specific gravity: 0.923 to 0.945

Optical rotation: 24° to 48°

Uses: Carminative, stimulant, aromatic, but rarely used alone; chiefly useful as an adjuvant or corrective. The seeds are helpful in indigestion and flatulence, giving a grateful but not fiery warmth. It is good for colic and disorders of the head.

Adulterants: Long wild native cardamom, Korarima cardamom.

Dill (Fig. 5.3.5)

Synonyms: Sanskrit—Misroya, Sthatapusphi; **English**—Dill, dill seed **Hindi**—Sowa; **Punjabi**—Soya; **Tamil**—Shatakupivirai.

Biological source: It consists of dried ripe fruits of *Peucedanum graveolens* belonging to family Compositae.

Habitat: Dill is a hardy annual, a native of the Mediterranean region and southern Russia. It grows wild among the corn in Spain and Portugal and upon the coast of Italy, but rarely occurs as a cornfield weed in northern Europe.

Botany

- Kingdom   Plantae
- Order   Apiales
- Family   Umbelliferae
- Genus   *Peucedanum*
- Species   *graveolens*

Part used: Dried ripe fruit

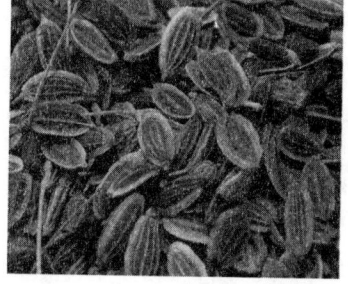

Fig. 5.3.5: Dill
(see also in colour Plate 5)

Organoleptic Characters

Color: Chocolate brown
Odor: Aromatic and spicy
Taste: Aromatic and spicy
Extra features: Dorsally compressed, mericarps are separated.

Microscopy of Dill Fruit

Epicarp: The epicarp is composed of a layer of colorless cells with uniform, well-marked cuticular striations.

Vittae: The brown fragments of the vittae, which are composed of thin-walled polygonal cells.

Mesocarp: The sclereids of the mesocarp occur in groups are composed of fairly thick-walled cells, square to rectangular. The occasional groups of reticulate parenchyma of the mesocarp are composed of elongated cells with fairly thick, lignified walls traversed by numerous conspicuous, rounded to oval pits. The innermost layer of the mesocarp is composed of yellowish-brown cells with thick walls which are usually lignified and have few indistinct pits.

Endocarp: The endocarp is composed of a layer of thin-walled lignified cells which are elongated and arranged in groups with the long axes of the adjacent groups approximately parallel to one another.

Testa: The testa is composed of a single layer of small, brown, thin-walled cells, polygonal.

Endosperm: The abundant endosperm is composed of thick-walled cells containing aleurone grains and microrosette crystals of calcium oxalate.

Fibrovascular bundle: The fragments of lignified fibrovascular tissue are composed of small groups of fibers and vessels showing spiral and annular thickening (Fig. 5.3.7).

Chemical constituents (Fig. 5.3.6): The fruit yields about 3.5% of the oil, which is a mixture of a paraffin hydrocarbon and 40 to 60% of d-carvone, with d-limonene.

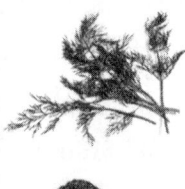

Fig. 5.3.6: Chemical constituents of dill

Staining Reagents

Phloroglucinol: HCl- 1:1 (lignified tissues are seen red/pink).

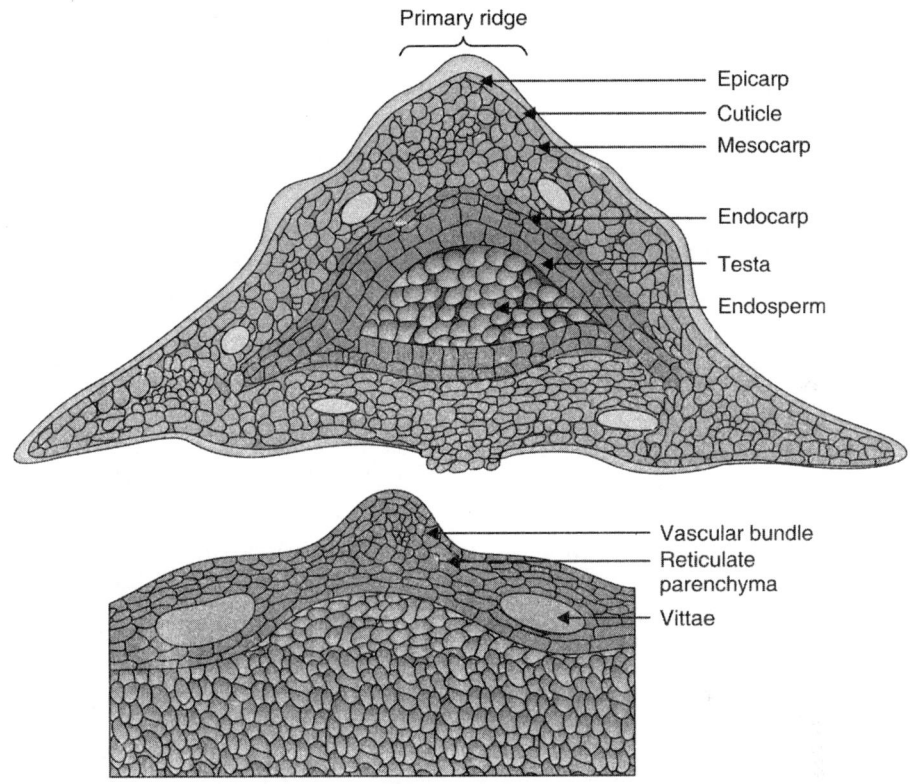

Fig. 5.3.7: Transverse section of dill plant

Alcoholic picric acid: Aleurone grain (yellow) Sudan red III- Cutin/cuticle (pink).

Chemical Test

Test for volatile oil: Soluble in 90% alcohol, filter paper is not permanently stained.
Uses: Dill possesses stimulant, aromatic, carminative and stomachic properties, making them of considerable medicinal value.
Substitutes: Indian dill (*Anethum sowa*, umbelliferae); cumin fruits (*Cuminum cyminum*, Umbelliferae).

Fennel (Fig. 5.3.8)

Synonyms: Sanskrit—Madhurika, Methica; **English**—Indian sweet fennel; **Hindi**—Badi or Bari Saunf; **Bengali**—Panmouri, Methi.

Biological source: It consists of dried ripe fruits of *Foeniculum vulgare*. It contains NLT 1.4% of volatile oil, family Umbelliferae.
Habitat: It grows wild in most parts of temperate Europe, but is generally considered indigenous to the shores of the Mediterranean, whence it spreads eastwards to India.

Botany

- Kingdom   Plantae
- Order   Apiales
- Family   Apiaceae
- Genus   *Foeniculum*
- Species   *vulgare*

Parts used: Seeds, leaves and roots.

Organoleptic Characters

Color: Greenish or yellowish brown

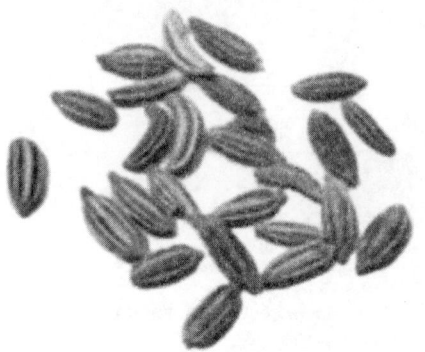

Fig.5.3.8: Fennel
(*see also in colour Plate 5*)

Odor: Sweet, aromatic and characteristic

Taste: Sweet, mucilaginous, aromatic and characteristic

Extra features: Fennel exhibits cremocarp. It consists of equal portions called as mericarps, connected by central stalks called as carpophore.

Microscopy of Fennel (Fig. 5.3.9)

Epicarp: The epicarp is composed of a layer of colorless, thin-walled cells, polygonal in surface view with a smooth cuticle. Stomata are found on some of the fragments but generally are not numerous.

Mesocarp: The innermost layer of the mesocarp, which is composed of slightly thick-walled cells, rounded to rectangular.

Vittae: The numerous brown fragments of the vittae are composed of thin-walled cells, polygonal in surface view.

Reticulate parenchyma: The reticulate parenchyma of the mesocarp is composed of ovoid or elongated, sub-rectangular cells. The walls are thickened and lignified and have conspicuous oval or rounded pits.

Endocarp: The endocarp is composed of a layer of thin-walled, lignified cells, elongated and arranged in groups of about six or more cells with their long axes parallel to one another.

Endosperm: The abundant endosperm is composed of moderately thick-walled cells containing aleurone grains and microrosette crystals of calcium oxalate.

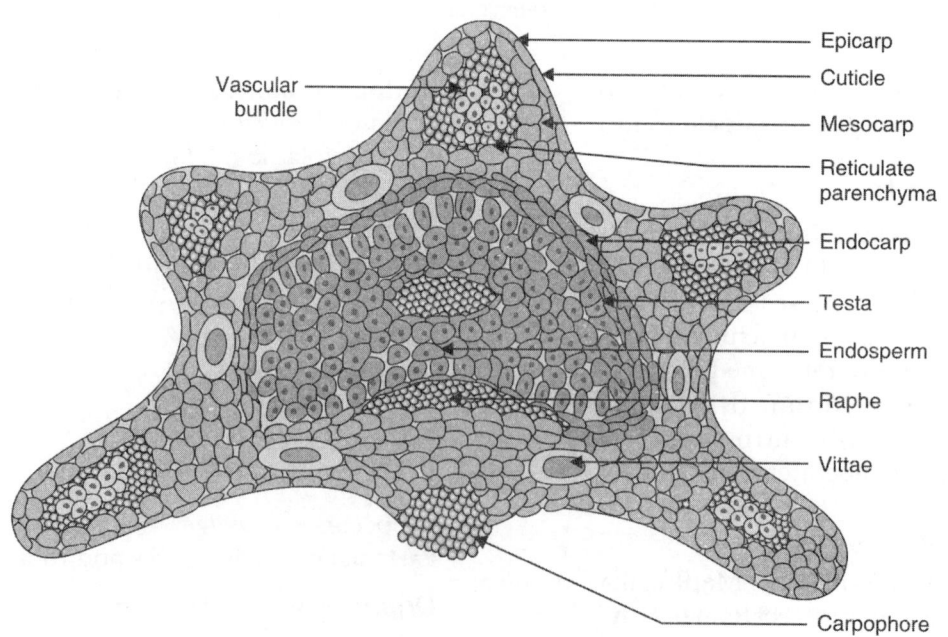

Fig. 5.3.9: Transverse section of fennel

Fibrovascular tissue: The are fragments of lignified fibrovascular tissue composed of small fibers, vessels and tracheids, and occasional larger vessels with reticulate thickening.

Staining Reagents

Phloroglucinol: HCl-1:1 (Lignified tissues are seen red/pink)
Alcoholic picric acid: Aleurone grain (yellow)
Sudan red III: Cutin/cuticles are seen pink.
Chemical constituent (Fig. 5.3.10): Volatile oil (4 to 6%), anethol (50 to 60% of volatile oil), d-fenchone (10% of volatile oil), fixed oil (12 to 18%), proteins (14 to 22%).

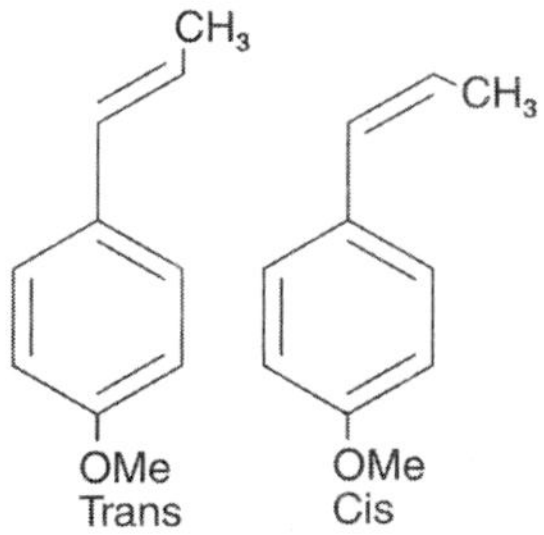

Fig. 5.3.10: Anethol

Chemical test: Test for volatile oil: Soluble in 90% alcohol, filter paper is not permanently stained.

Uses: Carminative, respiratory stimulant.

Adulterants: Exhausted fruit.

Caraway (Fig. 5.3.11)

Synonyms: Sanskrit—Ajaji, Jeeraka; **English**—Cumin seed, caraway seed; **Hindi**—Safed jeera, zira; **Gujrati**—Safed Jiraun.

Biological source: Caraway consists of dried ripe fruits of *Carm Carvi Linn* belonging to family umbelliferae.

Habitat: It is cultivated in central Asia, Europe and India especially north Himalayan region (Kashmir and Chamba).

Botany

- Kingdom   Plantae
- Order   Apiales
- Family   Apiaceae
- Genus   *Carum*
- Species   *carvi*

Part used: Fruit

Organoleptic Characters

Color: Brown

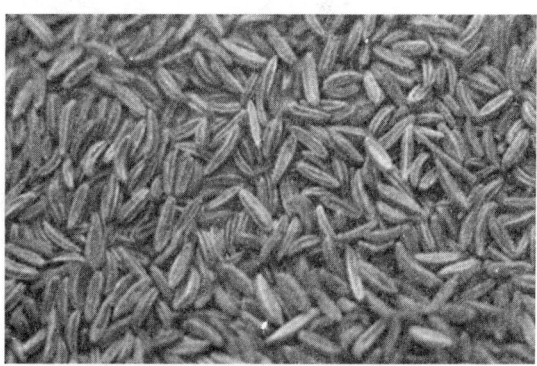

Fig.5.3.11: Caraway
(*see also in colour Plate 5*)

Odor: Characteristic and aromatic
Taste: Hot, spicy and characteristic.

Microscopy of Caraway (Fig. 5.3.12)

Epicarp: The epicarp is composed of colorless cells with a striated cuticle, stomata are fairly numerous and are parallel to those of the cells of the epicarp.

Vittae: The brown fragments of vittae are composed of thin-walled polygonal cells.

Mesocarp: The sclereids of the mesocarp are usually in a single layer with unlignified, thin-walled parenchymatous cells.

Endocarp: This layer is usually found adherent to fragments of the testa. The endocarp is composed of large cells with thin, slightly lignified walls. They appear rounded or radially elongated.

Testa: It is composed of a single layer of brown, thin-walled cells, polygonal, which is adherent to the endocarp.

Endosperm: The abundant endosperm containing aleurone grains and microrosette crystals of calcium oxalate.

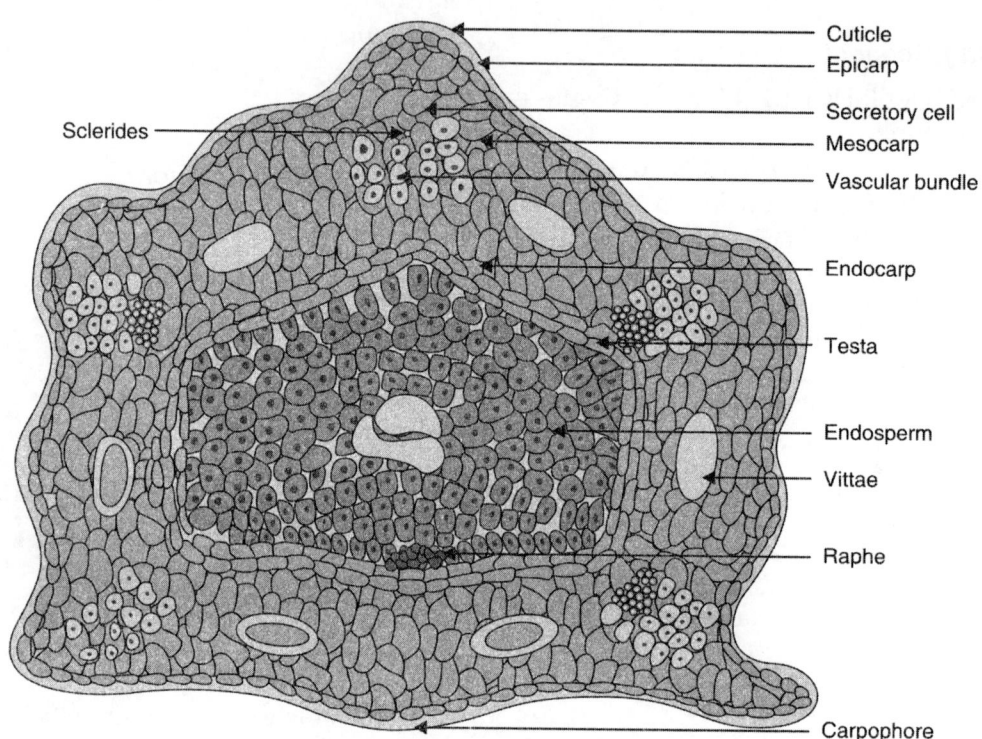

Fig. 5.3.12: Transverse section of caraway

Staining Reagents

Phloroglucinol: HCl- 1:1 (Lignified tissues are seen red/pink).
Alcholic picric acid: Aleurone grain (yellow).
Sudan red III: Cuticle are seen pink.

Chemical constituents (Fig. 5.3.13): It consists of volatile oil: Carvone, carveol, dihydrocarvone, limonene. It also contains protein, fat, fiber, carbohydrates, calcium, phosphorous, sodium, potassium, vitamins B_1, B_2, C, A.

Uses: Both fruit and oil possess aromatic, stimulant and carminative properties and used as spice for culinary purposes.

Adulterants: Exhausted fruit, caraway stalks, cummin fruits.

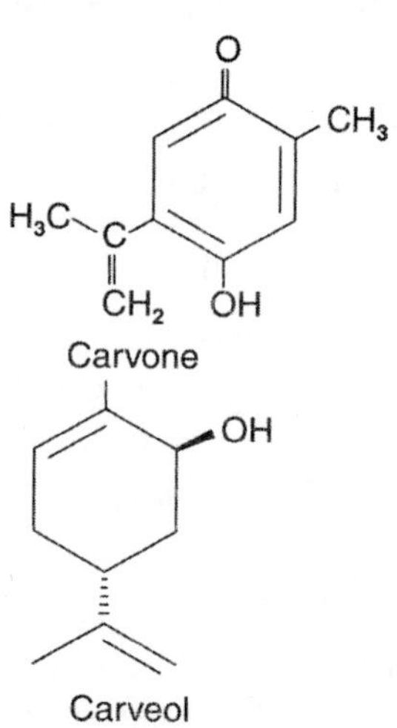

Fig. 5.3.13: Chemical constituents of caraway

Coriander Fruit (Fig. 5.3.14)

Synonyms: Sanskrit—Kustumbari, Dhanyaka; **English**—Coriander; **Hindi**—Kottmir, Dhania; **Bengali**—Dhane.

Biological source: It consists of dried ripe fruits of *Coriandrum sativum* belonging to family Umbelliferae. It should contain NLT 0.3% of volatile oil.

Habitat: Coriander, an umbelliferous plant indigenous to southern Europe, is found occasionally in Britain in fields and waste places, and by the sides of rivers. It is frequently found in a semi-wild state in the east of England.

Botany

- Kingdom   Plantae
- Order   Apiales
- Family   Apiaceae
- Genus   *Coriandrum*
- Species   *sativum*

Parts used: Fruits and leaves

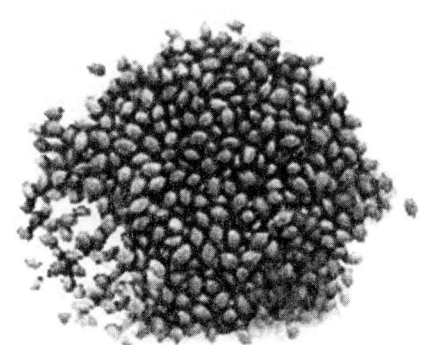

Fig. 5.3.14: Coriander
(*see also in colour Plate 5*)

Organoleptic Characters

Color: Brownish yellow
Odor: Aromatic
Taste: Spicy and characteristic

Extra features: The fruits (so-called seeds) are of globular form, beaked, finely ribbed, 1/5 inch in diameter, with five longitudinal ridges, separable into two halves (the mericarps), each of which is concave internally and shows two broad, longitudinal oil cells (vittae). The seeds have an aromatic taste and, when crushed, a characteristic odor.

Microscopy of Coriander (Fig. 5.3.15)

Epicarp: It is composed of a layer of polygonal, colorless, thin-walled cells, with a smooth cuticle. Most of the cells contain small prisms of calcium oxalate.

Mesocarp: The sclerenchyma of the mesocarp consist of two types of cell masses of very thick-walled, sinuous, fusiform cells with a narrow lumen and two or three layers of large, rectangular or polygonal cells with only slightly thickened walls.

Endocarp: The endocarp is composed of a layer of thin-walled, lignified cells, elongated. It is usually found adherent to the rectangular sclereids of the mesocarp.

Vittae: The brown fragments of the vittae composed of thin-walled cells, polygonal.

Testa: It is a single layer of brown, very thin-walled polygonal cells.

Endosperm: The endosperm is composed of thick-walled cells containing microrosette crystals of calcium oxalate and aleurone grains.

Staining Reagents

Phloroglucinol: HCl-1:1 (Lignified tissues are seen red/pink).

Alcoholic picric acid: Aleurone grain (yellow).
Sudan red III: Cuticles are seen pink.

Chemical constituents: Coriander fruit contains about 1% of volatile oil. It also contains coriandrol (d-Linalool—60–70%; Fig. 5.3.15), terpenes (20%), fixed oil (13 to 20%)

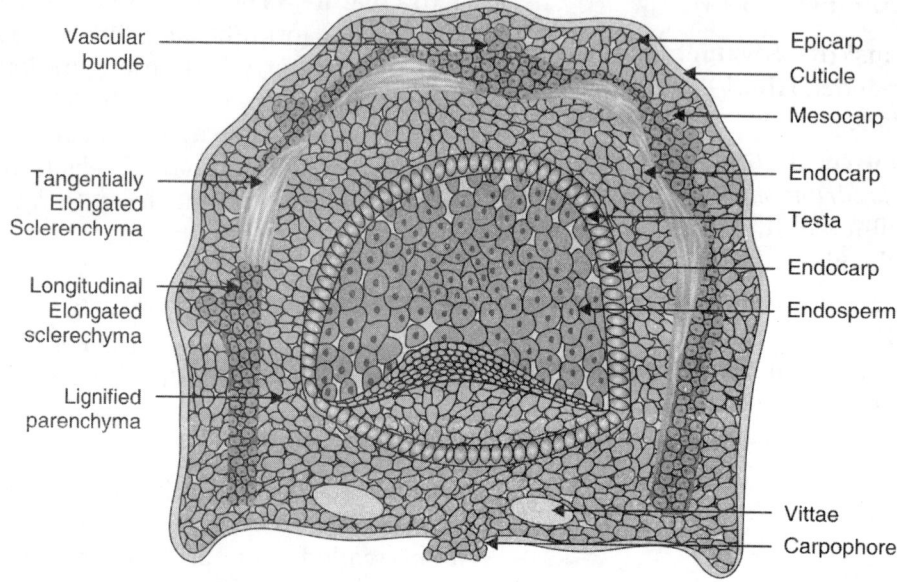

Fig. 5.3.15: Transverse section of coriander

and proteins (17%). The fruit yields about 5% of ash and contains also malic acid, tannin and some fatty matter.

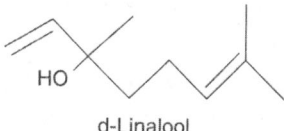

Fig. 5.3.16: d-Linalool

Uses: Stimulant, aromatic and carminative
Adulterants: Bombay coriander (less volatile oil, bigger and ellipsoidal in shape).

Cinnamon Bark

Synonyms: Sanskrit (Fig. 5.3.17): Gudatvak, Varangam; **English**—Cinnamon; **Telgu and Tamil**—Lowangapatta; **Bombay**—Dalchini, Taj.

Biological source: It consists of dried bark of *Cinnamomum zeylanicum,* belonging to family Lauraceae.

Habitat: Ceylon, but grows plentifully in Malabar, Cochin-China, Sumatra and eastern Islands. It has also been cultivated in the Brazils, Mauritius, India, Jamaica, etc.

Botany
- Kingdom   Plantae
- Division   Magnoliophyta
- Class   Magnoliopsida
- Order   Laurales
- Family   Lauraceae
- Genus   *Cinnamomum*
- Species   *verum*

Part used: Bark

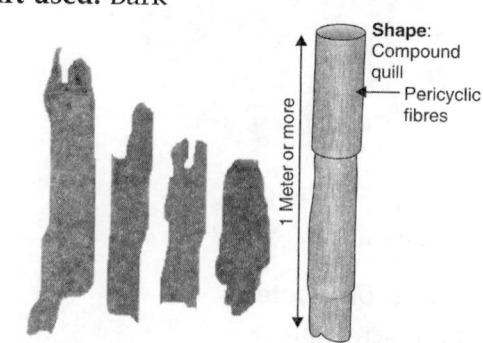

Fig. 5.3.17: Cinnamon bark (*see also in colour Plate 5*)

Organoleptic Characters

Color: Outer surface: Dull yellowish brown; Inner surface: Darker in color.

Odor: Fragrant

Taste: Warm, sweet and aromatic.

Extra Features: Fracture: Splintery.

Microscopy of Cinnamon Bark
(Figs 5.3.18 and 5.3.19)

Cork: It is very occasional fragments of cork.

Sclereids: They occur singly or in small groups but are usually more or less isodiametric, the walls of most of the cells are moderately thickened and occasional cells have very thick walls with a small lumen and striations are visible.

Fibers: The fibers are single, thick-walled and lignified with a small, uneven lumen. Some fibers are found with the sclereids of the pericycle, oil cells and parenchyma of the phloem.

Starch granules: The starch granules are small, simple or compound with up to four or more components are found scattered in the parenchymatous tissues and in the sclereids. Hilum (rounded or slit-shaped) is visible in some of the larger granules.

Oil cells: The thin-walled oil cells, frequently found associated with the parenchyma or fibers of the phloem; the cells are large, ovoid, and usually occur singly.

Parenchyma: The thin-walled parenchyma and medullary rays of the phloem contain numerous small, acicular crystals of calcium oxalate.

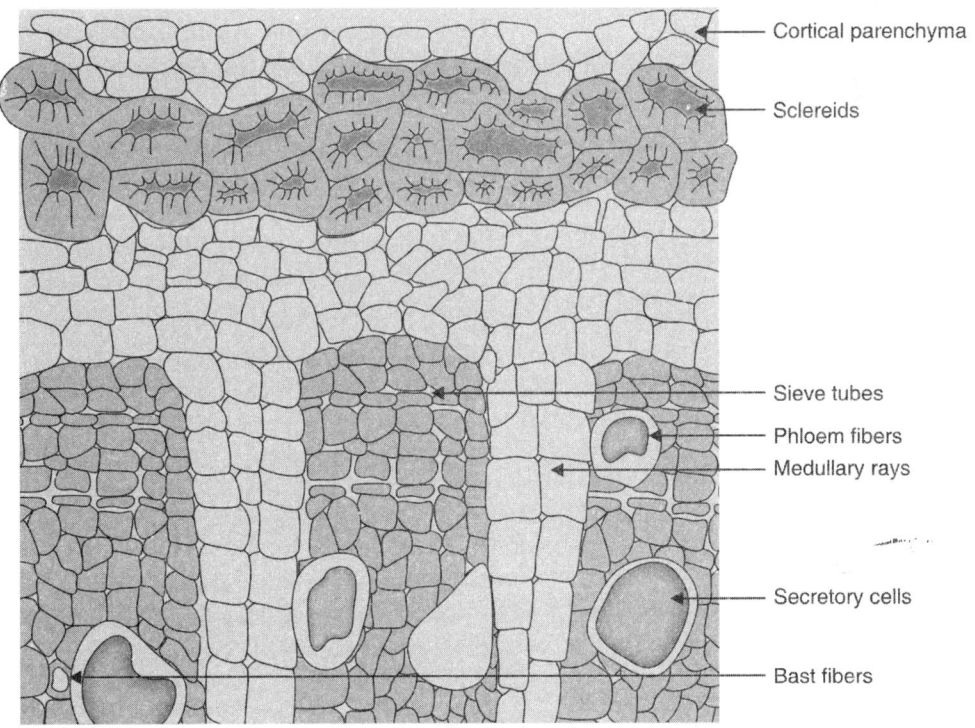

Fig. 5.3.18: Transverse section of cinnamon

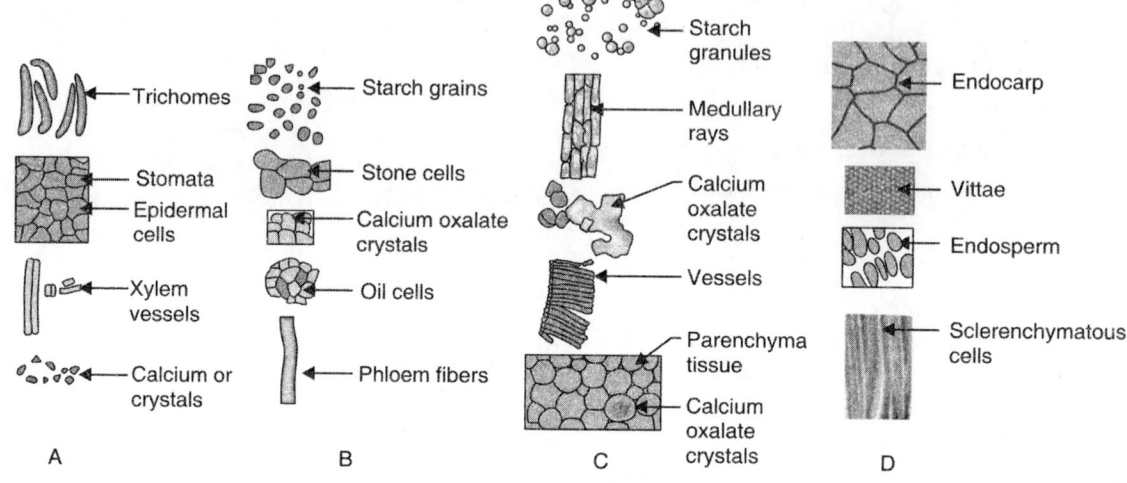

Fig. 5.3.19: Microscopy of powdered cinnamon

Staining Reagents

Phloroglucinol: HCl-1:1 (Lignified tissues are seen red/pink).

Iodine solution: Starch (blue).

Ruthenium red: Pink (mucilage cells)

Tincture of alkana: Volatile oil (red on standing)

Chemical constituents: 0 to 10% of volatile oil, cinnamic aldehyde (Fig. 5.3.20) (55 to 65%), eugenol (4 to 10%), terpenes, mucilage, starch, calcium oxalate, tannin, mucilage and sugar.

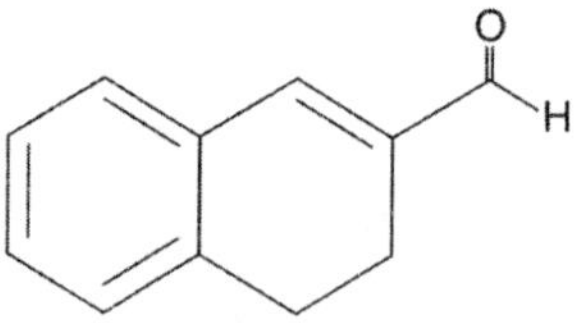

Fig. 5.3.20: Cinnamic aldehyde

Chemical Test

Test for volatile oil: Chloroform extract of volatile oil on slide treated with 10% aqueous phenyl hydrazine hydrochloride solution, rod-shaped crystals of cinnamic aldehyde are seen.

Test for tannins: Aqueous extract treated with ferric chloride, dark color indicates presence of tannins.

Uses: Carminative, astringent, stimulant, antiseptic; more powerful as a local than as a general stimulant. It stops vomiting, relieves flatulence, and given with chalk and astringents, is useful for diarrhea and hemorrhage of the womb.

Adulterants: Cassia bark, Chinese cinnamon.

Clove (Fig. 5.3.21)

Synonyms: English: Caryophyllum, clove flower and clove buds.

Biological source: It consists of dried flower buds of *Eugenia caryophyllus* belonging to family Myrtaceae. It contains NLT 15% v/w of clove oil.

Habitat: Molucca Islands, southern Philippines.

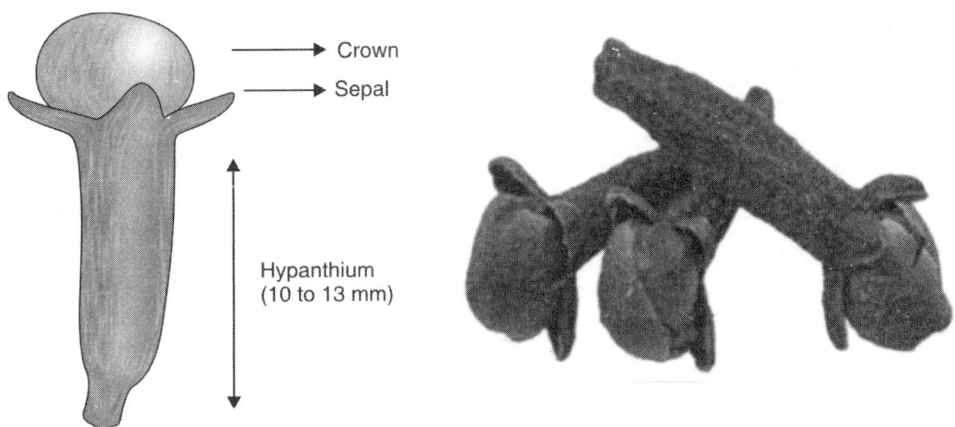

Fig. 5.3.21: Clove bud
(*see also in colour Plate 6*)

Botany

- Kingdom   Plantae
- Order   Myrtales
- Family   Myrtaceae
- Genus   *Syzygium*
- Species   *aromaticum*

Part used: Undeveloped flowers.

Organoleptic Characters

Color: Dark brown or crimson color

Odor: Aromatic

Taste: Spicy

Microscopy of Clove (Fig. 5.3.22)

Epidermis: The epidermis is composed of small, polygonal cells with slightly thickened walls; large, almost circular anomocytic stomata, the underlying tissue contains very large, brown, ovoid oil glands and occasional cluster crystals of calcium oxalate.

Parenchyma: The very abundant yellowish-brown parenchyma of the hypanthium in which the oil glands are embedded; the cells are frequently unevenly thickened and appear collenchymatous.

Calcium oxalate: The cluster crystals of calcium oxalate in the parenchymatous tissue but are rarely found scattered; they vary in size and are usually composed of a large number of small, sharply pointed components.

Fibers: The occasional fibers, are found singly or in groups of two or three cells; they are rather short and broad with bluntly pointed ends. The walls are lignified, usually strongly thickened.

Anther: The fragments of the fibrous layer of the anther are composed of rather small cells; in sectional view, the lignified thickening on the side walls of the cells appears as closely packed longitudinal bands and these are seen as small beads in surface view.

Pollen grains: The abundant pollen grains are small, biconvex with a rounded, triangular outline. A number of immature pollen grains also occur and these may be found in closely packed masses, frequently enclosed in the pollen sacs.

Aerenchyma: The occasional fragments of the aerenchyma of the hypanthium are composed of chains of two or three parenchymatous cells with moderately thickened walls; the contiguous walls of adjacent cells are traversed by numerous very small pits.

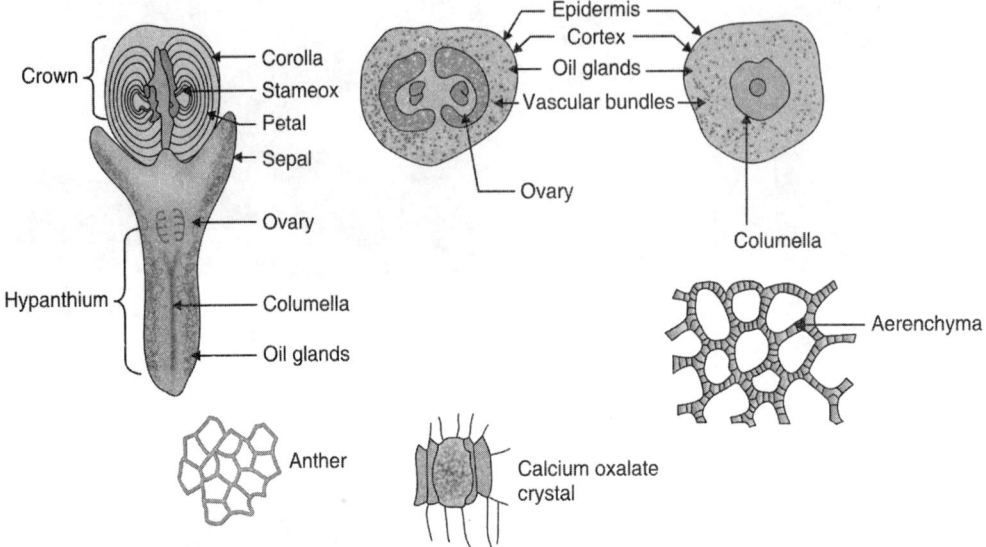

Fig.5.3.22: Transverse section of clove bud

Sclereids: The very occasional sclereids from the stalk; they are oval to subrectangular in outline with strongly thickened and striated walls which have numerous simple or branched pits; the lumen is frequently filled with brown contents.

Staining Reagents

Phloroglucinol: HCl- 1:1 (Lignified tissues are seen red/pink).
Sudan red III: Cuticles are seen pink.
Strong KOH: Needle-shaped potassium eugenate crystals (eugenol).

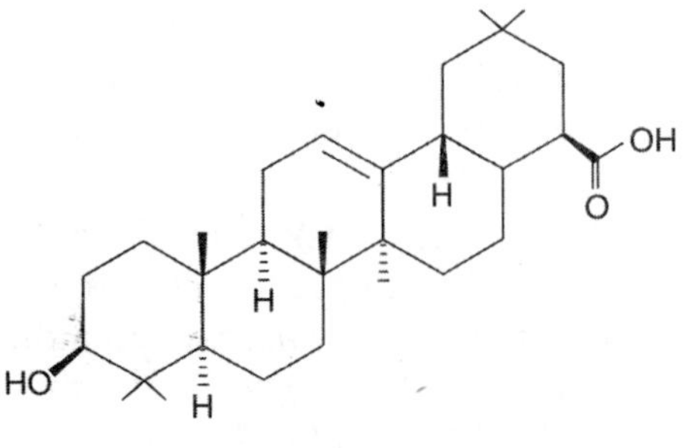

Fig. 5.3.23: Caryophyllin

Chemical constituents: Volatile oil, gallotannic acid, two crystalline principles caryophyllin (Fig. 5.3.23), which is odorless and appears to be a phylosterol, eugenin, gum, resin, fiber.

Chemical Test

Test for eugenol: Clove oil treated with alcohol and ferric chloride (5%) gives blue coloration.

Test for tannins: Aqueous extract treated with lead acetate solution gives white precipitate.

Uses: Stimulating and carminative given in powder or infusion for nausea emesis, flatulence, dental analgesic, flavouring agents, an anomatic antiseptic.

Adulterants: Exhausted cloves, mother cloves and clove stalks.

Ginger (Fig. 5.3.24)

Synonyms: Hindi—Sonth; **English**—Zingiber, rhizome zingiberis, Jamica ginger.

Biological source: It consists of rhizome of *Zingiber officinalis* Roscoe, family Zingiberaceae. Scrapped to remove outer skin and dried in the sun.

Habitat: Native to southeast Asia, cultivated mainly in Kerala, Andhra Pradesh, Uttar Pradesh, West Bengal, Maharashtra.

Botany

- Kingdom   Plantae
- Division   Angiosperma
- Class   Monocotyledoneae
- Order   Scitaminaea
- Family   Zingiberaceae
- Genus   *Zingiber*
- Species   *officinale*

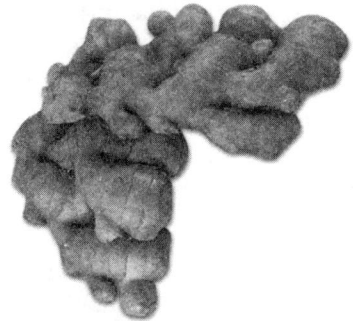

Fig. 5.3.24: Ginger
(*see also in colour Plate 6*)

Organoleptic Characters

Color: Externally, buff colored
Odor: Agreeable and aromatic
Taste: Agreeble, pungent and characteristic
Size: 3 to 6 cm
Shape: Irregular
Fracture: Short and fibrous
Extra features: Sympodial branching, horizontal rhizome, transversely cut surface shows well-marked endodermis and stele.

Chemical constituents (Fig. 5.3.25): Ginger contains usually 1–3% of volatile oil, pungent principles, viz. gingerols and shogaols and about 6–8 lipids and others. Ginger oil contains zingiberene and bisaboline as major constituents along with other sesqui and monoterpenes. Shogaols have been found to be twice as pungent as gingerols.

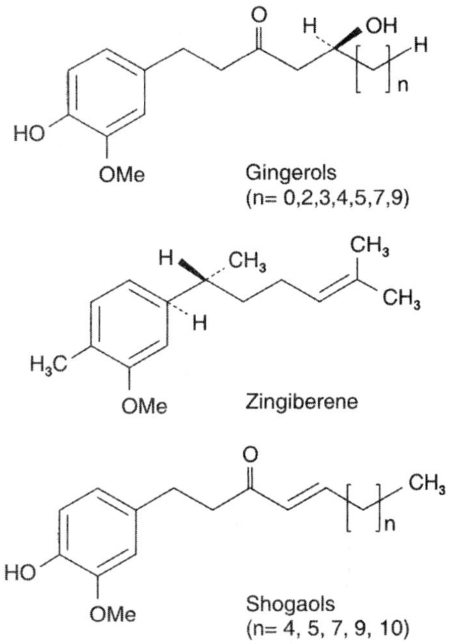

Gingerols (n= 0,2,3,4,5,7,9)

Zingiberene

Shogaols (n= 4, 5, 7, 9, 10)

Fig. 5.3.25: Chemical constituents of Ginger

Standards

- Foreign matter: NMT 1.0%
- Total ash: NMT 8.0%
- Acid insoluble ash: NMT 1.0%
- Moisture content: NLT 12.0%
- Alcohol-soluble extractive: NLT 7.0%
- Water-soluble extractive: NLT 14.0%
- Petroleum ether extractive: 1.5–2.5%
- Chloroform extractive: 3–5%
- Methanol extractive: 2–4%

Microscopy of the Ginger Rhizome
(Fig. 5.3.26)

Outer and inner cork: Few layers with irregularly arranged parenchymatous cells. The outer cork cells are dark-colored brown whereas inner cells are colorless.

Cortex with parenchymatous cells: The cortex is isodiametric with thin-walled parenchymatous cells.

Fibrovascular bundles: Collateral, conjoint and closed in nature.

Xylem vessels: The xylem vessel gives no reaction for lignin and they have reticulate or spiral thickening, and are often accompanied by narrow, thin-walled cells containing dark brown pigment; a few smaller, spirally or annularly thickened vessels also occur.

Fiber: Lignified, pitted and septate.

Starch: Starch abundant in the thin-walled ground tissue, as flattened, ovate to subrectangular, transversely striated, simple granules, each with the hilum in a projection towards one end.

Oleoresin cells: Bright yellow to reddish brown ovoid to spherical cells occurring in small groups in the parenchyma or singly.

Pigment and secretion cells: Pigment cells with dark reddish brown contents occurring either singly in the ground tissue or in axial rows accompanying the vascular bundles.

Sclereids and calcium oxalate crystals absent.

Chemical test: The drug is boiled with 50% KOH or alkali. Its pungency is destroyed.

Uses: Ginger is carminative, pungent, stimulant, used widely for indigestion, stomachache, malaria and fevers. It is used for abdominal pain, anorexia, arthritis, atonic dyspepsia, bleeding, cancer, chest congestion, chickenpox, cholera, chronic bronchitis, cold extremities, colic, colitis, common cold, cough, cystic fibrosis, diarrhea, difficulty in breathing, dropsy, fever, flatulent, indigestion, disorders of gallbladder, hyperacidity, hypercholesterolemia, hyperglycemia, indigestion, morning sickness, nausea, rheumatism, sore throat, throat ache, stomach ache and vomiting.

Adulterants: Spent or exhausted ginger, wormy ginger, unscraped ginger and capsicum powder.

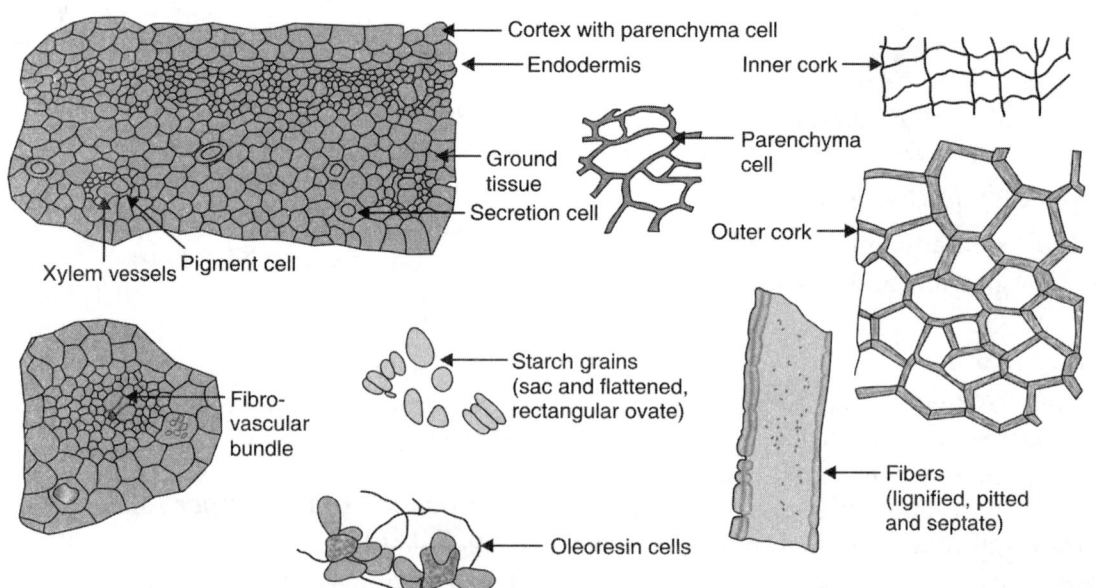

Fig. 5.3.26: Microscopic features of ginger rhizome

Turmeric (Fig. 5.3.27)

Synonyms: Curcuma, turmeric.

Biological source: It is obtained from rhizome of *Curcuma longa*, be longing to family Zingiberaceae.

Habitat: Cultivated extensively in India within tropical climate.

Botany

- Kingdom   Plantae
- Division   Magnoliophyta
- Class   Liliopsida
- Order   Zingiberales

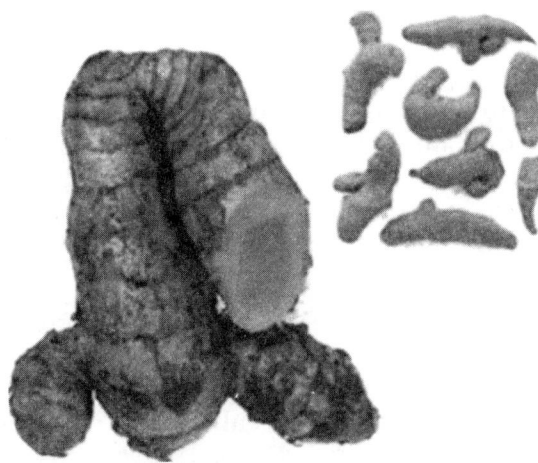

Fig. 5.3.27: Turmeric
(*see also in colour Plate 6*)

- Family   Zingiberaceae
- Genus   *Curcuma*
- Species   *longa*

Organoleptic Characters

Color: Yellowish brown
Odor: Characteristics
Taste: Slightly bitter
Shape: Oblong
Fracture: Horny

Extra features: Root scars and annulations are present.

Chemical constituents (Fig. 5.3.28): The active constituents of turmeric are the flavonoid curcumin and volatile oils including tumerone, atlantone, and zingiberone. Other constituents include sugars, proteins, and resins. The active constituent is curcumin, which comprises 0.3 to 5.4% of raw turmeric. It also consists of 1,8-cineole, 2-bornanol, 2-hydroxy-methyl-anthraquinone, 4-hydroxy-cinnamoyl-(Feruloyl)-methane, curcumene, curcumenol, curcumin, curdione, curlone and curzerenone.

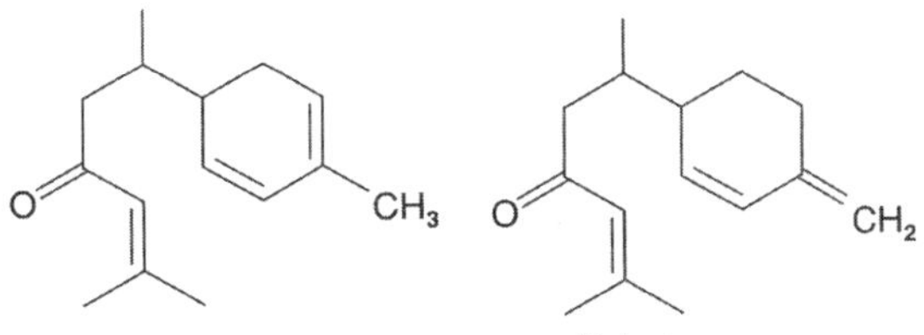

Alpha-turmerone   Beta-turmerone

Fig. 5.3.28: Chemical constituents of turmeric

Microscopy of Turmeric Rhizome
(Fig. 5.3.29)

Cork cells: The outer most surface consists of cork cells.

Parenchyma cells: Parenchyma cells are filled with gelatinized starch and yellow coloring matter.

Epidermis: Epidermis present on surface, it shows the presence of stoma and cicatrix.

Covering trichomes: It is present in turmeric.

Starch granules are also present.

Vessels: Spirally and reticulately thickened vessels.

Chemical Test

- Turmeric powder with sulphuric acid gives crimson color.
- Turmeric powder when treated with acetic anhydride and concentrated sulfuric acid,

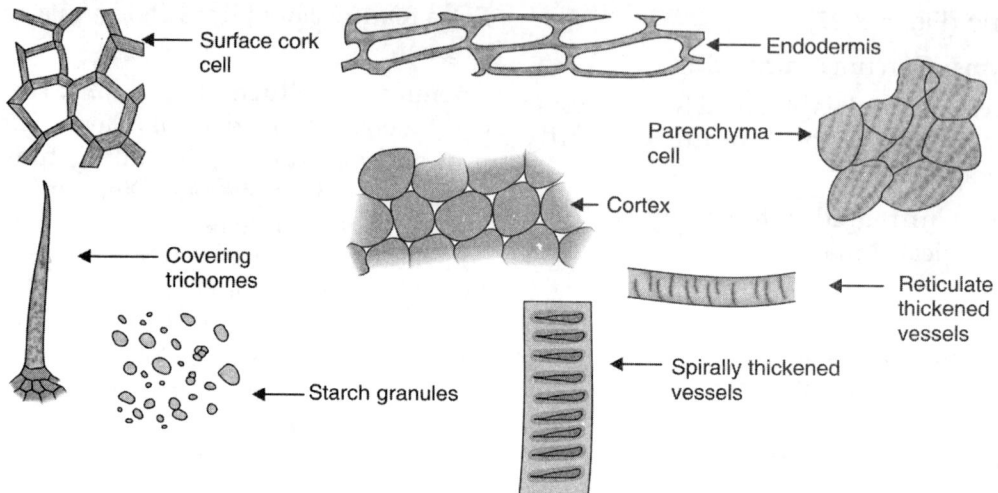

Fig. 5.3.29: Microscopic features of turmeric rhizome

it gives violet color (visible), red fluorescence (UV).

- Aqueous solution of turmeric powder with boric acid gives reddish brown color which turns to greenish blue on addition of alkali.

Uses: Used as a codimentor spice anti-inflammatory, antioxidant, anti-mutagenic, anti-cancerous, cholagogueue, depurative, diuretic, fumitory, hemostatic, hepatoprotective, lactagogue, stomachic, tonic, and vulnerary.

Substituents: C. aromatica, C.amada, C. zeodaria, C. xanthorrhiza.

Adulterants: Metanil yellow coloring.

When concentrated hydrochloric acid is added to a solution of turmeric powder, it turns magenta if metanil yellow is present.

5.4 ALKALOIDS

Definition

The term alkaloids or alkali was proposed by the pharmacist W. Meissner in 1819 for the basic nitrogen containing compounds or plants. The basic properties of alkaloids are due to the presence of nitrogen atom inside the ring. So the alkaloids are now generally defined as physiologically active basic compounds of plant origin, in which at least one nitrogen atom forms part of cyclic system.

The definition is not fully satisfactory because some compounds although alkaloids do not confine to the definition. While other compounds although not alkaloids confine to the definition.

Example: Adrenaline and ephedrine have nitrogen atom in the side chain, while thiamin (a vitamin) and purines are heterocyclic physiologically active nitrogenous bases but not regarded as alkaloids.

According to Landenberg "Alkaloids are defined as natural plant compounds that have a basic character and contain at least one nitrogen atom in a heterocyclic ring and having biological activities."

According to characteristic features, alkaloids are basic nitrogenous plant origin, mostly optically active and possessing nitrogen heterocycles as their structural units with physiological action. This definition not fully correct because not follow on all alkaloids, for example,

Colchicine: Colchicine is regarded as an alkaloid although it is not heterocyclic and is scarcely basic.

Thiamin: It is heterocyclic nitrogenous base but not as a alkaloid because it is universally distributed in living matter.

Nitrogen as side chain: Some compounds are classed as in alkaloids but they do not contain nitrogen in heterocyclic ring, but contain nitrogen inside chain, e.g. ephedrine, hordenine, betanine, choline, muscarine, strychnine and tryptamine, etc.

Naturally occurring open chain basic compounds: These compounds have physiological activity but do not class in alkaloids, e.g. cholines, amino acid, phenylethylamines, etc.

Piperine: It is neither basic character nor possessing any physiological activity but includes in alkaloids.

Those compounds, which fully satisfy the definitions, like physiologically active, heterocyclic basic nitrogenous ring, but they do not classed in alkaloids, e.g. thiamine, caffeine, purine, theobromine, and xanthenes.

Occurrence and Distribution (Table 5.4.1)

The number of structurally different alkaloids has been estimated to be 6000. Most of them occur in flora, ~1% in animals, and not more than 0.5% in fungi and bacteria. Most of alkaloids occur in plants but they do occur in animals, insects, marine organisms, microorganisms and lower plants, e.g. muscopyridine in muscle deer, castoranine in Canadian beaver, pyocyamine in bacteria (*Pseudomonas aeruginosa*), chanoclavin from fungi (Ergot) and lycopodine from the club moss. These alkaloid-containing plants are not statistically distributed over the genera; rather, they occur most abundantly in genera belonging to the dicotyledones and monocotyledones of the angiospermae (flowering plants). Alkaloids may occur in several parts of a plant (e.g. roots, stem, bark, leaves, fruits, seeds). In some cases (e.g. *Papaver somniferum, A. belladonna*), alkaloids are isolated from all parts, whereas in other cases they are found in only one part (e.g. the alkaloid of *Aphelandra squarrosa* is found only in the roots). It should

Table 5.4.1: Occurrence of alkaloids with its family

S.no.	Family	Typical	Typical alkaliods	Parts
1.	Apocynacaeae	Vinca	Vincristin, vinblastin	Leaves
		Rauwolfia	Reserpine	
2.	Liliaceae	Veretrum	Veritrine	Root
3.	Leguminosae	Scoparium	Spentine	Leaves and bark
4.	Loganiaceae	Nux vomica	Brucine, strychinine	Seeds
5.	Papaveraceae	Opium	Morphine, codeine, thiabine	poppy
6.	Solanaceae	Belladonna	Hyoscine	Roots
7.	Rubiaceae	Cinchona	Quinine, quinidine	Bark
8.	Baberidaceae	Berbaris	Berbarine	Fruit, leaves and bark
9.	Claviciptaceae	Ergot	Ergotanine	Fungal sclerotium
			Ergometrine	

be noted that the alkaloid-containing part of the plant may not necessarily be the site of alkaloid formation. The number of structurally different alkaloids varies from plant to plant. For example, *Catharanthus roseus* contains more than 100 alkaloids, whereas only 1 alkaloid has been detected in *A. squarrosa*. Quite often the ratio of the components of an alkaloid mixture is different in different parts of the plant. Other factors that influence the level and diversity of the alkaloid content are the age of the plant (e.g. investigated with *Adhatoda vasica*), the season (e.g. *P. somniferum*), the gathering time during the day (e.g. *Conium maculatum*), and the habitat (e.g. *Maytenus buxifolia*). The total amount of alkaloids in plants fluctuates between ~10% of quinine (*Cinchona* sp.) and ~5×10"6% of triabunnine in *Aristotelia peduncularis*, based on the dried weight of the drug.

Nomenclature

There is no systematic nomenclature. But there are some methods for nomenclature which are mentioned below.

1. **According to their source:** They are named according to the family in which they are found, e.g. papavarine, punarnavin, ephedrin.
2. **According to their physiological response:** They are named according to their physiological response. For example, morphine means God of dreams, emetine means to vomit.
3. **According to their discoverer:** They are named according to their discoverer, e.g. pelletierine group has been named its discoverer, P.J. Pelletier.
4. **Prefixes:** They are named by some prefixes which are fixed in nomenclature of alkaloids, e.g. epi- iso- neo- pseudo- nor-. CH_3 group not attach to nitrogen.

Classification

Alkaloids are classified as:

A. **Taxonomic based:** According to their family, e.g. solanaceous, papilionaceous without reference their chemical type of alkaloids present and another according to genus, e.g. ephedra, cinchona, etc.

B. **Pharmacological based:** Their pharmacological activity or response. For example:
1. Analgesic alkaloids
2. Cardioactive alkaloids, etc.

Do not have chemical similarity in their group.

C. **Bio-synthetic based:** According to this, alkaloids are classified on the basis of the type precursors or building block compounds used by plants to synthesize the complex structure, e.g. morphine, papaverine, narcotine, tubocurarine and colchicine in phenylalanine tyrosin derived base.

D. **Chemical classification:** This classification is universally adopted and depends on the fundamental ring structure. According to these, there are two main groups:

1. **Non-heterocyclic alkaloids:** In this group of alkaloids not has any one heterocyclic ring in their structure, e.g. hordinine (*Hordeum vulgare*), ephedrine (*Ephedra gerardiana*) genateceae.
2. **Heterocyclic alkaloids:** According to heterocyclic ring, the alkaloids are subdivide in following:
   a. **Pyrrole-pyrrolidine:** This type of alkaloids contains pyrole or pyrrolidine ring in their structure, e.g. hygrines, *Coca* sp.
   b. **Pyrrolizidine:** Alkaloids containing pyrrolizidine heterocyclic ring in their structure, e.g. seneciphylline, *Senecio* sp.

c. **Pyridine and piperidine:** Alkaloids containing pyridine heterocyclic ring in their structure, e.g. nicotine, lobaline, piperidine, ricinine.
d. **Piperidine (tropane):** Alkaloids containing tropone ring, e.g. hyoscyamine, atropine, hyoscine-Solanceae–Cocaine–Coca sp.
e. **Quinoline:** Those alkaloids containing quinoline ring in their structure, e.g. quinine, quinidine, (cinchona bark) cinchonine, cinchonidine and cusparin (cusparia bark).
f. **Isoquinoline:** Alkaloids containing isoquinoline ring in their chemical structure, e.g. papavarine, narceine, emetine and cephaline (Cephalis sp Rubiaceae).
g. **Reduced isoquinoline (aporphine):** The alkaloids contain reduced isoquinoline ring in their structure, e.g. Baldine (Peumus baldus) (Manioniaceae).
h. **Nor lupinane:** Alkaloids present in leguminoceae plants, e.g. spartine, lupanine.
i. **Indole alkaloids:** Alkaloids containing indole ring, e.g. yohimbine, aspidospermine (*Apocynaceae*), vinblasine, vincristine (*Catharanthus roseus*).

Properties

1. **Appearance:** Alkaliods are colorless, crystalline solids with a sharp melting point or decomposition range. Alkaloids of higher molecular weight sometimes with additional oxygen functions are usually colorless crystalline compounds, e.g. papaverine (from *Papaver somniferum*).

2. **Nature:** Some alkaloids are gums, while others like coniine, nicotine, etc. are liquid and volatile in nature. Low molecular weight amines, such as coniine (from *Conium maculatum*) and pelletierine (from *Punica granatum*) are colorless liquids. Other examples of liquid alkaloids are the *Nicotiana* alkaloids nicotine (from *N. tabacum*) and actinidine (from *Actinidia polygama*).

3. **Color:** Some alkaloids are colored in nature, e.g. the red-violet cryptolepine (from *Cryptolepis triangularis*). Betanidine is red, berberine is yellow and salts of sanguinarine are copper red in color.

4. **Solubility:** The majority of alkaloids are basic compounds. Whereas an alkaloid is usually soluble only in an organic solvent, such as ether, ethanol, toluene, or chloroform and mostly insoluble in water. Alkaloid salts (e.g. hydrochlorides, quaternary methochlorides) are soluble in water. Solubility in water is important for the therapeutic use of alkaloids.

Exceptions
a. Bases soluble in water: Caffeine, ephedrine, codeine, colchicine, pilocarpine and quaternary ammonium bases.

b. Bases insoluble or sparingly soluble in certain organic solvents: Morphine in ether, theobromine and theophylline in benzene.
c. Salts insoluble in water: Quinine monosulfate.
d. Salts soluble in organic solvents: Lobeline and apoatropine hydrochlorides are soluble in chloroform.

5. **Optical rotation** (Fig. 5.4.1): Most isolated alkaloids are optically active. The plane of polarized light passing through a solution of an optically active compound is rotated either to the left (counterclockwise, levorotatory) or to the right (clockwise, dextrorotatory). The value of deflection is given, for example, as the [α] D value. Optical activity is displayed by any molecule containing a carbon atom with four different sub-stituents (asymmetric carbon atom).

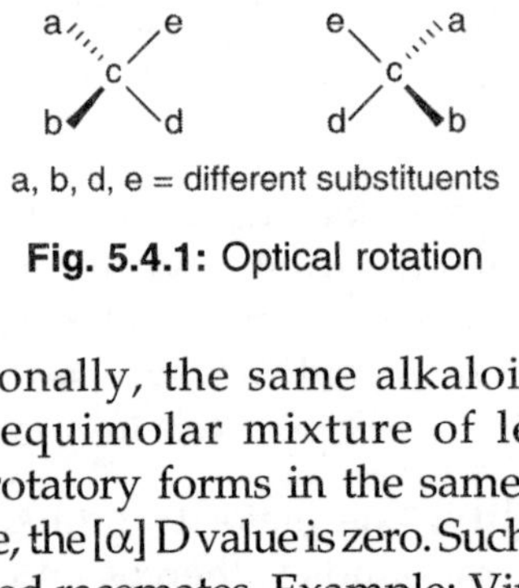

a, b, d, e = different substituents

Fig. 5.4.1: Optical rotation

Occasionally, the same alkaloid occurs as an equimolar mixture of levo- and dextrorotatory forms in the same plant. In this case, the [α] D value is zero. Such mixtures are called racemates. Example: Vincadifformine was isolated from different plants (Fig. 5.4.2).

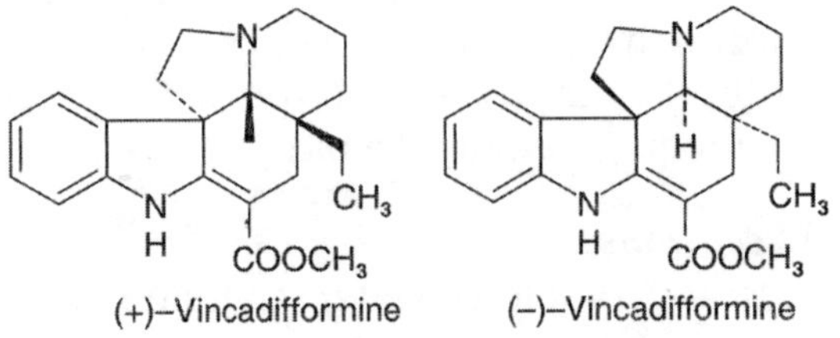

(+)-Vincadifformine   (–)-Vincadifformine

Fig. 5.4.2: Optical rotation of vinca

Optically active isomers may show different physiological activities.
a. *l*-ephedrine is 3.5 times more active than *d*-ephedrine.
b. *l*-ergotamine is 3–4 times more active than *d*-ergotamine.
c. *d*-tubocurarine is more active than the corresponding *l*-form.
d. Quinine (*l*-form) is antimalarial and its *d*-isomer quinidine is antiarhythmic.
e. The **racemic** (optically inactive) *dl*-atropine is physiologically active.

Chemical Nature

1. **Nitrogen:** The alkaloids may contain one or more number of nitrogen and they may exist in the form as:
   a. Primary amines R–NH_2, e.g. muscaline, norephedrine.
   b. Secondary amines R_2–NH, e.g. ephedrine
   c. Tertiary amines R_3–N, e.g. atropine.
   d. Quaternary ammonium salts R_4–N, e.g. *d*-tubocurarine chloride.

2. **Basicity:**
   a. R_2–NH > R–NH_2 > R_3–N saturated hexacyclic amines are more basic than aromatic amines.

2. **Oxygen:** Most alkaloids contain oxygen and are solid in nature, e.g. atropine. Some alkaloids are free from oxygen and are mostly liquids, e.g. nicotine, coniine.

3. **Stability:**
   i. **Effect of heat:** Alkaloids are decomposed by heat, except **strychnine** and **caffeine** (**sublimable**).
   ii. **Reaction with acids:**
   1. Salt formation.
   2. Dilute acids hydrolyze ester alkaloids, e.g. atropine.

4. **Effect of alkalies:** 1-Dilute alkalies liberate most alkaloids from their salts, e.g. NH_3. They may cause isomerization (racemization) of

alkaloid as the conversion of hyoscyamine to atropine. They also can form salts with alkaloids containing a carboxylic group, e.g. narceine.

5. **Strong alkalis:** Such as aqueous NaOH and KOH form salts with phenolic alkaloids. They can cause hydrolysis of ester alkaloids (e.g. atropine, cocaine and physostigmine) and amide alkaloids (colchicines).

Classification of Alkaloidal Precipitating Reagent

1. **Reagents that form double salts:**
   a. Mayer's reagent: Potassium mercuric iodide.
   b. Dragendorff's reagents: Potassium iodobismethate.
   c. Gold chloride.
2. **Reagents containing halogens:**
   a. Wagner's reagent: Iodine/potassium iodide.
3. **Organic acids:**
   a. Hager's reagent: Picric acid
   b. Tannic acid.
4. **Oxygenated high molecular weight acids:**
   a. Phosphomolybdic acid
   b. Phosphotungestic acid
   c. Silicotungestic acid

Color Reagents

1. **Froehd's reagent:** Phosphomolybdic acid
2. **Marqui's reagent:** Formaldehyde/conc. H_2SO_4.
3. **Mandalin's reagent:** Sulphovanidic acid.
4. **Erdmann's reagent:** Conc. HNO_3/conc. H_2SO_4.
5. **Mecke's reagent:** Selenious acid/conc. H_2SO_4.
6. **Shaer's reagent:** Hydrogen peroxide/conc. H_2SO_4.
7. **Rosenthaler's reagent:** Potassium arsenate/conc. H_2SO_4.
8. **Conc. HNO_3.**

Extraction and Isolation

Purification or isolation of alkaloids from a plant is always difficult process because an alkaloids-bearing plant generally contains a complex mixture of several alkaloids with glycoside organic acid also complicate the process. Following steps are involved in isolation process.

Extraction: The plant is dried, then finally powdered and extracted with boiling methanol. The solvent is distilled off and the residue treated with inorganic acids, when the bases (alkaloids) are extracted as their soluble salts. The aqueous layer containing the salt of alkaloids and soluble plant impurities is made basic with NaOH. The insoluble alkaloids are set free precipitate out. The solid (ppt.) is then extracted with ether when alkaloid pass into solution and impurity left behind (Fig. 5.4.3).

Separation of alkaloids: After extraction, the next step is separation of a relatively small percentage of alkaloids from large of crude drugs, e.g. opium contains 10% morphine, chincona contains 5–8% quinine, Belladona-0.2% of hyoscyamine. The required alkaloid is separated from the mixture from fractional, crystallization, chromatography and ion exchange method.

INDOLE ALKALOIDS

Ergot (Fig. 5.4.4)

Synonyms: English—Ergot of rye, fungus of rye; **Ayurveda**—Annamaya, Sraavikaa.
Biological source: A fungal sclerotium of *Claviceps purpurea* in ovary of rye plant *Secale*

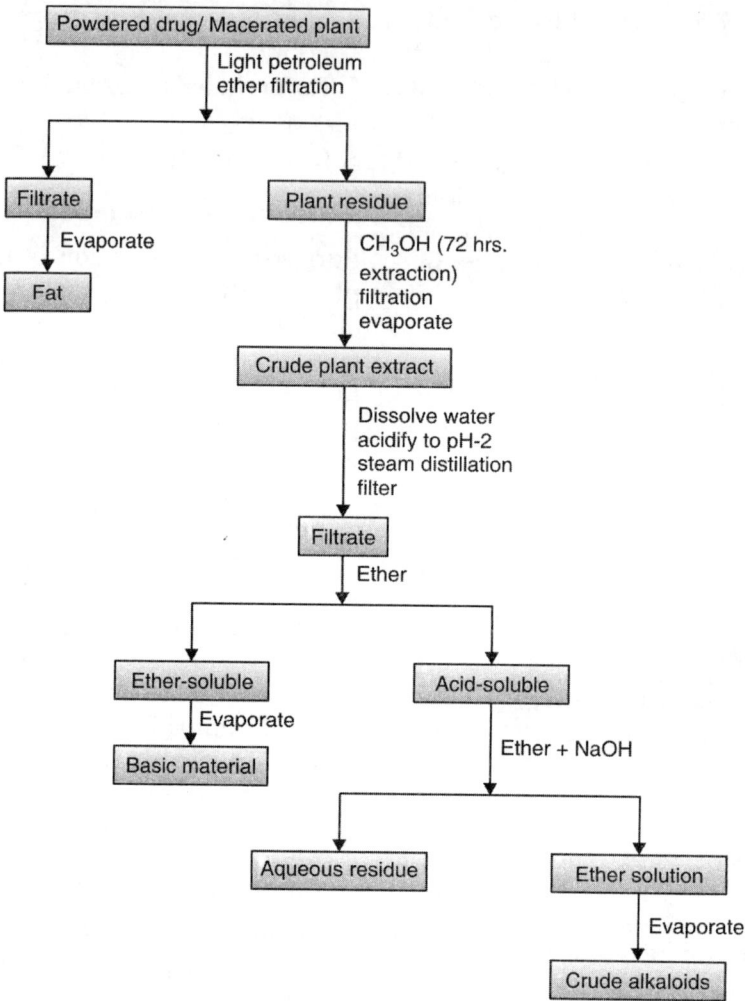

Fig. 5.4.3: Extraction of alkaloids

cereale. Family of fungus Clavicipitaceae; family of rye Gramineae.

Habitat: It is cultivated in Switzerland, Yugoslavia, Hungary and Czechoslovakia.

Life cycle: The parasitic life cycle of the ergot fungi begins in the spring, with wind-borne ascopores landing on susceptible host plants. Hyphae invade and colonize the ovary, producing masses of anamorphic spores that are exuded into a syrupy fluid (honeydew). Insect vectors, rainsplash, or head-to-head contact transfer this honeydew to other blooming florets, allowing the spread of the ergot fungi in a field. When the sclerotia begin to form, production of honeydew and condition cease, and the sclerotia mature in about 5 weeks. The number and size of sclerotia produced on each spike of cereal by *C. purpurea* varies according to grain, with rye usually bearing a considerable number, while wheat has relatively few. The sclerotia are considered as the early stage of sexual differentiation of Claviceps. In autumn, the ripe pigmented sclerotium leaves the spike and falls to the ground, ultimately producing asci and nonseptate ascospores, thereby completing the cycle.

Botany

- Kingdom   Fungi
- Division   Ascomycota
- Order   Hypocreales
- Family   Clavicipitaceae
- Genus   *Claviceps*
- Species   *purpurea*

Part used: Fungal sclerotium

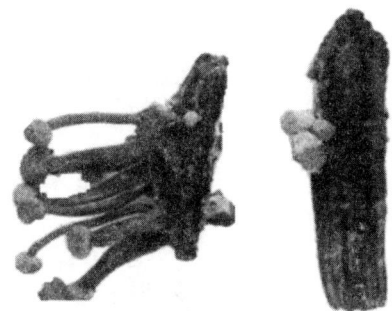

Fig. 5.4.4: Ergot
(*see also in colour Plate 6*)

Organoleptic Characters

Macroscopic characters

Color: Dark violet to black (externally)
Whitish to pinkish white (internally)

Odor: Disaggreable and faint

Taste: Unpleasant and bitter

Shape: Triangular, fusiform and usually tapering at both ends.

Size: 1 to 3 cm in length; 1 to 5 mm in width

Microscopy of ergot (Figs 5.4.5 and 5.4.6)

The ergot consists of three distinct parts:
1. The *internal part* or *body* of the ergot is composed of the hexagonal or rounded cellular tissue. The cells have the shape and regularity of the normal cells of the albumen, but they are considerably smaller.
2. The *violet* or *blackish* coat of the ergot consists of a layer of longitudinally elongated delicate cells.
3. The *bloom*, which to a greater or less extent covers the violet coat of the ergot; resembles the bloom of plums, and may be readily wiped off (Fig. 5.4.6).

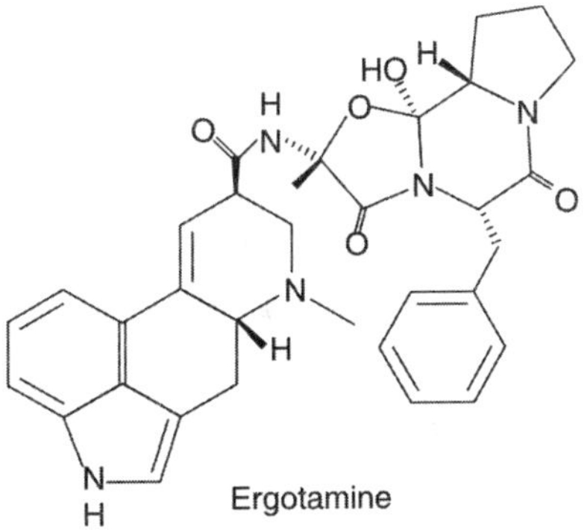

Ergotamine

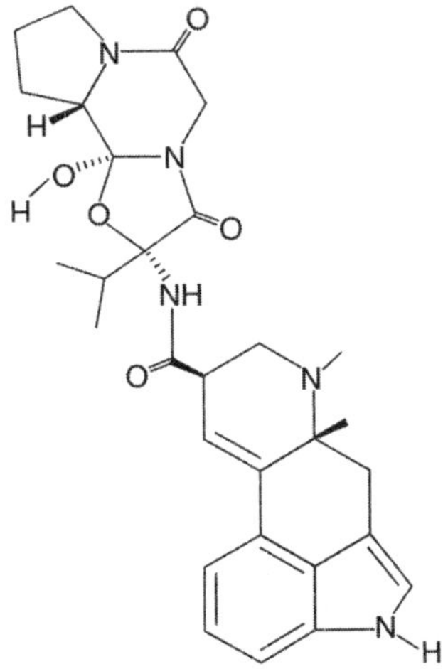

Ergotoxine

Fig. 5.4.5: Chemical constituents of ergot

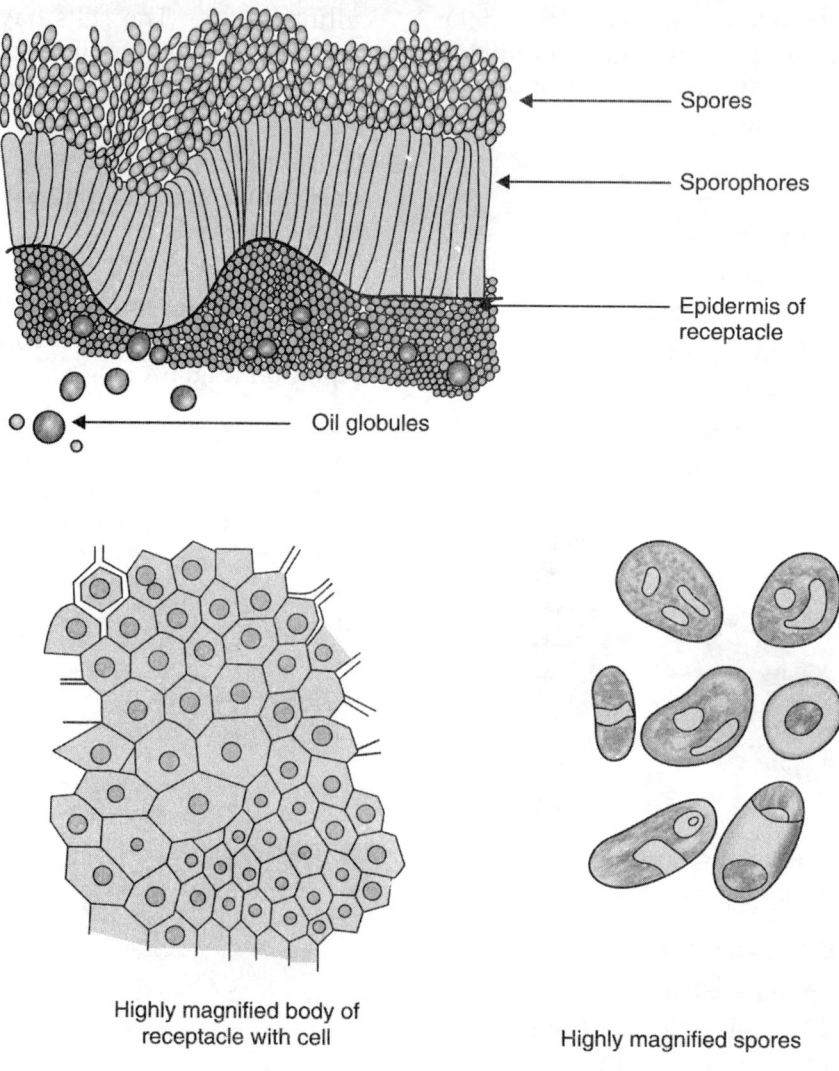

Fig. 5.4.6: Microscopy of ergot of rye

Chemical constituents (Fig. 5.4.5.): Ergot owes its activity to specific complex alkaloids, ergotoxine and ergotamine; in good Ergots, the alkaloidal content may be 0.02, fatty oil, (30 to 35%), and red coloring matter, sclererythrin. The drug also contains mannitol, partly combined as a glucoside, and the sugar trehalose. About 3% of ash is yielded. The ergometrine or ergonovine group includes ergometrine and ergometrinine. The ergotamine group includes ergotamine and ergotaminine. The ergotoxine group includes ergocristine, ergocristinine, ergocryptine, ergocryptinine, ergocornine and ergocorninine. The fungus also contains histamine, tyramine and other amines, sterols and acetylcholine.

Chemical Test

1. Ergot powder gives blue color with p-dimethylaminobenzaldehyde.
2. Ergot is treated with solvent ether and sulfuric acid and the filtrate shows red violet color in aqueous layer, when treated with saturated solution of sodium bicarbonate.

Uses: Ergot stimulates plain muscle, directly and indirectly throughout the body; its action on the uterus is like that on other plain muscle, and it is employed almost entirely to excite uterine contraction in the final stages of parturition. It has a strongly sedative action on the central nervous system and has proved a useful remedy in delirium tremens and spinal congestion and has been employed in certain forms of asthma, hysteria, amenorrhea and in menstrual disorders. It increases the secretion of milk and is used to check the night-sweats of phthisis.

Nux Vomica (Fig. 5.4.7)

Synonyms: English—Nux vomica, poison; nut, **Hindi**—Jahar; **Tamil**—Yetti; **Malayalam**—Kanjiram.

Biological source: It consists of dried seeds of *Strychnos nuxvomica* Linn., family Loganiaceae. It should contain NLT 1.2% of total alkaloids calculated as strychnine.

Botany

- Kingdom   Plantae
- Family   Loganiaceae
- Genus   *Strychnos*
- Species   *nuxvomica*

Habitat: It is indigenous to east India and largely collected from the forest of Sri Lanka, northern Australia and India.

Part used: Seeds

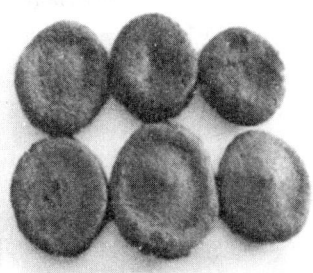

Fig. 5.4.7: Nux vomica
(see also in colour Plate 6)

Organoleptic Characters

Macroscopic characters

Color: Mouse-colored or greenish

Odor: Characteristic

Taste: Extremely bitter

Shape: Button-like seeds

Size: An inch in diameter by one-fourth inch thick

Extra features: Seeds are albuminous, very hard, tough, horny, round, flat, slightly convex on one surface and concave on the other, and covered with short silky hairs, of an ash-gray or yellowish color, which are directed from the center toward the circumference. Maceration in water, especially hot water, softens the albumen.

Microscopy of Nux Vomica (Fig. 5.4.8)

The seed-coat is very thin and consists of a narrow layer of brown, collapsed parenchyma covered with an epidermis, the cells of which have developed into hairs. Basically, seed is divided into four parts: Testa, endodermis, cavity and Hilum. The testa consists of lignified trichomes which are thick-walled, bent and twisted. Second layer of testa consists of single layer, large thick walled linear pits. Final layer is collapsed parenchyma. The endosperm consists of large cells with very thick walls of cellulosic parenchymatous cells, which swell in boiling water or in solution of potassium hydroxide. These cells contain the alkaloids.

In powdered, nux vomica consists of lignified trichomes and endosperm with oil globules and aleurone grains.

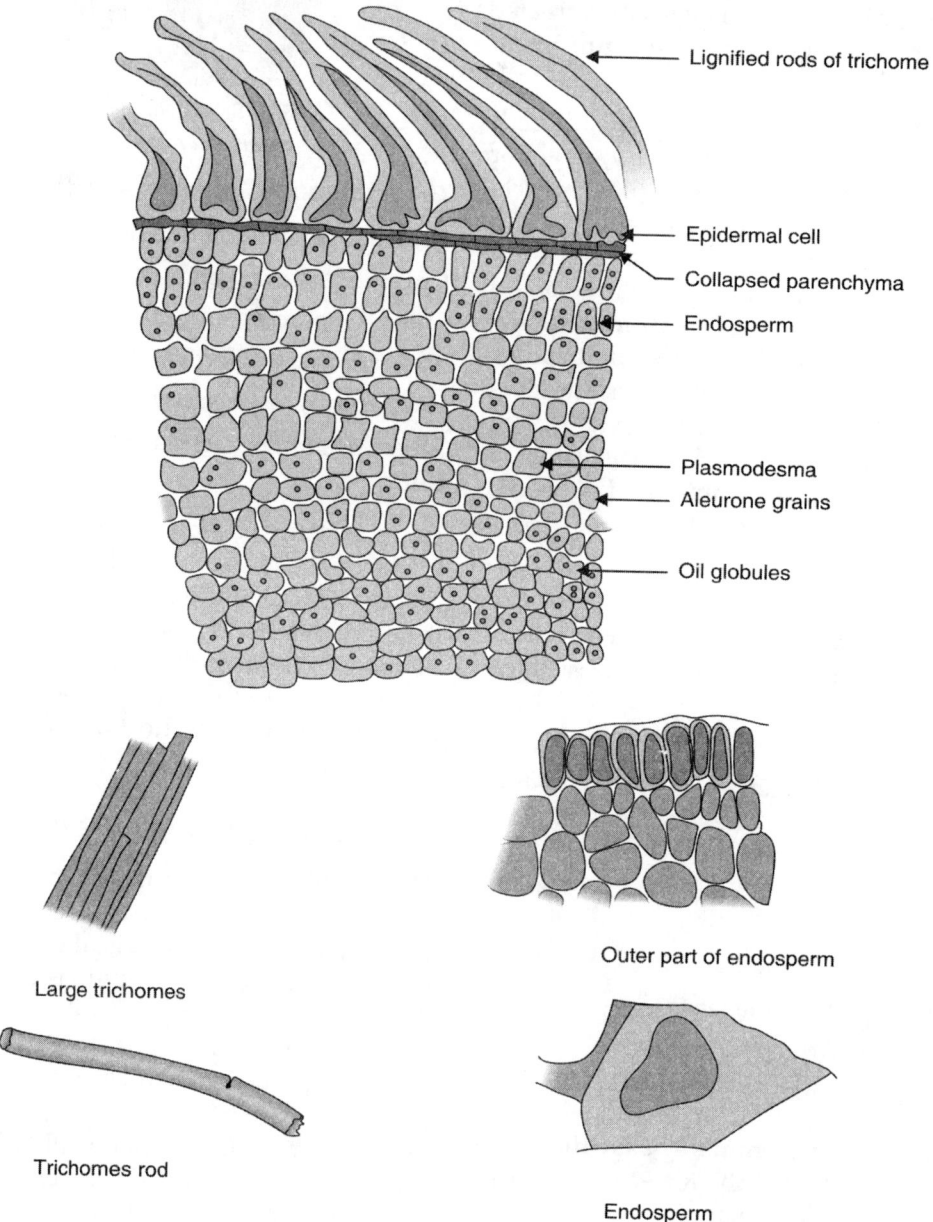

Fig. 5.4.8: Transverse section of nux vomica and its powder microscopy

Chemical Constituents (Fig. 5.4.9)

The seeds contain indole alkaloids, the major one is strychnine (approx. 50% of the alkaloids); others include strychnine N-oxide, brucine and its N-oxide, alpha- and beta-colubrine, condylocarpine, diaboline, geissoschizine, icajine, isostrychnine, nor-macusine, novacine, pseudobrucine, and pseudo-alpha-colubrine. The alkaloidal content of the seeds ranges from 1.8 to 5.3%. The leaves contain strychnine and brucine (together 1.6%), strychnine 0.025%; vomicine is the major constituent of leaves. The bark contains 9.9% total alkaloids (brucine 8%, strychnine 1.58%); pseudostrychnine, pseudobrucine and beta-colubrine in small amounts. The roots contain 0.99% alkaloids (brucine 0.28%, strychnine 0.71%).

Chemical test: In hydrochloric acid solution of brucine and strychnine, potassium ferrocyanide solution is added, the brucine precipitates, while the strychnine remains dissolved, the mixed alkaloids can be quite closely separated by alcohol 0.97 sp. g., which freely dissolves brucine, but scarcely dissolves strychnine.

Uses: The properties of nux vomica are substantially those of the alkaloid strychnine. The tincture of nux vomica is often used in mixtures for its stimulant action on the gastrointestinal tract. In the mouth, it acts as a bitter, increasing appetite; it stimulates peristalsis in chronic constipation due to atony of the bowel. It is often combined with cascara and other laxatives with good effects. Seeds are used in emotional disorders, insomnia, hysteria, epilepsy, paralytic and neurological affections, retention or nocturnal incontinence of urine, spermatorrhea, sexual debility and impotence, general exhaustion; as antidote to alcoholism; GIT disorders. Bark juice given in acute dysentery, diarrhea and colic. Root is given in intermittent fevers.

Physostigma

Synonyms: English—Calabar bean (Fig. 5.4.10) and ordeal bean

Biological source: It is dried seed of *Physostigma venenosum*, belonging to family Leguminosae. It contains NLT 0.15% of alkaloids of physostigma.

Botany

- Kingdom   Plantae
- Division   Magnoliophyta
- Class   Magnoliopsida
- Order   Fabales
- Family   Fabaceae
- Genus   *Physostigma*
- Species   *venenosum*

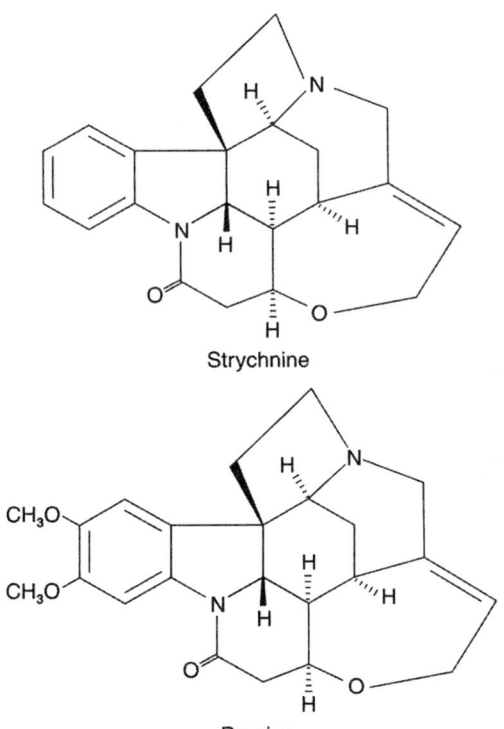

Fig. 5.4.9: Chemical constituents of nux vomica

Habitat: Gulf of Guinea, West Africa
Part used: Seeds

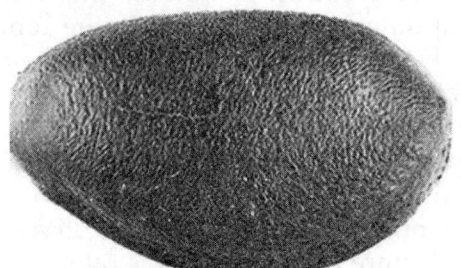

Fig. 5.4.10: Calabar bean (*see also in colour Plate 6*)

Organoleptic Characters

Macroscopic characters
Color: Brown-colored
Odor: Ordorless
Taste: Bean-like
Shape: Flattened and reinform, extremely hard
Size: 25 to 30 mm (1 to 1¼ inch) long, 15 to 20 mm (3/5 to 3/4 inch) broad, and 10 to 15 mm (2/5 to 3/5 inch) thick.

Chemical constituents: Calabar bean contains starch (48%), mucilage, albumen (23%), fatty oil (2.5%), and salts, mainly potassium phosphate. The chief active principle of physostigma is the alkaloid *physostigmine* (Fig. 5.4.11), with which are associated small quantities of eseridine and eseramine. Physostigmine forms large crystals melting at 105 to 106°; it is tasteless, levorotatory, sparingly soluble in water, readily in alcohol, ether, chloroform, benzene, or carbon bisulphide. The seeds also contain the phytosterol stigmasterol, and abundance of starch; and yield about 4% of ash. Calabar bean an alkaloid, *eseridine* ($C_{15}H_{23}N_3O_3$), distinguished by its property of liberating iodine from iodic acid.

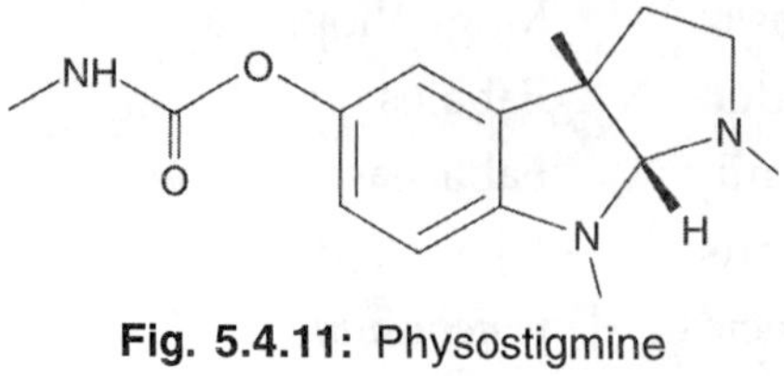

Uses: Chiefly used for diseases of the eye. It causes rapid contraction of the pupil and disturbed vision. It is also used as a stimulant to the unstriped muscles of the intestines in chronic constipation. Its action on the circulation is to slow the pulse and raise blood-pressure; it depresses the central nervous system, causing muscular weakness; it has been employed internally for its depressant action in epilepsy, cholera, etc. and given hypodermically in acute tetanus.

Substituents: Antiaris, (*Upas antiar*). A gummy-resinous exudate from *Antiaris toxicaria*.

Rauwolfia (Figs 5.4.12 and 5.4.13)

Synonyms: Sanskrit—Chandrika, Sarpagandha; **Hindi**—Chota chand; **Bengali**—Chandra; **Telgu**—Patala-gandhi; **Tamil**—Chivan melpodi.

Biological source: It consists of dried roots of the plant *Rauwolfia serpentine*, belonging to family Apocynaceae. It contains NLT 0.14% of reserpine.

Botany

- Kingdom   Plantae
- Division   Magnoliophyta
- Class   Magnoliopsida
- Order   Fabales
- Family   Fabaceae
- Genus   *Physostigma*
- Species   *venenosum*

Habitat: It is produced in India, Sri Lanka, Myanmar and America
Part used: Roots

Fig. 5.4.11: Physostigmine

Drugs Derived from Natural Sources

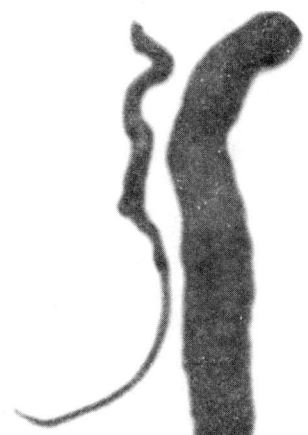

Fig. 5.4.12: Rauwolfia
(*see also in colour Plate 6*)

Organoleptic Characters

Macroscopic characters:

Color: Grayish in color

Odor: Odorless

Taste: Bitter and pungent

Shape: Cylindrical, slightly tapering and tortuous

Size: 10 to 18 cm long, 2 cm in diameter.

Chemical constituents (Fig. 5.4.14): The major alkaloids present in Rauwolfia is reserpine and rescinnamine. The root contains an alkaloid ophioxylin, an orange-colored crystalline principle, resin, starch and wax. The total alkaloid yield is 0.5%. Five crystalline alkaloids isolated are ajmaline, ajmalicine, serpentine, serpentinine and yohimbine. Other constituents are phytosterol, oleic acid and unsaturated alcohols. The root also contains a lot of resin and starch and when incinerated leaves about 8% of ash consisting mainly of potassium carbonate, phosphate, silicate and traces of iron and manganese.

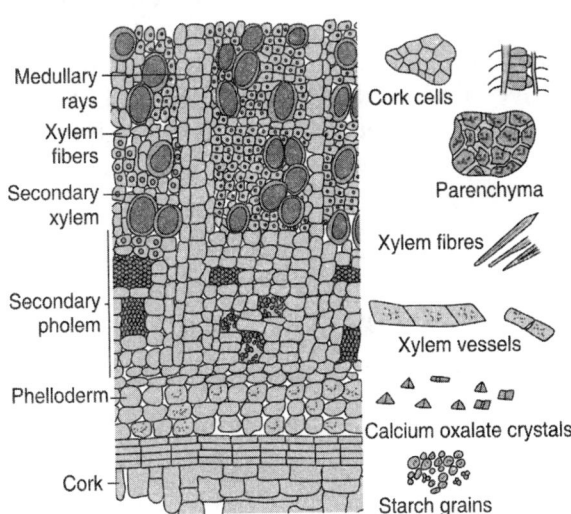

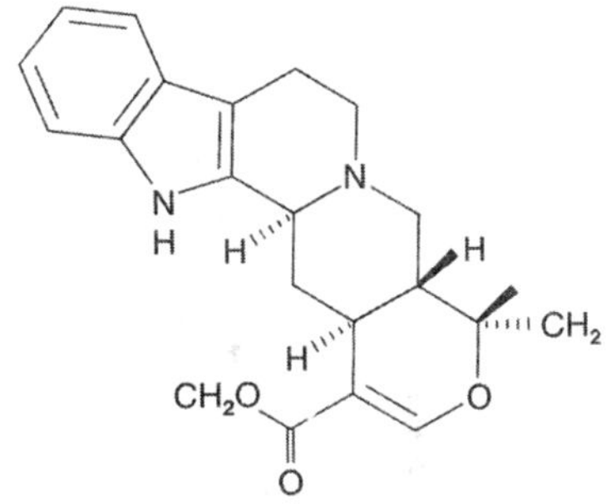

Fig. 5.4.13: Transverse section of roots of Rauwolfia

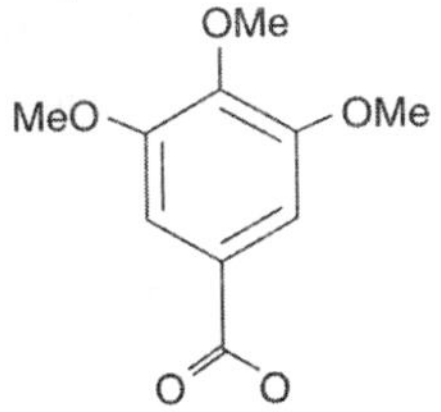

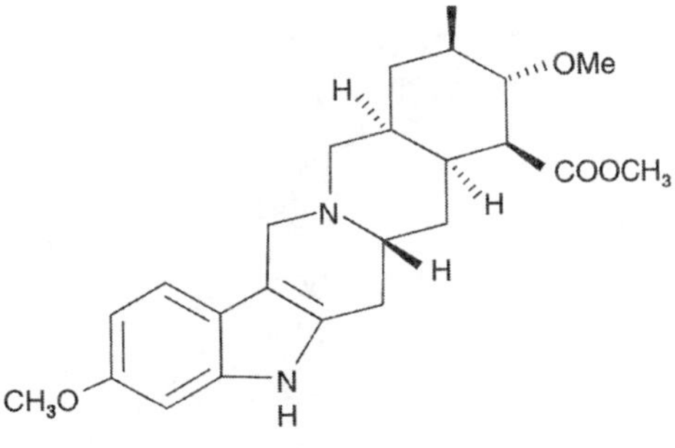

Fig. 5.4.14: Chemical constituents of Rauwolfia

Uses: The major uses of Rauwolfia is that it is antihypertensive drug. Sarpagandha is seldom used externally. In chronic fever, the root powder is given by itself. In serpant bite, the powder of its roots is given orally, as well as, applied topically on the site of bite. Sarpagandha, being an uterine stimulant, is beneficial in dysmenorrhea and is salutary in the delivery of the placenta and to augment the uterine contractions (labor pains). In males, it is used to suppress the excessive sexual vigor, as it depresses the libido. The juice of the leaves is used as a remedy for the removal of opacities of the cornea seed in gastrointestinal maladies like anoresia, dyspepsia, worms and abdominal pain.

Vinca (Fig. 5.4.15)

Synonyms: Folk—Ainskati, Nayantra, Rattanjot, Sada bahar; **English**—Madagascar periwinkle (*Vinca major* L. Pich. and *Vinca minor* Linn. are known as greater periwinkle and lesser periwinkle, respectively)

Biological source: It is obtained from leaves of *Catharanthus roseus* (L.) G. Don, family Apocynaceae.

Habitat: It is cultivated in India, Europe, USA, Australia and South Africa.

Botany (Table 5.4.2)

- Kingdom   Plantae
- Division   Magnoliophyta
- Class   Magnoliopsida
- Family   Apocynaceae
- Genus   *Catharanthus*
- Species   *roseus*

Part used: Whole plant

Table 5.4.2: Botanical trait of vinca

Nature	Perennial herb
Appearance	An erect bushy perennial herb and evergreen shrub
Height	Grows to a height of 90 centimetre with a spread of one metre
Stem	Erect
Leaves	Simple, opposite, exstipulate, petiolate.
Inflorescence	Racemose
Flowers	Soft pink, tinged with red
Petals	Five petals appearing in spring and autumn.
Varieties	There are three varieties rose purple flowers, white flower, white flowers with a rose purple spot in the centre

Organoleptic Characters

Chemical constituents: It consists of indole alkaloids mainly vincristine (Fig. 5.4.16), vinblastine, vireolidine and vincrelbine. Vinblastine (Fig. 5.4.17) contains indole alkaloids part called catharanthine and dihydroindole alkaloid part called vindoline. The other alkaloids are ajmalicine, lochnerine, serpentine and tetrahydroalstonine.

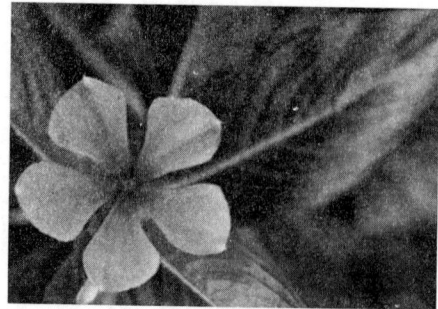

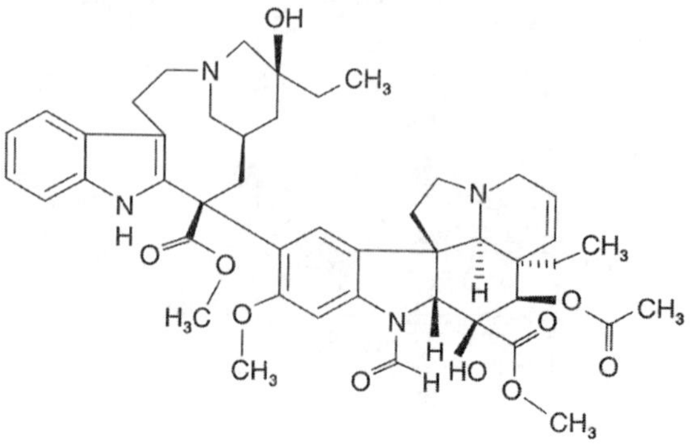

Fig. 5.4.15: Vinca
(*see also in colour Plate 6*)

Fig. 5.4.16: Vincristine

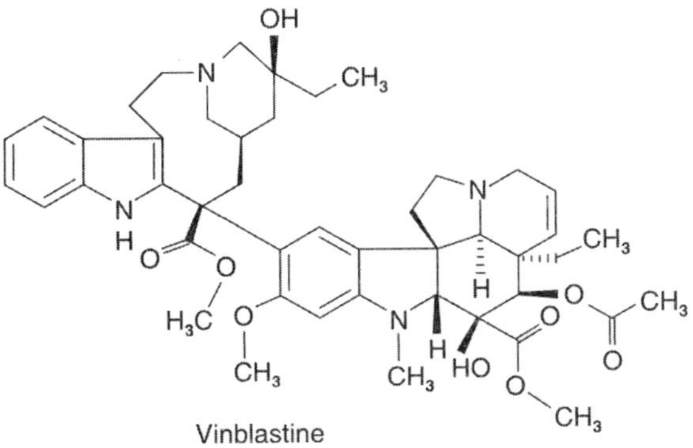

![Vinblastine structure]

Fig. 5.4.17: Vincristine

Uses: It is used as cytostatic, anti-neoplastic, slows down growth of cells by suppressing immune response. Vinblastine and vincristine to prolong remission of leukemia to more than five years. These chemotherapeutic agents are toxic to the nervous system. Vinblastine is also used for breast cancer and Hodgkin's disease. *Vinca major* L. (greater periwinkle): astringent, anti-hemorrhagic; used for menorrhagia and leukorrhea. It contains indole alkaloids including reserpine and serpentine; tannins.

Vinca minor Linn. (lesser periwinkle): astringent; circulatory stimulant. Leaves are stomachic and bitter. Roots are hypotensive. Used for gastric catarrh, chronic dyspepsia, flatulence; also for headache, dizziness, behavior disorders.

ISOQUINOLINE ALKALOIDS

Opium

Synonyms: Hindi—Ajim; **Gujrati**—Afin; **English**—Raw opium.

Biological source: It is obtained from flowering plant *Papaver somniferum* Linn of the family Papaveraceae. It contains NLT 9.5% of morphine.

Habitat: Native to Asia; now grown in Uttar Pradesh, Punjab, Rajasthan and Madhya Pradesh.

Botany

- Kingdom   Plantae
- Family   Papaveraceae

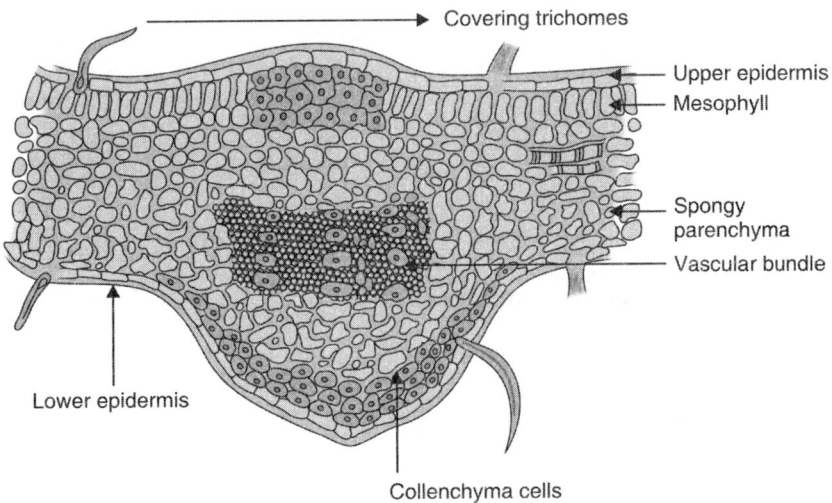

Fig. 5.4.18: Transverse section of vinca leaves

- Genus   *Papaver*
- Species   *somniferum*

Part used: Capsule

Organoleptic Characters

Macroscopic characters

Color: Olive-brown or olive-gray

Odor: Strong characteristic

Taste: Bitter

Shape: More or less rounded, oval, brick-shaped or elongated

Size: 8–15 cm in diameter.

Extra features: It tends to be plastic when fresh, but becomes more dense and tough on storage.

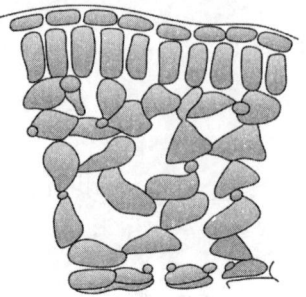
Upper epidermis

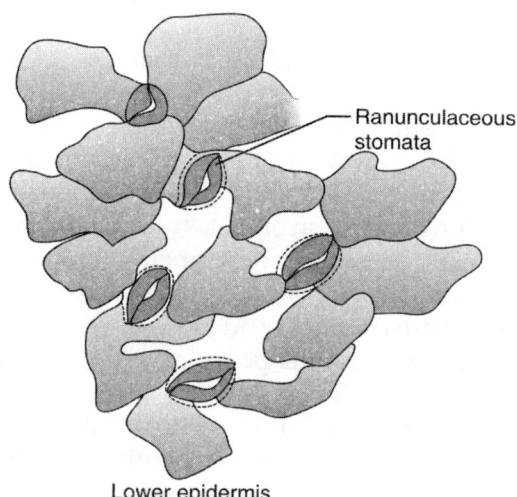
Lower epidermis

Fig. 5.4.20: Microscopy of opium leaf

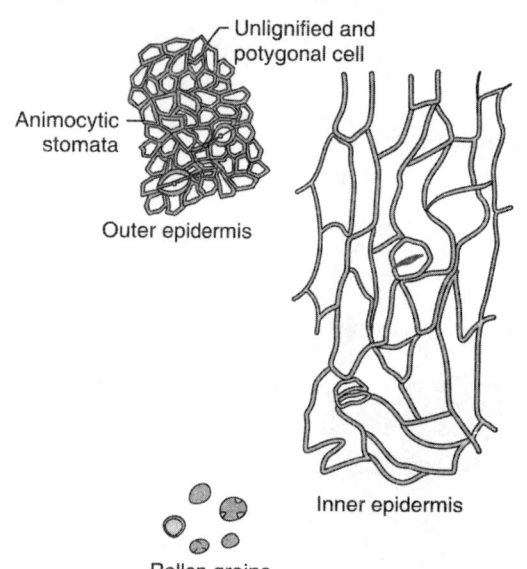

Fig. 5.4.19: Powder microscopy of opium capsule

Chemical constituents: Opium poppy contains over 40 opium alkaloids, including codeine (about 1%) (Fig. 5.4.22), morphine (up to 20%) (Fig. 5.4.23), narcotine (about 5%), and papaverine (about 1%). It also contains meconic acid, albumin, mucilage, sugars, resin, and wax.

Microscopy (Figs 5.4.19 and 20): Microscopic examination of powdered opium demonstrates the presence of amorphous latex masses, leaf and epicarp fragments, brown stone cells, narrow spiral vessels or pieces of vessels, parenchyma, starch grains and refringent crystals.

Fig. 5.4.21: Morphine

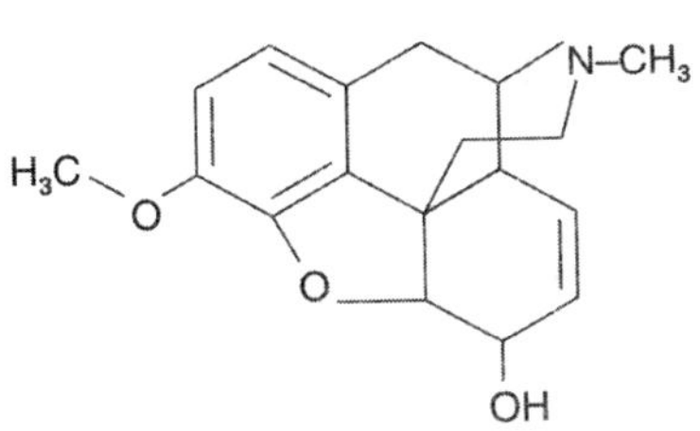

Fig. 5.4.22: Codeine

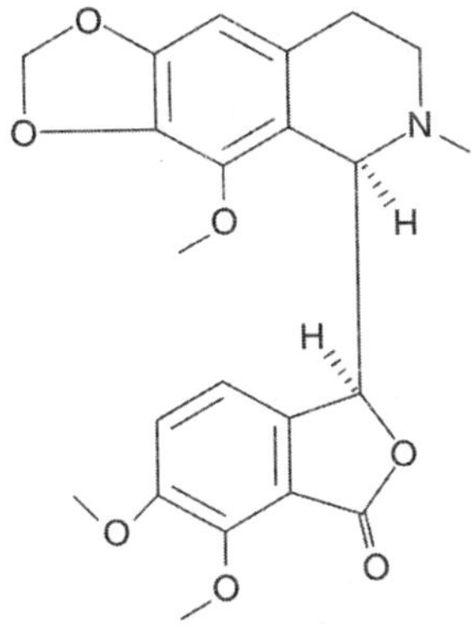

Fig. 5.4.23: Narcotine

Uses: Opium poppy has also been used as a base for powerful synthetic opiates. Its form of dried latex has been used as a powerful narcotic, analgesic, and antispasmodic. In herbal tradition, opium is considered to be an excellent 'cold' remedy, because of its ability to reduce physical function, and to sedate and suppress coughs, nervous activity, including pain.

Curare

Synonyms: South American arrow poison, curare, D-tubocurarine, ourari, tubocurarine.

Biological source: It consists of dried extracts of Stems and leaves of various plants from families Loganiaceae and Menispermaceae. Some of prominent members yielding curare is *Chondrodendron tomentosum, Strychnos castelnaea, S. crevauxii, S. toxifera.*

Habitat: It is available in Brazil, Columbia, Peru and Guiana.

Botany
- Kingdom   Plantae
- Family   Loganiaceae
- Genus   *Chondrodendron*
- Species   *tomentosum*

Parts used: Leaf, root, bark, stems, seeds.

Chemical constituents: Curare is of a bitter taste, soluble in cold water the extract also contains poisonous substance known as curarine ($C_{18}H_{35}N$) (Fig. 5.4.24). It is colorless or white, of a bitter taste, deliquescent to a certain extent in moist air, soluble in water, and in alcohol, less soluble in chloroform, and insoluble in pure ether, benzol, oil of turpentine, and disulphide of carbon. It has an alkaline reaction, and unites with acids to form crystallizable salts.

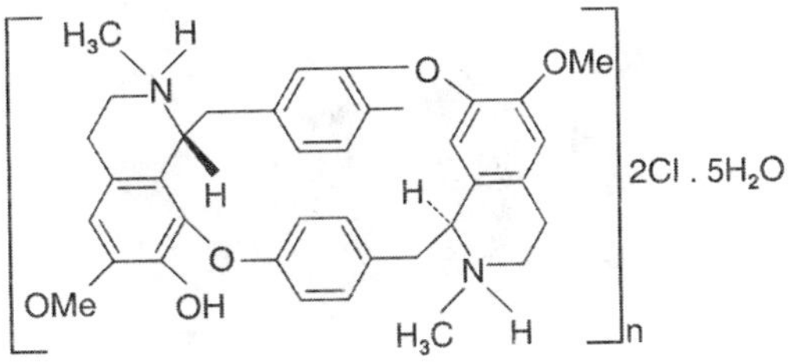

Fig. 5.4.24: Curarine

Uses: Arthritis, bacterial and fungal infection, black widow spider bite therapy, contraceptive, cautery, diagnosis of Myasthenia gravis, facilitates larynogoscopy and esophagoscopy, general anesthesia: skeletal-muscle relaxant drug (particularly of the abdominal wall), orthopedic procedures, parasitic, poison (arrow), poliomyelitis, shock therapy, snakebite, stomach problems, uterine stimulant.

Ipecacuanha (Fig. 5.4.25)

Synonyms: English—Ipecac, ipecacuanha.

Biological Source: It consists of dried roots or the rhizomes of *Cephelis ipecacuanha* or *Cephaelis acuminate*, both belonging to family Rubiceae.

Habitat: Native to tropical America now cultivated in Darjeeling, Assam, in the Nilgiris, and in Sikkim.

Botany

- Kingdom   Plantae
- Order   Gentianales
- Family   Rubiaceae
- Genus   *Cephelis*
- Species   *ipecacuanha*

Parts used: Dried roots and rhizomes

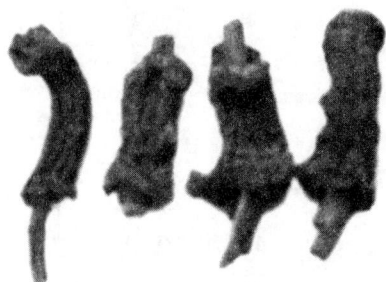

Fig. 5.4.25: Ipecacuanha
(see also in colour Plate 6)

Organoleptic Characters

Macroscopic Characters:

1. Brazilian ipecacuanha

a. Root:

Color: Dark brick red to brown.

Odor: Faint.

Taste: Bitter.

Shape: Tortuous pieces.

Size: 150 mm in length and 6 mm in thickness.

Extra features: Fracture is short and pith is absent.

b. Rhizome:

Color: Brick red to dark brown.

Shape: Cylindrical

Size: 2 mm in diameter and short, attached to roots.

Extra features: Wrinkled longitudinally and shows presence of prominent pith.

2. Cartagena ipecacuanha

Color: Greyish brown to reddish brown

Odor: Faint.

Taste: Bitter.

Shape: Cylindrical

Size: 9 mm in thickness

Extra features: Characterized by absence of annulation and presence of transverse ridges at interval of 1 to 3 mm.

Microscopy (Fig. 5.4.26)

Below the narrow cork is a largely developed cortex consisting of thin-walled parenchymatous cells most of which are filled with starch, but

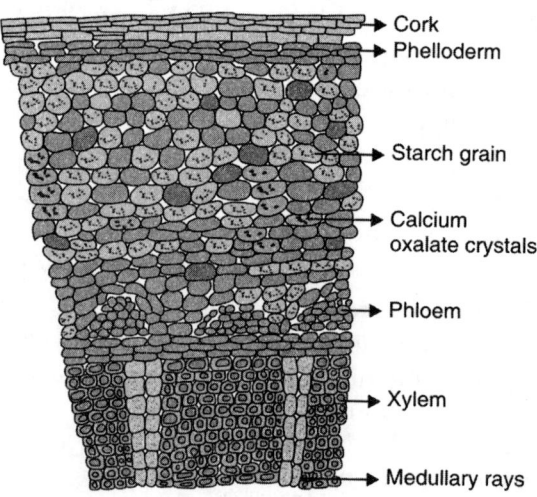

Fig. 5.4.26: Transverse section, showing dense wood of ipecacuanha

a few contain acicular calcium oxalate. The bast ring is narrow, and both this and the cortex are free from sclerenchymatous cells and fibers and from cells containing coloring matter. The wood is composed of tracheids, wood fibers, and parenchyma and is free from typical vessels. The tracheids, when isolated, exhibit moderately thick walls, and often near the pointed extremities a large perforation.

The powder is characterized by the starch grains which are either oval or rounded (not over 15 µ) or compound with 2 to 5 constituent grains, by the acicular calcium oxalate, by the characteristic tracheids and by the absence of sclerenchymatous cells, spiral vessels (ipecacuanha stem), cells containing colouring water, calcium oxalate in other than acicular crystals, and typical sclerenchymatous fibers or vessels.

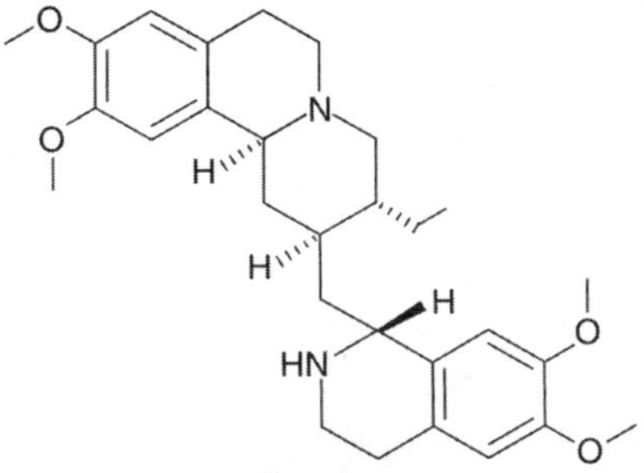

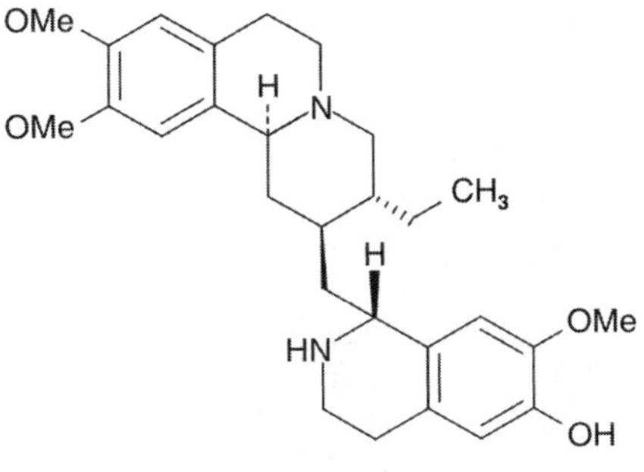

Fig. 5.4.27: Chemical constituent of ipecacuanna

Chemical constituents: Ipecacuanha root contains three alkaloids; two of which, emetine and cephaline, whilst the third, psychotrine, which occurs in much smaller quantity. These alkaloids exist in good root to the extent of 2 to 3%, and are contained chiefly in the bark, the wood yielding only about 1% Ipecacuanha also contains about 0.4%, of a crystalline glucoside. Ipecacuanhin, which is sparingly soluble in cold water, more freely in hot, and insoluble in ether; it is apparently devoid of marked physiological action.

Uses: Ipecacuanha root is emetic; in smaller doses, diaphoretic and expectorant, and in still smaller, stimulating to the stomach, intestines and liver, exciting appetite and facilitating digestion.

TROPANE ALKALOIDS

Belladonna (Fig. 5.4.28)

Synonyms: English: Deadly nightshade; **Hindi**—Sag-angur or Angurshefa; **Bengali**—Yebruj; **Bombay**—Girbuti.

Biological source: Dried leaves and flowering tops of *Atropa belladonna*, family Solanaceae.

Habitat: It is available in central and southern Europe; in England, it is confined chiefly to the southern counties; it also widely cultivated not only in this country but also on the continent, in India, in the United States, etc.

Botany

- Kingdom   Plantae
- Order   Solanales
- Family   Solanaceae
- Genus   *Atropa*
- Species   *belladonna*

Parts used: Dried leaves, fruits and flowering top

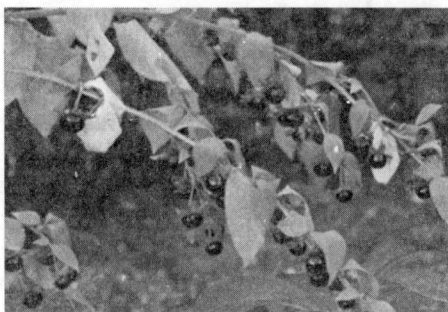

Fig. 5.4.28: Belladonna
(see also in colour Plate 7)

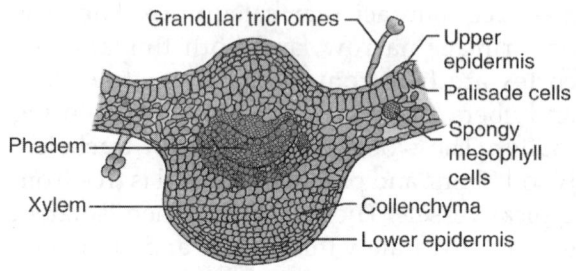

Fig. 5.4.29: Transverse section of Belladenna leaves

Organoleptic Characters

Macroscopic character:

Color: Leaves: Dull green color
Fruits: Green to brown
Flowers: Purple to yellowish brown
Odor: Slight and characteristic
Taste: Bitter and acrid.
Shape: Leaves: Ovate and lanceolate
Fruits: Subglobular in shape
Flowers: Campanulate
Size: Leaves: 5 to 25 cm long and 2.5 to 12 cm wide
Fruits: 10 cm in diameter
Flowers: Corolla 2.5 cm long and 1.5 cm wide.

Microscopical Characters
(Figs 5.4.29 and 5.4.30)

Leaf: Epidermal cells consists of conical and glandular trichomes with unicellular hand, followed by single layer of palisade parenchyma and spongy mesophyll containing calcium oxalate crystals. The midst shows tricollateral vascular bundles.

Root: The microscopy section of root consists of four to seven layers of cork cells. The cork cells are followed by phellogen (single layer). The other characteristic parts in the section are cambium, xylem fibers and parenchyma cells.

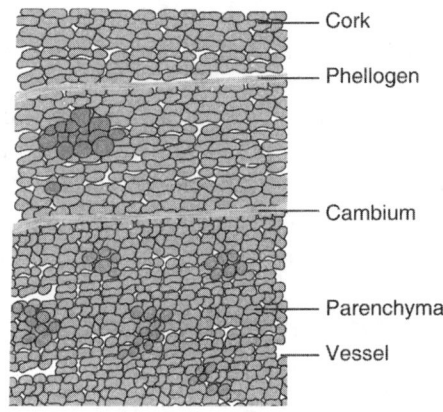

Fig. 5.4.30: Transverse section of Belladonna root

Powder microscopy: The dark green powder of lamina contains multicellular uniserate covering trichomes, anisocytic stomata, crystal of calcium oxalate, annular and spindly thickened vessels.

Constituents: The chief constituents of the drug are the alkaloids, hyoscyamine and atropine. It contains about 0.4%, of total alkaloid, but as much as 1%, has (exceptionally) been found. The alkaloids are contained in all parts of the plant (Table 5.4.3); in the calices and young ovaries 0.79%, in the ripe seeds 0.83%, in the root 05%, and in fresh fruit 0.12%. The main alkaloid is (S)-hyoscyamine 87.6% in leaves and 68.7% in roots. The other alkaloids are apoatropine 6.7%, tropine 3%, scopolamine 1.9%, aposcopolamine 0.5%, 3-α-phenyl-acetoxytropane 0.3%, tropinone 0.2%. Belladonna leaves also contain a fluorescent substance, β-methyl-sesculetin (scopoletin, chrysatropic acid), and yield about 14%, of ash.

Hyoscyamine

Uses: Belladonna acts as a local anesthetic and anodyne, and is used externally to relieve pain. Internally, it is given to check the sweating in phthisis, as a sedative to the respiratory nerves, to relieve spasmodic cough, and in numerous other cases.

Adulterants

1. The leaves of *Scopola carniolica*, Jacquin, a Solanaceous plant, closely resemble belladonna leaves, but are more lanceolate, more translucent, brighter in color, and with more distinct veinlets; the crystal cells are less numerous, hairs are absent, and stomata occur on the under surface only.

2. The leaves of *Phytolacca decandra*, Linne; may be distinguished by containing acicular crystals of calcium oxalate, and by the epidermal cells which are elongated and straight-walled.

3. The leaves of *Ailanthus glandulosa*, Desfontaines (N.O. Simaru-beai); have cluster-crystals of calcium oxalate along the veins.

Datura (Fig. 5.4.31)

Synonyms: Sans: Krishna dhatura; **Hindi and Bengali**—Kala dhatura; **Tamil**—Karu-umattai.

Biological source: It consists of dried leaves and flowering tops of *Datura metel* var *fastuosa*, family Solanaceae.

Habitat: It is found in India, England and other tropical and subtropical regions.

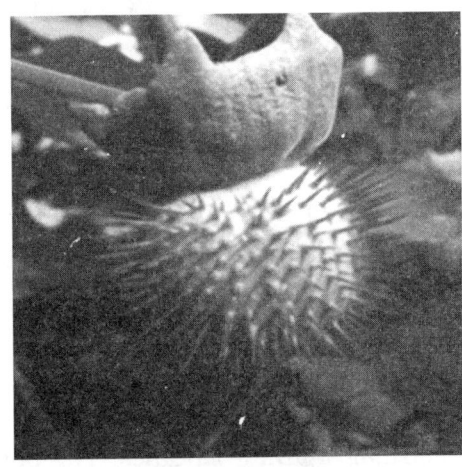

Fig. 5.4.31: Datura
(see also in colour Plate 7)

Botany

- Kingdom Plantae
- Order Solanales
- Family Solanaceae
- Genus *Datura*
- Species *metel*

Parts used: Dried leaves and Flowering tops

Organoleptic Characters

Macroscopic characters

Color:	Leaves: Green
Flower:	Reddish purple on outer side, Whitish on inner side
Odor:	Unpleasant odor
Taste:	Bitter
Shape:	Leaves: Unequal at base with acute apex and glabrous lamina

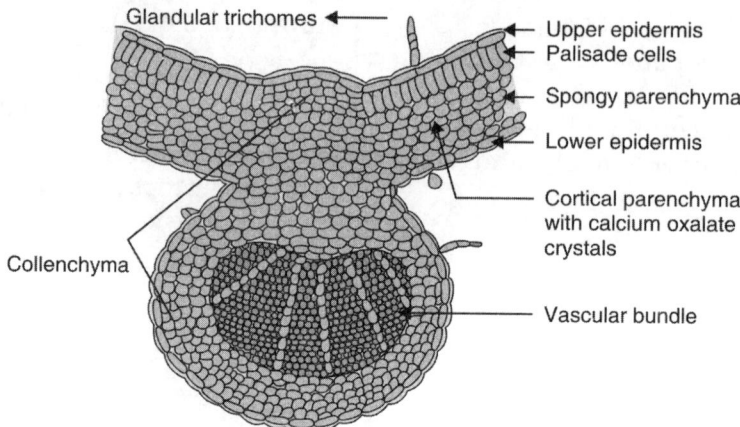

Fig. 5.4.32: Transverse section of datura leaf

Flower: Funnel-shaped
Size: Leaf: 9–18 cm in length, 8–13 cm in width

Microscopic characters (Fig. 5.4.32): It shows dorsiventral character. The epidermal cell shows anisocytic stomata. The cells are covered with thin cuticle and glandular and nonglandular simple trichomes. The parenchymatous cells are present. The spongy parenchyma consists of calcium oxalate crystals.

Chemical constituents (Fig. 5.4.33): It consists of scopolamine (hyoscine), little hyoscyamine, and atropine, fatty oil 11%; palmintic acid, 6.18%; oleic acid, 60.80%; d-linolic, 23.55%; β-linolic acid, 2.92%; capronic acid and 1%; phytosterin.

Uses: The whole plant, but especially the leaves and seed, is anaesthetic, anodyne, antiasthmatic, antispasmodic, antitussive, bronchodilator, hallucinogenic, hypnotic and

Table 5.4.3: Total alkaloid content of plant	
Part of plant	Total alkaloids%
Leaves	0.25 – 0.55
Fruit	0.12
Seeds	0.23 – 0.50
Roots	0.10 – 0.22
Stems	0.208 – 0.440
Flowers	0.485 – 0.550
Immature seeds	0.248
Mature seeds	0.393 – 0.589
Immature fruit	0.131 – 0.409
Mature fruit	0.175 – 0.380
Mature pods	0.076 – 0.327

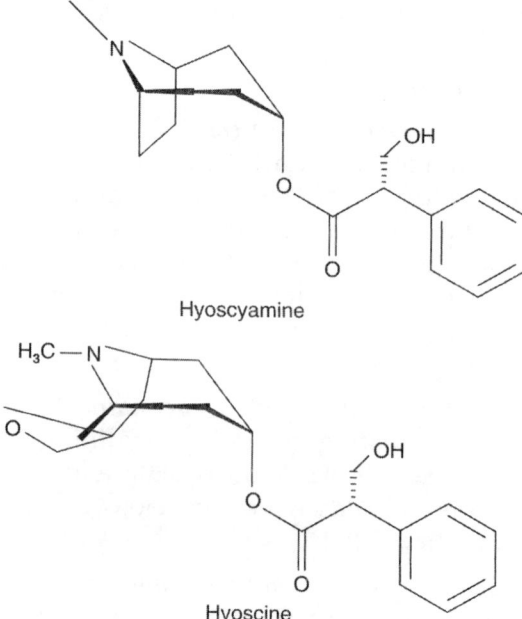

Fig. 5.4.33: Chemical constituents of Datura

mydriatic. It has a wide range of applications in India, including in the treatment of epilepsy, hysteria, insanity, heart diseases, fever with catarrh, diarrhea, skin diseases, etc.

Note: Great caution is advised in the use of this plant since excess doses cause hallucinations, severe intoxication and death

Hyoscyamus (Fig. 5.4.34)

Synonyms: English—Henbane, hyoscyamus herb.

Biological source: It consists of the dried leaves and flowering tops of *Hyoscyamus niger*, belonging to family Solanaceae.

Habitat: It is originated in Eurasia though it is now globally distributed and is cultivated in United States, South America, France, Germany and Hungary.

Botany

- Kingdom   Plantae
- Order   Solanales
- Family   Solanaceae
- Genus   *Hyoscyamus*
- Species   *niger*

Parts used: Dried leaves and flowering tops

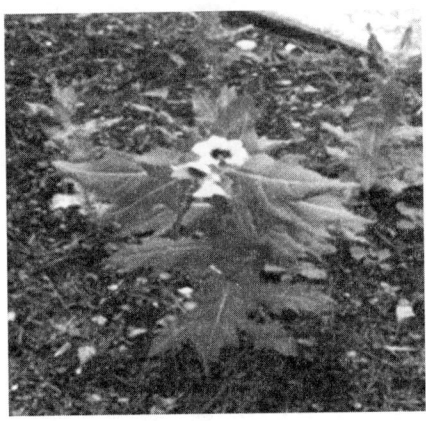

Fig. 5.4.34: Hyoscyamus (*see also in colour Plate 7*)

Organoleptic Characters

Macroscopic characters of leaves

Color: Pale greenish green

Odor: Disagreeable, fetid odor

Taste: Bitter and somewhat acrid

Shape: Ovate, or ovate-oblong

Size: 25 cm (10 inches) long and 10 cm (4 inches) broad

Extra features: The leaves are large, oblong, acute, alternate, coarsely and unequally sinuated, occasionally somewhat decurrent, stem-clasping at the base, pale dull-green, and slightly pubescent, with long, glandular hairs upon the midrib. The flowers are numerous, axillary, subsolitary, nearly sessile, and embosomed in the uppermost leaves, than which they are much shorter. The fruit is an ovate, 2-celled capsule, opening transversely by a convex lid. The seeds are many, small, obovate, and brownish.

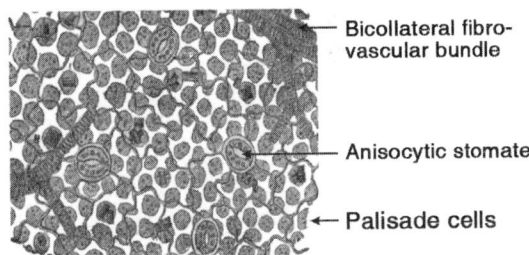

Fig. 5.4.35: Transverse section of epidermis of hyoscyamus leaf

Microscopic Characters (Fig. 5.4.35)

The leaf is dorsiventral. Epidermis is covered by glandular trichomes. Palisade cells contains prismatic or cluster layer of calcium oxalate crystals. Anisocytic stomata are present in epidermal layer. Mid-rib shows the presence of Bicollateral vascular bundles.

Chemical constituents (Fig. 5.4.36): The chief constituents of hyoscyamus seeds, besides fixed oil and fatty matter, gum, starch, albuminous matter, etc. are two alkaloids, *hyoscyamine* and *hyoscine*. Pure *hyoscyamine* crystallizes in tufts or stellate, has silky needles of an acrid, and has unpleasant taste; when impure it is an amorphous, deliquescent mass, having a nauseating, narcotic, tobacco-like smell. It dissolves sparingly in cold water, more readily in hot water, is soluble in alcohol, ether, chloroform, benzol, and amyl alcohol. Its melting point is 108.5°C (227.3°F). *Hyoscyamine* is strongly basic and forms crystallizable salts with acids. It is an isomer of *atropine* yielding the same decomposition products (*tropine* and *tropic acid*) as atropine when heated with diluted hydrochloric acid.

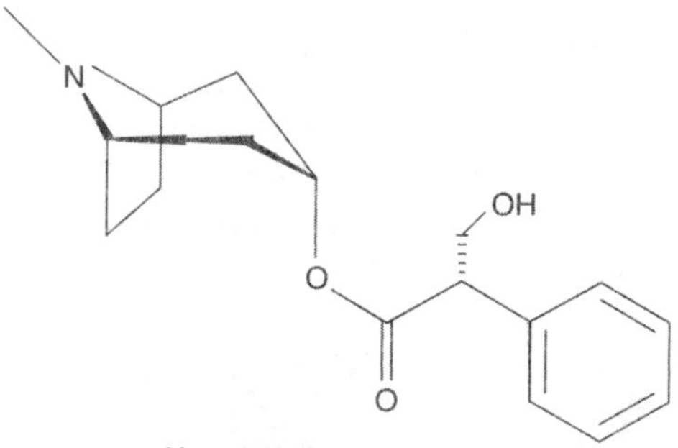

Hyoscyamine

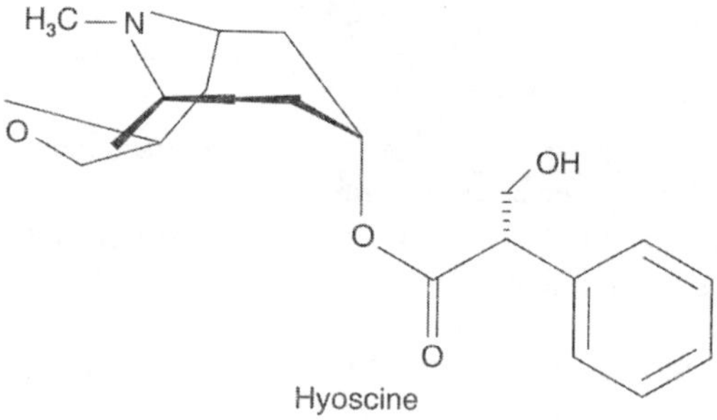

H₃C—N

Hyoscine

Fig. 5.4.36: Chemical constituents of Hyoscyamus

Uses: Henbane has a very long history of use as a medicinal herb. It is used extensively as a sedative and pain killer and is specifically used for pain affecting the urinary tract, especially when due to kidney stones. Its sedative and antispasmodic effect makes it a valuable treatment for the symptoms of Parkinson's disease, relieving tremor and rigidity during the early stages of the disease.

QUINOLINE ALKALOIDS

Cinchona (Fig. 5.4.37)

Synonyms: English—Cinchona bark; Jesuit's bark; peruvian bark

Biological source: It consists of the dried bark of cultivated trees of *Cinchona calisaya, C. ledgeriana, C. officinalis,* and *C. succirubra* (Rubiaceae), or of hybrids of these containing not less than 6% of total alkaloids.

Habitat: It is found in India, Bolivia, Columbia, Indonesia and Sri Lanka it is cultivated in Nilgiri hills and Tamil Nadu.

Botany

- Kingdom   Plantae
- Order   Gentianales
- Family   Rubiaceae
- Genus   Cinchona
- Species   *calisaya, ledgeriana, officinalis, succirubra.*

Part used: Bark

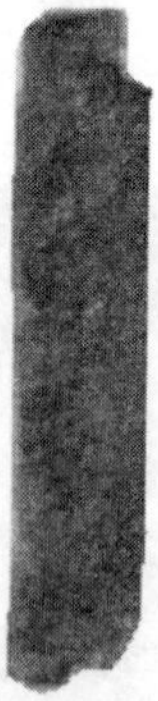

Fig. 5.4.37: Cinchona bark
(*see also in colour Plate 7*)

Organoleptic Characters

Odor: Slight and characteristic
Taste: Bitter

Drugs Derived from Natural Sources

Table 5.4.4: Macroscopic characters of types of cinchona

Characters	C. calisaya	C. ledgeriana	C. officinalis	C. succirubra
Color	Cinnamon brown	Cinnamon brown	Yellow	Reddish brown
Size	12–25 mm in diameter and 2–5 mm thick	12–25 mm in diameter and 2–5 mm thick	12 mm in diameter and 1.5 mm thick	20–40 mm in diameter and 2–5 mm thick
Total alkaloids (%)	3–7	5–8	5–14	6–16
Quinine content (%)	0–4	2–7.5	3–13	4–14

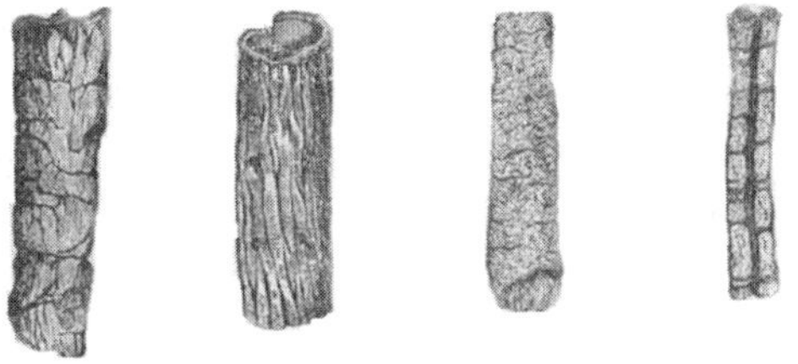

C.calisaya C.succirubra C.officinalis C.ledgeriana

Fig. 5.4.38: Types of Cinchona
(*see also in colour Plate 7*)

Types of Cinchona
(Fig. 5.4.38 and Table 5.4.4)

C. calisaya **Weddell:** It is tall, and trunk is often more than two feet in diameter. Leaves petiolate, the blade ovate-oblong to slightly obovate, 7 to 17.5 cm long by 2.5 to 7 cm broad, and obtuse.

C. ledgeriana **Moens:** It is formerly recognized as a variety of *C. calisaya*, differs from the type chiefly in its thicker, narrower, oblong leaves, with attenuate base, often bluish-green below. It yields a thick and remarkably rich bark, and is probably the most valued of all the cinchonas.

C. succirubra **Pavon, Mas:** It is of extreme size, petiole pubescent, leaf ovate to oval, acute with a very short point, the base more or less narrowing, often 6 by 9 inches, dark green and smooth.

C. officinalis **Hooker fil:** Petioles smooth, cylindrical, and, like the veins, reddish; blade 10 to 12.5 cm long, varying from broadly oval to lanceolate, acute at both ends.

The cinchona bark consists of cork cells followed by phellogen. The cortex consists of several secretory channels and phloem fibres. Medullary rays with radially arranged cells are present. The starch grains and stone cells are also present.

Microscopic Characters (Fig. 5.4.39)

Chemical constituents (Fig. 5.4.39): The principal dried barks, used for the production of the salts of the cinchona alkaloids, are: red cinchona bark, from *C. succirubra*, yielding

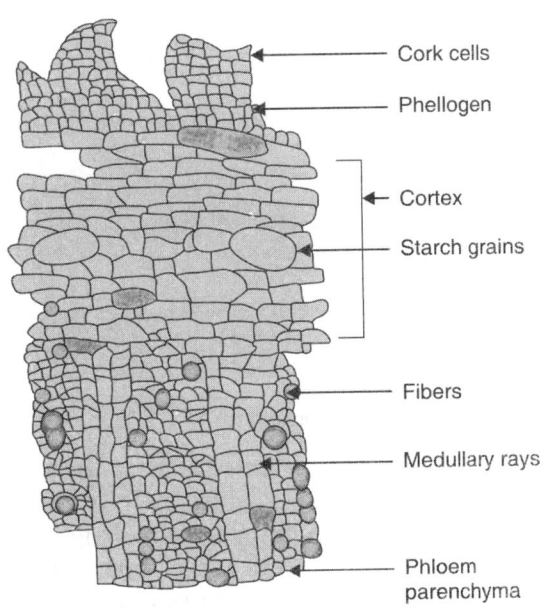

Fig. 5.4.39: Transverse section of cinchona bark

6 to 9% of total alkaloids; yellow cinchona bark, from *C. calisaya*, yielding 6 to 7% of alkaloids, 3 to 4% being quinine; pale cinchona bark (crown or Loxa bark), from *C. officinalis*, yielding about 6% of alkaloids half being quinine; ledger bark, from *C. ledgeriana*, yielding 10 to 14% of quinine. Hybrid bark, usually a hybrid between *C. ledgeriana* and *C. succirubra*, forms a large proportion of the bark of commerce and yields a high percentage of quinine.

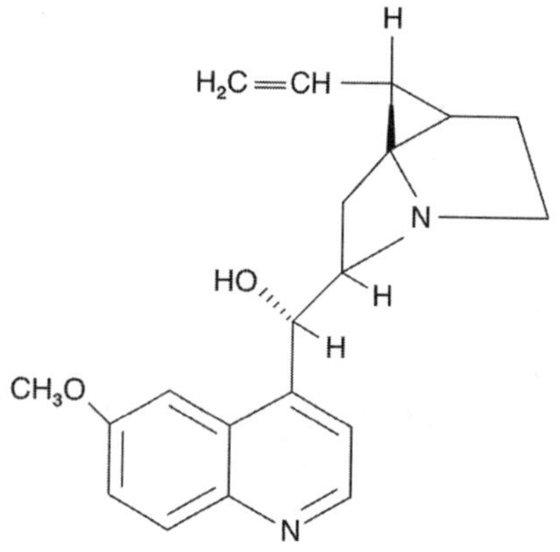

Fig. 5.4.40: Chemical constituents of cinchona

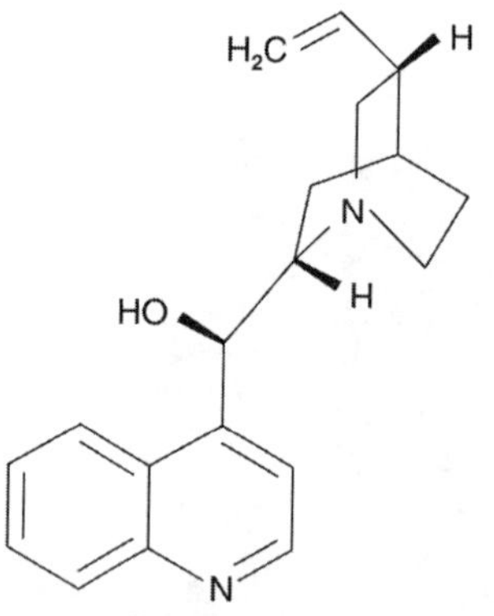

Chemical test: Heat the powered drug in dry test tube with glacial acetic acid purple vapors are produced in upper part of test tube.

Uses: Cinchona is a bitter stomachic and has astringent properties. It may sometimes cause vomiting and if taken over long periods may give rise to symptoms of cinchonism. It is used as an antimalarial, bitter digestive aid, antiparasitic, antispasmodic, febrifuge (reduces fever).

AMINO ALKALOIDS

Ephedra (Fig. 5.4.41)

Synonyms: Ma-Huang

Biological source: It consists of dried stems of *Ephedra gerardiana* and *E. nebrodensis*, belonging to family Gnetaceae (Ephedraceae).

Habitat: The main source is Australia, China, Kenya and Pakistan.

Botany

- Kingdom   Plantae
- Family   Ephedraceae
- Genus   *Ephedra*
- Species   *gerardiana, nebrodensis*

Parts used: Stems, root

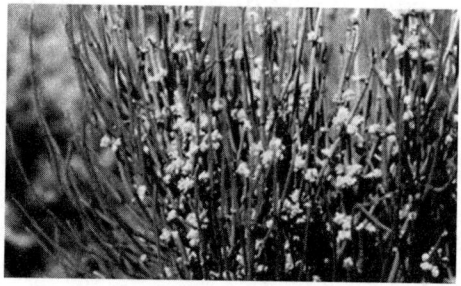

Fig. 5.4.41: Ephedra
(*see also in colour Plate 7*)

Organoleptic Characters

Macroscopic characters (Fig. 5.4.42)
Color: Greenish green
Shape: Woody, cylindrical
Size: 5 mm in diameter
Extra features: It is gymnospermous plant bearing stems. It shows internodes at distance of about 3 to 3.5 cm.

Ephedra species include methylephedrine, methyl-pseudoephedrine, pseudoephedrine, nor-pseudoephedrine (cathine), norephedrine, ephedine, ephedroxane, and pseudoephedroxane. Other compounds include a volatile oil, ephedrans, catechin, gallic acid, tannins, flavonoids, inulin, dextrin, starch, pectin and some common plant acids, sugars, and trace minerals. The root contains ephedradines, feruloylhistamine, moakonine, and mahuannins. The woody stems contain the alkaloids, which are almost always absent from the fruit and root.

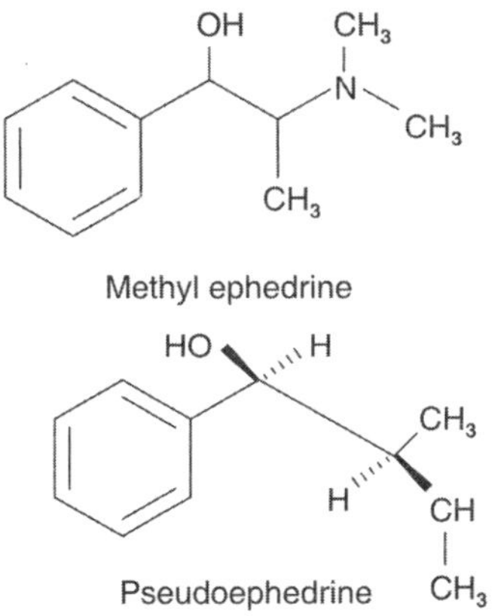

Chemical test: Ephedrine shaken with solvent ether shows purple color and aqueous layer shows blue color.

Uses: Ephedra has been used for arthralgia, bronchial asthma, chills, colds, coughs, edema, fever, flu, headaches, and nasal congestion. In the West, it is commonly used for its CNS stimulant properties ("natural ecstasy") and as an appetite suppressant ("natural fenphen"). Ephedrine produces mydriasis, enhances myocardial contraction and increases heart rate, causes bronchodilation, decreases GI motility, and stimulates peripheral vasoconstriction with an associated elevation in blood pressure.

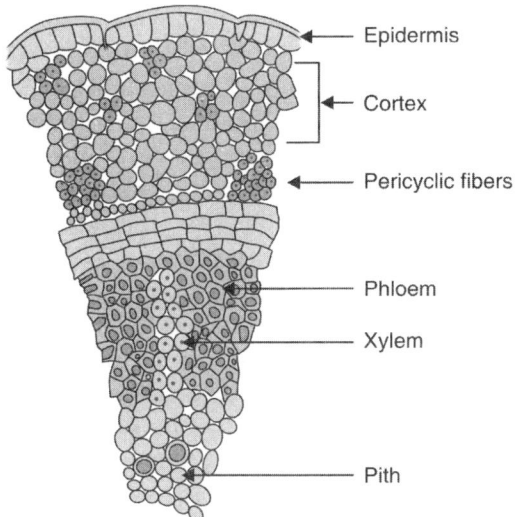

Fig. 5.4.42: Transverse section of ephedra

Microscopic Characters

The T.S. of ephedra shows unicellular epidermis, stomata and chlorenchymatous cortex with non-lignified hypodermal fibers and lignified pericyclic fibers. It also contains crystals of parenchyma.

Chemical constituents (Fig. 5.4.43): The primary active ingredient is the alkaloid ephedrine 0.5 to 2.5%. *E. equisetina* contains the most ephedrine, whereas the American species, *E. nevadensis* and *E. trifurea*, lack the agent. Other alkaloids commonly found in

Fig. 5.4.43: Chemical constituents of ephedra

5.5 TANNINS

Tannins are astringent, bitter plant polyphenols that either bind and precipitate or shrink proteins and various other organic compounds including amino acids and alkaloids. Tannins are distributed in species throughout the plant kingdom. They are commonly found in both gymnosperms as well as angiosperms. Botanically, tannins are mainly physically located in the vacuoles or surface wax of plants. These storage sites keep tannins active against plant predators. Tannins are found in leaf, bud, seed, root, and stem tissues.

There are three major classes of tannins:
1. Hydrolyzable tannins

2. Non-hydrolyzable tannins or condensed tannins
3. Pseudotannins

Hydrolyzable Tannin

Hydrolyzable tannins are mixtures of polygalloyl glucoses and/or polygalloyl quinic acid derivatives containing in between 3 up to 12 gallic acid residues per molecule. Hydrolyzable tannins are hydrolyzed by weak acids or weak bases to produce carbohydrate and phenolic acids. They are tannins on heating with hydrochloric or sulphuric acids yield gallic or ellagic acids. While hydrolyzable tannins and most condensed tannins are water soluble. Examples of gallotannins are the gallic acid esters of glucose in tannic acid ($C_{76}H_{52}O_{46}$), found in the leaves and bark of many plant species.

Non-hydrolyzable or Condensed Tannin

Condensed tannins, also known as proanthocyanidins, are polymers of 2 to 50 (or more) flavonoid units that are joined by carbon-carbon bonds, which are not susceptible to being cleaved by hydrolysis. They on heating with hydrochloric acid yield phlobaphenes, like phloroglucinol. Some very large condensed tannins are insoluble.

Condensed tannins from *Lithocarpus glaber* leaves have been analyzed through acid-catalyzed degradation in the presence of cysteamine and have a potent free radical scavenging activity.

Pseudotannins

Pseudotannins are low molecular weight, compounds associated with other compounds. They do not answer gold beater skin test unlike hydrolyzable and condensed tannins.

Properties of Tannins

Hydrolyzable tannins are yellow-brown amorphous substances which dissolve in hot water to form colloidal dispersions. They are astringent and have the ability to tan hide. Chemically speaking, they are esters which can be hydrolyzed by boiling with dilute acid to yield a phenolic compound, usually a derivative of gallic acid, and a sugar. These are often referred to as pyrogallol tannins.

Condensed tannins are polymers of phenolic compounds related to the flavonoids and are similar in general properties to the hydrolysed tannins but are not very soluble in water and following treatment with boiling dilute acid red-brown insoluble polymers known as phlabaphenes or tannins-red are formed.

Chemical Test of Tannins

Gelatin-block test: This test employs aqueous extract prepared from 80% ethanol extracted plant material. A sodium chloride solution is added to one portion of the test extract, of 1% gelatine solution to a second portion, and the gelatin salt reagent to a third portion. Precipitation with the latter reagent or with both the gelatine and gelatine-salt reagents is indicative of the presence of tannins. If precipitation is observed only with the salt solution, a false-positive test is indicated. Positive test is confirmed by the addition of ferric chloride solution to the extract and should result in a blue, blue-black, green or blue-green color and precipitate.

Gambier fluorescein test: The powdered drug is boiled with alcohol and filtered, and to the filtrate solution, NaOH is added, stirred and few ml of light petroleum is added. The petroleum layer shows green fluorescence.

Extraction of Tannins

The process used to extract tannins is the hydrosolubilization. Because this process operates with temperatures around 100°C, the extraction process motives a hydro cracking of sugar and other organic compounds with a darkening of the final product. The supercritical extraction process as alternative procedure to obtain the natural raw material to leather tannage. In which, supercritical carbon dioxide and polar or non-polar co-solvents were used as solvents.

The advantages of supercritical extraction process with regard to hydrosolubilization and solvent extraction are low extraction temperature, short extraction time and absence organic solvent concentration in the extract.

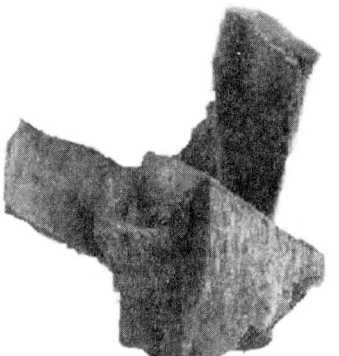

Fig. 5.5.1: Arjuna bark
(see also in colour Plate 7)

Arjuna Bark (Fig. 5.5.1)

Synonyms: Sanskrit—Arjuna; **English**—Arjuna myrobalan; **Hindi**—Arjun, Kahu; **Guj.**—Sajadan.

Biological Source: Arjuna is dried bark of *Terminalia arjuna*, family Combretaceae.

Origin: *Terminalia arjuna* is common throughout India especially in the sub-Himalayan tracts and eastern India.

Botany

- Kingdom   Plantae
- Division   Magnoliophyta
- Class   Magnoliopsida
- Order   Myrtales
- Family   Combretaceae
- Genus   *Terminalia*
- Species   *arjuna*

Organoleptic Characters

Color: Externally, it is pink or flesh colored with mealy coating and internal surface is reddish brown.

Odor: None

Taste: Gritty and astringent

Fracture: Fibrous

Size: Varying size with 5 to 10 mm thickness

Extra features: 40 meters high deciduous tree. Leaves are simple, 4–6' long oppositely arranged, rectangular or oval. At the base of the lamina, two glands are present. Flower: Green and star-like spikes, calyx smooth. Fruit: Truncate.

Chemical constituents: The bark contains specific medicinal active constituents namely triterpene glycosides like arjenetosides I, II, III, IV, arjunine and arjunetin (Fig. 5.5.2). It is also rich in saponins, natural antioxidants (flavonoids—arjunone, arjunolone, leteilin) gallic acid, ellagic acid, oligomeric proanthocyanidins, phytosterols, rich in minerals like calcium, magnesium, zinc and copper.

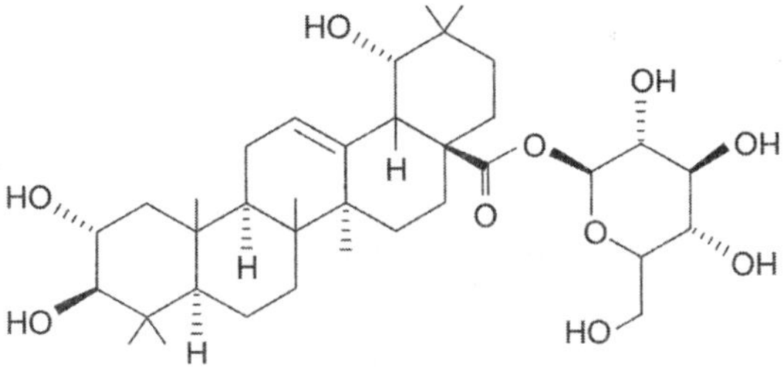

Fig. 5.5.2: Arjunetic

Chemical Test (Table 5.5.1)

Fluorescence analysis: The fluorescence analysis is carried out with 10% extract of ether and petroleum ether in UV chamber.

Table 5.5.1: Comparative chemical test		
Chemicals	T. arjuna	T. tomentosa
Ether	Pinkish white	Pale blue
Petroleum Ether	Bright pinkish red	Pale white blue

Uses: The bark is astringent, sweet, acrid, cooling, aphrodisiac, cardiotonic, urinary astringent, expectorant, alexiteric and is useful in fractures, ulcers, cirrhosis of the liver, hyperhidrosis, otalgia and hypertension.

Adulterants: *Terminalia tomentosa* (dried bark). It is distinguished by Arjuna bark by fluorescence test.

Ashoka Bark (Fig. 5.5.3)

Synonyms: Sanskrit—Ashoka; **English**—Ashoka tree; **Gujrati**—Asupala; **Telegu**—Asok.

Biological source: Ashoka is dried bark of *Saraca indica*, family Leguminosae.

Habitat: India, abundantly found in central and eastern Himalayas and extending up to Burma.

Botany

- Kingdom   Plantae
- Division   Magnoliophyta
- Class   Magnoliopsida
- Order   Fabales
- Family   Fabaceae/leguminosae
- Genus   *Saraca*
- Species   *indica*

Organoleptic Characters

Color: Outer surface: Rough, rusty brown in color; Inner surface: Smooth, reddish-brown in color.

Odor: Indistinct

Taste: Astringent

Size: 40 cm in length, 3–6 cm wide, and 5–8 mm thick.

Fracture: Short and fibrous

Chemical constituents: It contains condensed tannins, catechol (Fig. 5.5.4), sterol, ketosterol and organic calcium compound.

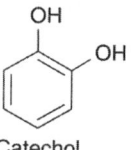

Fig. 5.5.4: Catechol

Chemical Test

1. With ferric chloride, it shows green color.
2. With bromine water, it gives ppt.
3. With vanillin: Alcohol: Dil HCl (1:10:10), it gives red color.

Uses: Menorrhagia (scant menses), dysmenorrhea (painful menses, menstrual cramps), depression, bleeding hemorrhoids, uterine fibroids, considered a uterine sedative and tonic.

Adulterants: Bark of *Polyalthia longifolia* (Anonaceae).

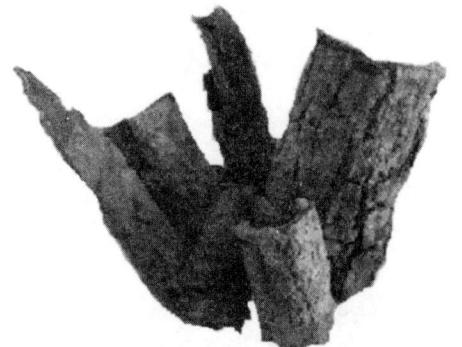

Fig. 5.5.3: Ashoka bark
(*see also in colour Plate 8*)

Amla (Fig. 5.5.5)

Synonyms: **Sanskrit**—Dhatri-pala; **English**—Indian gooseberry, emblic myrobalan; **Hindi**—Amla, Amlika.

Biological source: It consists of fruits of *Emblica officinalis*, belonging to family Euphorbiaceae.

Origin: It is found throughout India till the height of 4500 feet.

Botany

- Kingdom   Plantae
- Division   Flowering plant
- Class   Magnoliopsida
- Order   Malpighiales
- Family   Phyllanthaceae
- Tribe   Phyllantheae
- Subtribe   Flueggeinae
- Genus   *Phyllanthus*
- Species   *emblica*

Parts used: Fresh fruit, dried fruit, the nut or seed, leaves, root, bark and flowers. Ripe fruits used generally fresh, dry also used.

Organoleptic Characters

Color: Green when unripe and light yellow when mature.

Odor: None

Taste: Sour, slightly bitter.

Size: 1.3–1.6 cm in diameter.

Extra features: Fruits are globose and depressed six-lobed, hard and smooth in appearance.

Chemical constituents (Fig. 5.5.6): The major chemical constituents of Amla are phyllemblin, ascorbic acid (vitamin C), gallic acid, tannins, pectin, etc. It contains 81.2% moisture, 0.5% proteins, 0.1% fats, carbohydrates 14.1%, calcium 0.05%, phosphorus 0.02%, iron 1.2 mg and nicotinic acid 0.2 per 100 gm.

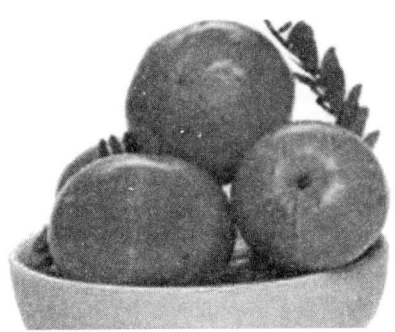

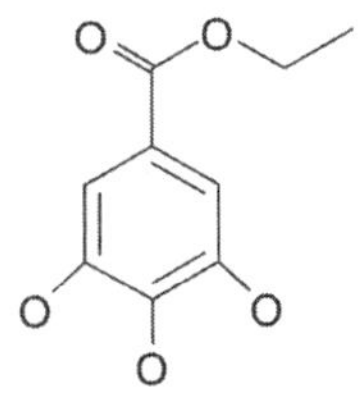

Fig. 5.5.5: Amla fruit
(*see also in colour Plate 8*)

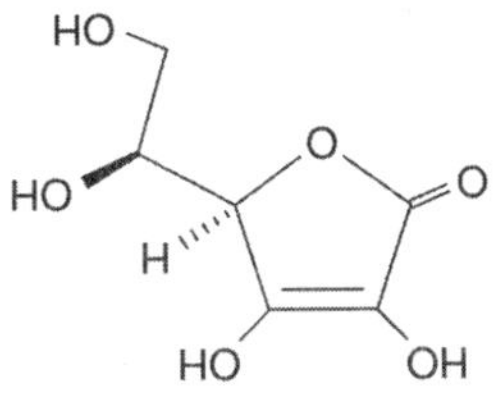

Fig. 5.5.6: Chemical constituents of amla

Chemical Test

1. To 0.5 g of powder, add 10 ml of hot water, allowed to stand for 5 min, shake frequently and filter. Add 1% gelatin containing 10% NaCl to 5 ml of filtrate; milky white color is produced.

2. To the aqueous solution of amla, add lead acetate or gelatin, remove precipitate by filtration. To the filtrate, add solution of 2, 6 dicholorophenol indophenol, colors disappear.

Standards

- Foreign matter: NLT 3.0%
- Total ash: NMT 5.0%
- Acid-insoluble ash: NMT 2.0%
- Alcohol-soluble extractive: NLT 40.0%
- Water-soluble extractive: NLT 40.0%

Uses: Amla is a wonder herb with numerous indications. Due to its sheet virya potency, it is widely used in diseases caused by *pitta* disorders. It has found an esteemed place in ayurvedic preparations. *Chawanprash, triphala* and *amlaki rasayan* possess dominance of Amla. It is used to substitute vitamin C in disease like scurvy. It has actions on all the systems of the body.

Bahera (Fig. 5.5.7)

Synonyms: Sans.—Vibhitaki; **Hindi**—Bahera, Bhaira; **Ben.**—Bohera,

Biological source: It is obtained from fruits of *Terminalia belerica*, family Combretaceae.
Habitat: A tree common in Indian forest and plant.

Botany

- Kingdom   Plantae
- Family   Combretaceae
- Genus   *Terminalia*
- Species   *belerica*

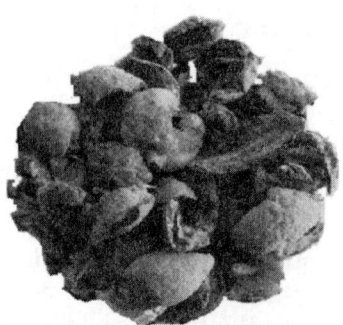

Fig. 5.5.7: Bahera fruits
(*see also in colour Plate 8*)

Organoleptic Characters

Color: Grey-velvetty wooly hairs with a hard thick-walled light yellow putamen
Odor: Offensive
Taste: Astringent in taste, sweet in the post-digestive effect and has hot potency
Size: 1.3 to 1.9 cm in diameter
Shape: Dry fleshy drupe, globose or ovoid
Extra features: Fruit is hard due to its endocarp and it exhibits a yellow internal surface projecting threads which represents vascular bundles.

Chemical constituents: The fruit contains moisture 6%, tannin 21% (which comprises both condensed and hydrolysable types), water extractable 44%. Fruits contain a green fixed oil, saponin, tannins, a resitious residue and three amorphous and hygroscopic glycosidal compounds. The fruit pulp contains a non-nitrogenous crystalline substance. Kernles yield yellow fatty oil containing fatty acids. The seeds contain protein and oxalic acid, while bark contains tannin. Its oil contains palmitic, oleic and linoleic acids as major fatty acids. A new cardiac glycoside-bellericnin isolated which yielded glucose and galactose (2:1) sitosterol, gallic acid (Fig. 5.5.8), ellagic acid, ethyl gallate, galloyl glucose and chebulagic acid isolated from fruits.

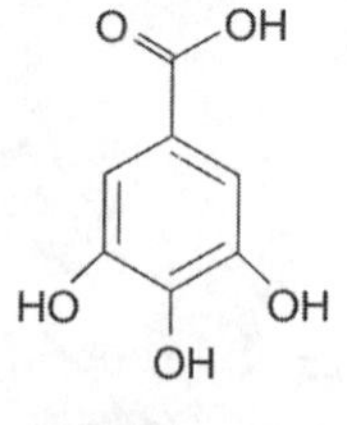

Fig. 5.5.8: Gallic acid

Chemical Test

Test for gallic acid: It gives blue color when treated with ferric chloride solution
Uses: The fruits are useful in stomach disorder, such as indigestion, diarrhea. It is

given also as a brain tonic and is applied on eyes as a soothing lotion. Baheda is useful in piles, leprosy, dropsy and fever. The half-dried fruits are considered to be purgative but the ripe and dried fruits have the opposite property. The Baheda fruit is one of the three constituents of the *Triphala*.

Myrobalan (Fig. 5.5.9)

Synonyms: Bengali—Haritaki, Harida; **Hindi**—Harad, Harar; **English**—Chebulic myrobalan.

Biological source: It consists of dried, ripe and fully matured fruits of *Terminalia chebula* Retzr belonging to family Combretaceae.

Habitat: Organic chebula is found all over India from eastern to western region.

Botany

- Kingdom   Plantae
- Division   Magnoliophyta
- Class   Magnoliopsida
- Order   Myrtales
- Family   Combretaceae
- Genus   *Terminalia*
- Species   *chebula*

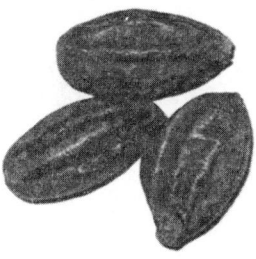

Fig. 5.5.9: Myrobalan fruits
(*see also in colour Plate 8*)

Organoleptic Characters

Color: Yellowish brown
Odor: Odorless
Taste: Astringent, slightly bitter and sweetest at the end.

Size: 20 to 25 mm long and 15 to 25 mm wide.
Shape: Ovate and wrinkled longitudinally.
Extra features: The fruits are hard and stony with single seed which is yellow in color and 15 to 320 mm in length. The pulp of fruit is non-adherent to the seed.

Chemical constituents: Myrobalan fruits are the important source of tannin. The tannins of myrobalan are pyrogallol type (hydrolyzable tannin). Choplogic acid, chebulinic acid (Fig. 5.5.10) and corilagin are the hydrolyzable tannin while cherubic acid, ellagic acid and gallic acid are the other contents. It is also contain glucose, orbital, gentiobiose and other sugars in traces.

Standards

- Foreign matter: NMT 2.0%
- Total ash: NMT 5.0%
- Acid-insoluble ash: NMT 2.0%
- Alcohol-soluble extractive: NLT 35.0%
- Water-soluble extractive: NLT 32.0%
- Loss on drying: NMT 11.0%

Chemical test: Alcoholic/aqueous solution of myrobalan treated with 10% ferric chloride gives deep blue color and with lead acetate gives white precipitate.

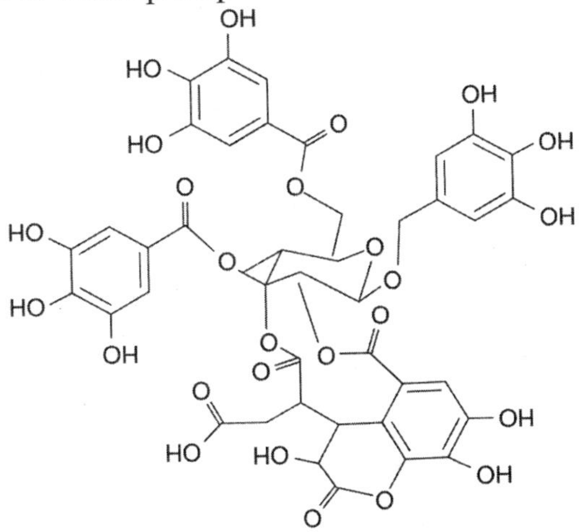

Fig. 5.5.10: Chebulinic acid

Uses: *Terminalia chebula* is used to treat many diseases such as digestive diseases, urinary diseases, diabetes, skin diseases, parasitic infections, heart diseases, irregular fevers, flatulence, constipation, ulcers, vomiting, colic pain and hemorrhoids. It promotes wisdom, intellect and eyesight. *Terminalia chebula* has a strong effect against the herpes simplex virus (HSV), has antibacterial activity and exhibits strong cardiotonic properties. It is good antioxidant also.

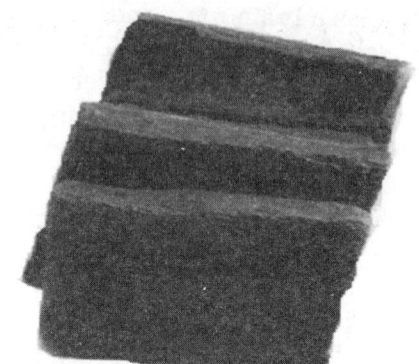

Fig. 5.5.11: Catechu
(see also in colour Plate 8)

Catechu (Fig. 5.5.11)

Synonyms: Hindi—Katha, Khair; **Bengali**—Khayera; **Gujarati**—Kher; **Telegu**—Kachu.

Biological source: Black catechu consists of dried bark or dried aqueous extract of heartwood of *Acacia catechu* belonging to family Leguminosae.

Pale catechu consists of leaves and young shoots of *Uncaria gambier* Rox, family Rubiaceae. The pale catechu is differentiated from black by its pale color and light weight.

Habitat: Widely distributed in East Africa, Andhara Pradesh, Bihar, Punjab and Himalayas.

Botany

- Kingdom   Plantae
- Division   Magnoliophyta
- Class   Liliopsida
- Order   Arecales
- Family   Leguminosae
- Subfamily   Arecoideae
- Genus   *Acacia*
- Species   *catechu*

Organoleptic Characters

Color: Light brown to black
Odor: None

Taste: Astringent
Shape: Cubes or irregular fragments
Size: 2 to 5 cm
Extra features: Pieces are friable, porous with vegetable debris, fracture short soluble in water and alcohol.

Chemical constituents (Fig. 5.5.13): Main chemical constituents of heartwood are tannins—condensed tannins, catechin (2–12%), catechuic acid, pyrocatechin, epicatechin, dicatechin, phloroglucin, protocatechuic acid, quercetin, gum, kaempferol, gossyptin and mineral.

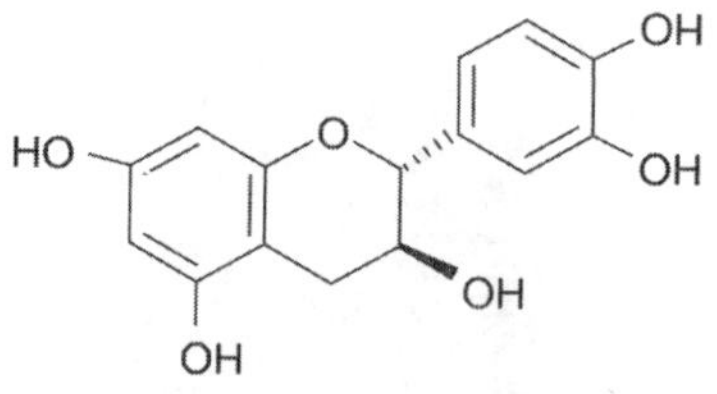

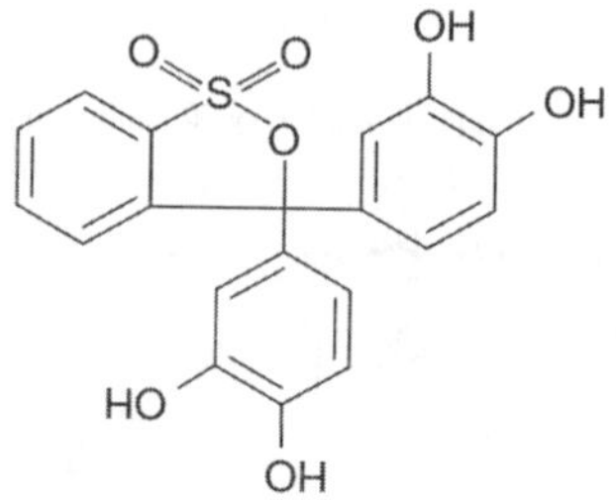

Fig. 5.5.12: Chemical constituents of catechin

Chemical Test

- **Gambier fluorescein test:** The powdered drug is boiled with alcohol and filtered and to the filtrate solution of NaOH is added stirred and a few ml of light petroleum is added. The petroleum layer shows green florescence. Black catechu does not respond to this test.
- Catechu gives bluish black color with ferric chloride solution.
- Pink and red color with vanillin and HCl.
- Brown color with lime water.

Standards

- Total ash: NMT 6.0%
- Acid-insoluble ash: NMT 3%
- Alcohol-soluble extractive: NLT 40.0%
- Water-soluble extractive: NLT 50.0%

Uses

1. It is useful in stomach problems, like diarrhea, dysentery, colitis and gastric cancer.
2. It is used as mouthwash for mouth, gum and throat diseases like gingivitis, stomatitis.
3. It is used in high blood pressure.
4. It is used as astringent and helpful in pharyngitis, and hemorrhages.

Substitutes and adulterants: *Rhizovhora mangle* Linn, *Ceriops candolleana* Arnold, family Rhizophoraceae.

5.6 LIPIDS, FATS AND WAXES

LIPIDS (Table 5.6.1)

Lipids contain the elements carbon, hydrogen and oxygen but have a lower proportion of oxygen in the molecule than carbohydrates. With the exception of glycerol they are insoluble in water, but dissolve in organic solvents such as ether, chloroform and benzene. They are lighter (less dense) than water.

Table 5.6.1: Functions of lipids with examples

S.no.	Functions of lipids	Examples
1.	Cell membrane components	Phospholipids, glycolipids, cholesterol
2.	Fat transporters	Lipoproteins (e.g. like high density and low-density lipoproteins)
3.	Storage of excess energy	FAs in TAGs
4.	Thermal insulation	Nonpolar lipids
5.	Major source of caloric energy	
	Energy source as a mobile respiratory substrate	Glycerol, fatty acids
	Energy store as a insoluble respiratory substrate	Fats in animal, oils in plants (seeds).
6.	Essential for normal growth and function	Docosahexaenoic acid (DHA for brain development)
7.	Precursors of hormones, coenzymes and chemical mediators prostaglandins,	Vitamins (A, D, E, K), thromboxanes, prostacyclins
8.	Bioeffectors/bioregulators	Phosphatidylinositol
9.	Others	As enzyme cofactors in electron carriers as light absorbing pigments, as fat, soluble vitamins (terpenes). Intracellular messengers and hydrophobic anchors which provide buoyancy in aquatic animals (fats). Waxes act as an water-proofing material on the surface of leaves and insects

Classification of Lipids

1. Simple Lipids

Esters of fatty acids with various alcohols.

a. **Fats and oils:** Chemically, fats are triesters of glycerols and fatty acids. Fats may be either solid or liquid at room temperature.

Oils are fats that are in liquid state at normal room temperature.

b. **Waxes:** Chemically, waxes are esters of fatty acids with higher molecular weight monohydric alcohols as cetyl alcohol ($C_{16}H_{33}OH$) or cholesterol. They are a mixture of long-chain apolar lipids forming a protective coating (cutin in the cuticle) on plant leaves and fruits and also in animals.

Example: Cetyl, meryl, merecyl alcohol.

2. Compound (or Complex) Lipids

Esters of fatty acids with alcohol containing additional groups, such as phosphate, nitrogenous base, carbohydrates or protein, etc.

a. **Phospholipids:** Chemically, glycerol forms ester links with two fatty acid molecules and with one phosphate group. The phosphate group can ionize (become polarized) and so becomes water-soluble but the fatty acid tails are non-polar and remain water-insoluble. The possession of both hydrophilic and hydrophobic groups is a very important biological property. Sphingophospholipids are phospholipids with sphingosine as alcohol, e.g. sphingomyeline.

b. **Glycolipids (glycosphingolipids):** Glycolipids (molecular complexes of lipid and polysaccharides) are found on the outside of cell membranes as the glycocalyx. This is involved in cell to cell recognition and communication, particularly during growth and development. They may also be used as infection sites by viruses and bacteria.

3. **Derived lipids:** These include by-products of metabolic processes like fatty acids, glycerol, mono- and diacylglycerols, lysophosphatides, fatty aldehydes, ketone bodies.

4. **Steroid lipids:** Steroids are lipids because they are hydrophobic and insoluble in water, but they do not resemble lipids Example: Cholesterol, cholesteryl esters, cholesterol derivatives: bile acids, steroid hormones, vitamin D, phytosterols. Because they are uncharged, also they are termed **neutral lipids**.

5. **Miscellaneous lipids:** Aliphatic hydrocarbons, carotenoids, squalene, terpenes (composed of isoprene units), vitamin E and K, glycerol ether, glycosyl glycerols (in plants).

Analytical Parameters for Fats and Oils

- *Physical constants:* Viscosity, specific gravity, refractive index, solidification point.
- *Chemical constants:* Iodine value, acid value, peroxide value, saponification value, unsaponifiable matter.

The brief idea of some analytical parameters of chemical constant is as follows:

Iodine value: Iodine number is the determination of the amount of unsaturation contained in fatty acids. The iodine value (or "iodine adsorption value" or "iodine number" or "iodine index") is the mass of iodine in grams that is consumed by 100 grams of a chemical substance.

Acid value: Acid value (or "neutralization number" or "acid number" or "acidity") is the mass of potassium hydroxide (KOH) in milligrams that is required to neutralize one gram of chemical substance. The acid number is a measure of the amount of carboxylic acid groups in a chemical compound, such as a fatty acid, or in a mixture of compounds.

$$\text{Acid value} = \frac{\text{Volume (ml) of 0.1 Mol/l ethanolic potassium hydroxide consumed}}{\text{Weight (g) of the sample}} \times 5.611$$

Peroxide value: Peroxide value is defined as the milliequivalents of peroxidises per kilogram of sample. It is used as a measurement of the extent to which rancidity reactions have occurred during storage.

Saponification value: Saponification value (or "saponification number") represents the number of milligrams of potassium hydroxide or sodium hydroxide required to saponify 1 g of fat under the conditions specified. It is a measure of the average molecular weight (or chain length) of all the fatty acids present.

$$\text{Saponification value} = \frac{(a-b) \times 28.05}{\text{Weight (g) of the sample}}$$

Where,
a = volume (ml) of 0.5 mol/l hydrochloric acid consumed in the blank test
b = volume (ml) of 0.5 mol/l hydrochloric acid consumed in the test.

Unsaponifiable matter: Unsaponifiables are components of an oily (oil, fat, wax) mixture that fail to form soaps. It includes sterols, oil-soluble vitamin, hydrocarbons and higher alcohols.

Ester value: The ester value is the number of mg of potassium hydroxide (KOH) required to saponify the esters in 1 g of a sample.

Ester value = Saponification value × Acid value

Hydroxyl value: The hydroxyl value is the number of mg of potassium hydroxide (KOH) required to neutralize acetic acid combined to hydroxyl groups.

$$\text{Hydroxyl value} = \frac{(a-b) \times 28.05}{\text{Weight (g) of the sample}} + \text{acid value}$$

Where,
a = volume (ml) of 0.5 mol/l ethanolic potassium hydroxide consumed in the blank test.
b = volume (ml) of 0.5 mol/l ethanolic potassium hydroxide consumed in the test.

Castor Oil (Fig. 5.6.1)

Synonyms: Palma christi. castor oil bush

Biological source: Castor oil is obtained from seeds of *Ricinus communis*, Family: Euphorbiaceae.

Habitat: It has been distributed throughout not only all tropical and subtropical regions, but also in many of the temperate countries of the globe.

Botany
- Kingdom   Plantae
- Phylum   Magnoliophyta
- Class   Magnoliopsida
- Order   Malpighiales
- Family   Euphorbiaceae
- Subfamily Acalyphoideae
- Genus   *Ricinus*
- Species   *communis*

Part used: Processed seed oil

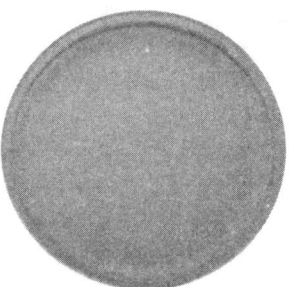

Fig. 5.6.1: Castor oil
(*see also in colour Plate 8*)

Organoleptic Characters

Color: Viscid fluid, almost colorless
Odor: Slight odor
Taste: Nauseous and disagreeable taste
Specific gravity: 0.96
Solubility: It dissolves freely in alcohol, ether and glacial acetic acid

Chemical constituents (Fig. 5.6.2): Castor oil consists chiefly of the glycerides of ricinoleic, isoricinoleic dihydroxystearic, and other acids. **Ricinolein** (Fig. 5.6.2) is the chief constituent of castor oil and is the triglyceride of ricinoleic acid (Table 5.6.2).

Table 5.6.2: Average composition of castor seed oil/fatty acid chains

Acid name	Average percentage range
Ricinoleic acid	85 to 95%
Oleic acid	6 to 2%
Linoleic acid	5 to 1%
Linolenic acid	1 to 0.5%
Stearic acid	1 to 0.5%
Palmitic acid	1 to 0.5%
Dihydroxystearic acid	0.5 to 0.3%
Others	0.5 to 0.2%

Chemical test: 10 ml of castor oil with 5 ml of light petroleum shows a clear solution. If light petroleum is increased to 15 ml, the mixture becomes turbid.

Uses: Castor oil is a well-known cleansing laxative and purgative. It is sometimes used to treat food poisoning. Externally, it is used for warts, fibroid cysts, appendicitis, sores, abscesses, and neuralgia. Castor oil is also the source for undecylenic acid, a natural fungicide.

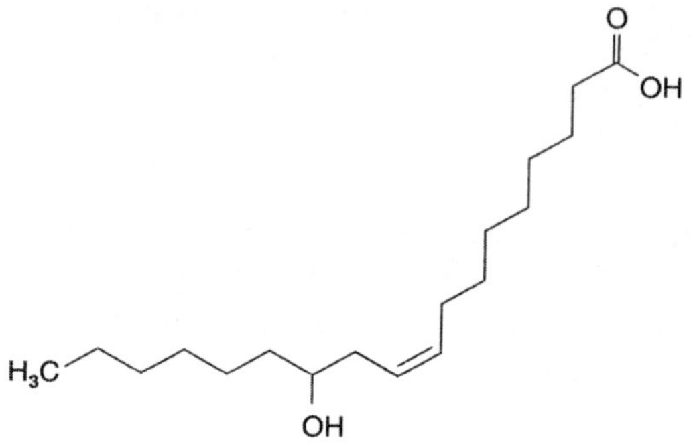

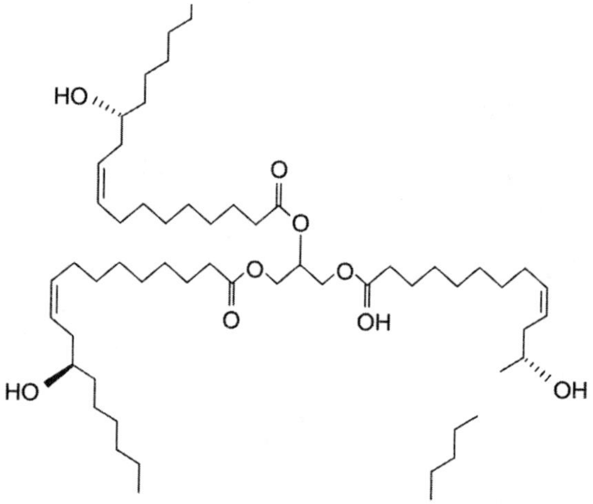

Fig. 5.6.2: Chemical constituents of castor oil

Linseed oil (Table 5.6.3)

Synonyms—Hindi: Alsi; **English**—Flax seeds

Biological source: It consists of dried ripe seeds of *Linum usitatissimum* Linn, containing NLT 25% of fixed oil, family Linaceae.

Habitat: Linseed is cultivated in many sub-tropical countries, such as South America, India, USA, Canada, England, Russia, Greece, Italy and Spain.

Botany

- Kingdom — Plantae
- Division — Magnoliophyta
- Class — Magnoliopsida
- Order — Malpighiales
- Family — Linaceae

- Genus   *Linum*
- Species   *usitatissimum*

Part used: Dried ripe seeds

Organoleptic Characters

Color: Brown

Odor: Odorless

Taste: Mucilaginous, oily

Size: 4–6 mm long, 1–2 mm thick

Shape: Elongated-ovoid, flattened

Extra features: Testa is hard, smooth and glossy in appearance.

Characters of Oil

- **Color:** Pale yellow clear liquid.
- **Taste:** Disagreeable but bland taste.
- **Solubility:** Slightly soluble in alcohol, soluble in organic solvents, insoluble in water.
- **Acid value:** NMT 4
- **Unsaponifiable matter:** NMT 1.5
- **Iodine value:** 160–200
- **Saponification value:** 188–195
- **Specific gravity:** 0.977 to 0.931
- **Refractive index:** 1.478 to 1.482

Chemical constituents: Linseed seeds contain fixed oil (30–40%), mucilage (6%), protein (25%), small amount of enzyme lipase and linamarin (Fig. 5.6.3). Carbohydrates present are sucrose, raffinose, cellulose and mucilage.

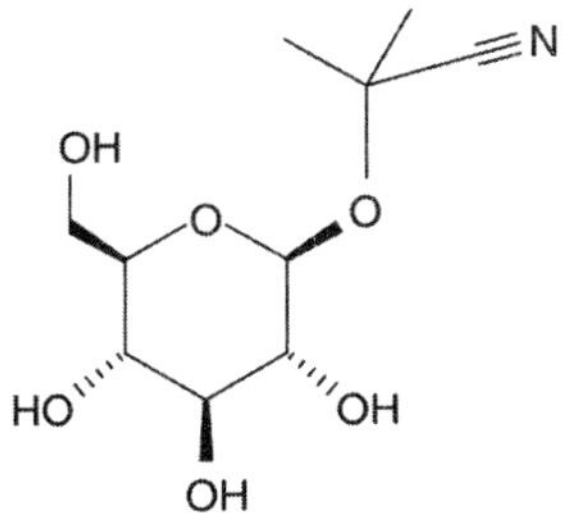

Table 5.6.3: Average composition of linseed oil

Acid name	Average % range
Palmitic acid	6%
Oleic acid	18.5 to 22.6%
Stearic acid	2.5%
Arachidic acid	0.5
Linoleic acid	24.1
Alpha-linolenic acid	47.4
Other	0.5

Chemical test: With ruthenium red, it gives red color.

Uses: It is used to make demulcent and in constipation. Linseed oil has emollient, expectorant, diuretic, demulcent and laxative properties. Treated linseed oil is also added to things, like paints, resins, varnishes, and inks. Painters use linseed oil as a carrier oil for their paints.

Adulterants: Linseed oil is adulterated with vegetable oils, such as rape, cottonseed, soyabean, sunflower and candlenut.

Fig. 5.6.3: Linamarin

Olive Oil

Synonyms: Salad oil, sweet oil, oleum olival.

Biological source: Olive oil is a fixed oil obtained by expression of ripe fruits of *Olea europaea* Linn, family Oleaceae.

Habitat: California, Southern Australia.

Botany

- Kingdom   Plantea
- Order   Lamiales
- Family   Oleaceae
- Genus   *Olea*
- Species   *europaea*

Part used: Ripe fruits

Organoleptic Characters

Color: Yellowish to greenish yellow
Odor: Slight and characteristic
Taste: Bland and faintly acrid
Size and shape: Liquid

Chemical constituents (Fig. 5.6.4): It contains mixed glycerides of oleic acid (83.5%), palmitic acid (9.4%), linoleic acid (7%), stearic acid (2%) and arachidic acid (0.9%), along with traces of squalene (up to 0.7%) and sterols (about 0.2%, phytosterol and tocosterols. Olive oil contains a group of related natural products with potent antioxidant properties and esters of tyrosol and hydroxytyrosol, including oleocanthal and oleuropein.

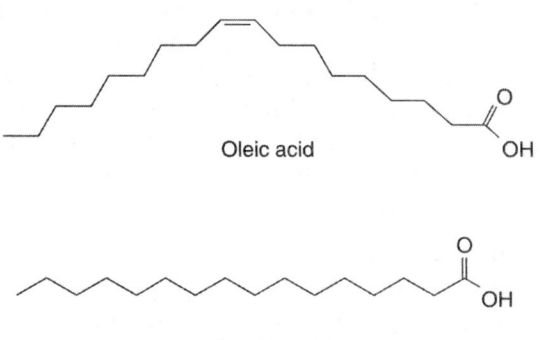

Fig. 5.6.4: Chemical constituents of olive oil

Characters of Olive Oil

- **Color:** Pale yellow or light greenish yellow
- **Taste:** Bland and acrid taste.
- **Odor:** Acrid odor
- **Solubility:** Slightly soluble in alcohol, miscible with ether, chloroform and carbon disulfide.
- **Acid value:** 0.2–2.8
- **Iodine value:** 79–90
- **Saponification value:** 187–196
- **Specific gravity:** 0.914 to 0.919
- **Refractive index:** 1.478 to 1.482

Chemical test: Under ultraviolet radiation, it gives deep yellow coloration.

Uses: Emollient and soothing agent, demulcent, mild laxative and nutritive.

Cod Liver Oil

Synonyms: Latin—Oleum Morrhuae; English—Codliver oil

Biological source: It is fixed oil obtained from the fresh livers of *Gadus morrhua* and other species of Gadus., family Gadidae.

Habitat: Oil is produced mainly in western Europe, including Germany and Denmark.

Botany

- Kingdom — Animalia
- Phylum — Chordata
- Class — Actinopterygii
- Order — Gadiformes
- Family — Gadidae
- Genus — *Gadus*
- Species — *morrhua*

Organoleptic Characters

Color: Pale yellow
Odor: Fishy odor
Taste: Fishy taste

Chemical constituents (Fig. 5.6.5): It has high levels of the omega-3 fatty acids, EPA and DHA, and very high levels of vitamin A, vitamin D and vitamin E. It also contains unsaturated acid (85%) and saturated acid (15%).

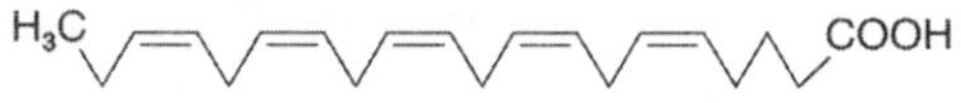

Eicosapentaenoic acid (EPA)

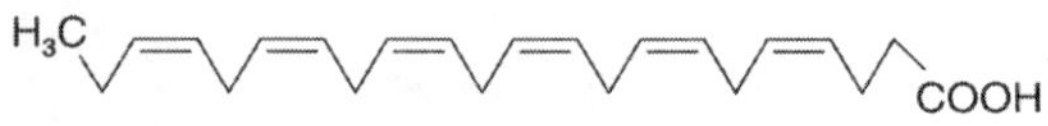

Docosahexaenoic acid (DHA)

Fig. 5.6.5: Chemical constituents of codliver oil

Characters of Cod Liver Oil

- Color: Pale yellow
- Taste: Slightly fishy
- Odor: Fishy and not rancid
- Solubility: Sparingly soluble in alcohol, readily soluble in ether and chloroform.
- Iodine value: 159–173

Chemical Test

Test for vitamin A: In 1 ml of chloroform, dissolve the quantity equal to 10–15 units of vitamin A and add 5 ml of antimony trichloride solution, a transient blue color is produced.

Test for vitamin D: In 1 ml chloroform, dissolve the quantity equal to 1000 units of vitamin D and add 10 ml of antimony trichloride solution, a pinkish red color appears.

Uses: Emollient, nutrient, tonic, alterative. It is employed in the treatment of tuberculosis, chronic bronchitis, rachitis, etc. and used externally for chronic skin diseases, as eczema.

Adulterants and substitutes: Cod liver oil is adulterated with other fish-liver oils and seal oil. Halibut liver oil is a fixed oil prepared from the livers of Halibut, *Hippogolossus vulgaris*, Family: Pleurnectidae. It has lot of vitamins A and D.

Neem oil

Synonyms: Margosa, Neem, Nim tree

Biological source: Neem oil is botanical oil, extracted from seeds and kernels of Neem tree (*Azadirachta indica*), a member of the Meliaceae family.

Habitat: South-east Asia, India, Pakistan, Sri Lanka, Burma and Malaya.

Parts used: Seeds and kernels

Organoleptic Characters

Nature: Hydrophobic
Color: Light to dark brown
Odor: Strong odor (like peanut and garlic)
Taste: Bitter
Solubility: Slightly soluble in water
pH: 6.5 to 7.5
Extra characters: It boils at more than 200°C and freeze at 13°C.

Chemical constituents: It comprises mainly triglycerides and large amounts of triterpenoid compounds, which are responsible for the bitter taste. Neem oil also contains steroids (campesterol, beta-sitosterol, and stigmasterol) and a plethora of triterpenoids. Most active compound in neem oil is azadirachtin A and B, out of which azadirachtin A is more active and is in abundance (Fig. 5.6.6). Active ingredients in neem oil include nimbin, meliantriol, salanin, meldenin, azadiradione, azadirone, isonimolicinolide, mahmoodin, nimbidinin, nimbonin, vepinin, etc.

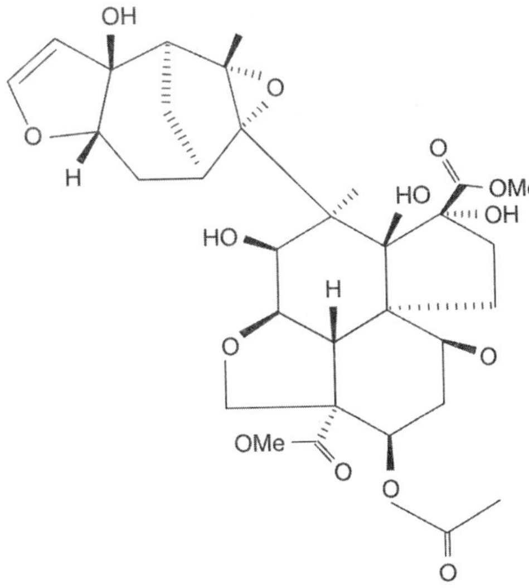

Fig. 5.6.6: Azadirachtin

Methods of extraction: The methods used for extraction is pressing (expelling) or solvent extraction. The oil can be obtained through pressing (crushing) of the seed kernel through cold pressing. Neem seed oil can also be obtained by solvent extraction of the neem seed, fruit, oil, cake or kernel.

Chemical Test

Test for terpenoids (Salkowski test): Five ml of oil mixed in 2 ml of chloroform, and concentrated H_2SO_4 (3 ml) added to form a layer. A reddish brown coloration of the interface will be formed to show positive results for the presence of terpenoids.

Uses

1. Neem oil is widely used in crop protection against insects, pests, nematodes, fungi, and virus.
2. Neem oil is used as veterinary medicines for pets.
3. Neem oil is used for preparation of various cosmetic and toiletries.

Cocoa Butter (Theobroma Oil) (Fig. 5.6.7)

Synonyms: Cocoa butter, semina theobromatis.
Biological source: Theobroma oil is obtained by expression of ground kernels of *Theobroma cacao* Linn (family Sterculiaceae).
Habitat: The chocolate tree (cocoa tree) is a native of tropical America and cultivated in Ecuador, Mexico, Central America, Sri Lanka, South India and Orissa.

Botany

- Kingdom   Plantae
- Order   Malvales
- Family   Malvaceae
- Genus   *Theobroma*
- Species   *cacao*

Part used: Seeds

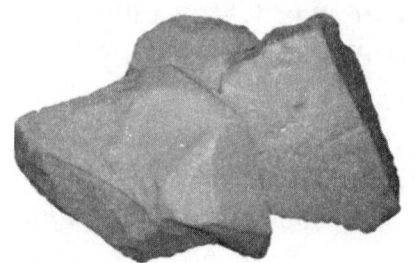

Fig. 5.6.7: Cocoa butter
(*see also in colour Plate 8*)

Organoleptic Characters

Color: Seed coat is chocolate brown in color
Odor: Chocolate
Taste: Chocolate
Size: 15 mm wide and 7 mm thick
Shape: Flattened-ovoid
Extra features: The kernel consists of two irregularly folded, chocolate-colored cotyledons.

Extraction of cocoa butter: Cocoa beans are ground into chocolate liquor and pressed to separate the cocoa butter from the cocoa solids. Cocoa butter can alternately be extracted from whole beans by the broma process. It is most often deodorized to remove its strong and undesirable taste.

Characters of Cocoa Butter

- **Color:** Yellowish white solid
- **Taste:** Chocolate
- **Odor:** Chocolate
- **Solubility:** Slightly soluble in alcohol, soluble in boiling alcohol, very soluble in ether, benzene and chloroform.
- **Melting point:** 30°–35 °C

Chemical constituents: Cocoa butter consists of the glycerides of stearic (34%), palmitic (26%), arachidic, oleic (37%) and other acids. The seeds contain fixed oil (35–50%), starch

(15%), theobromine (1–4%), caffeine (0.36%), proteins (15%), sugar, cacoa-red, volatile odorous principle and ash.

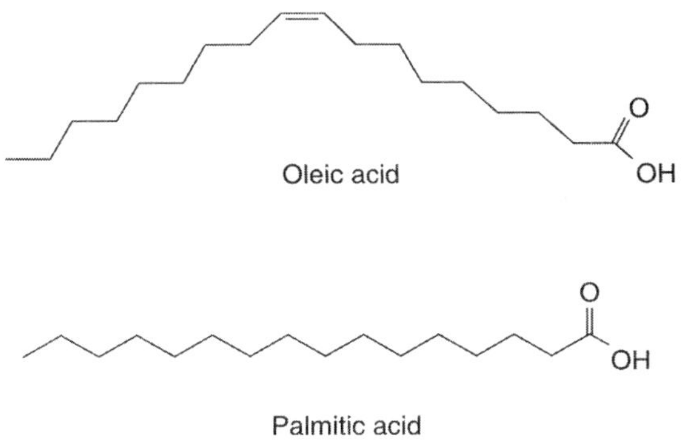

Oleic acid

Palmitic acid

Fig. 5.6.8: Chemical constituents of cocoa butter

Chemical test: Dissolve 1 gm of theobroma oil in 3 ml of ether in a test tube at temperature 17°C. Immerse the test tube in cold water. The solution does not become turbid or deposit while flexes in less then 3 minutes. After congealing range, the temperature up to 15°C, clear liquid is gradually formed.

Uses: Because of the low melting point of cocoa butter, it is often used in pharmaceuticals as a base for suppositories. Cocoa butter is one of the most stable fats known, containing natural antioxidants. The smooth texture, sweet fragrance and emollient property of cocoa butter make it a popular ingredient in cosmetics.

Adulterants: Waxes, stearin like coconut stearin or animal and vegetable tallows.

Wool Fat

Synonyms: Adeps lanae, wool wax, wool fat, anhydrous wool fat or wool grease

Biological source: Wool fat is a fatty, purified and anhydrous waxy substance secreted by the hairs constituting the fleece of the sheep *Ovis aries* Linn, Family Bovidae.

Habitat: Australia, USA, India (lesser extend)

Botany

- Kingdom   Animalia
- Phylum   Chordata
- Class   Mammalia
- Order   Artiodactyla
- Family   Bovidae
- Genus   *Ovis*
- Species   *aries*

Extraction of wool fat: Wool fat is extracted with hot water, and allowing the emulsion thus produced to stand, when impure wool fat rises as a cream. This can be cleansed by repeatedly mixing with water and separating by centrifugation, the resulting wool fat being subjected to a final process of purification.

Characters of Wool Fat

- **Color:** Pale yellow
- **Taste:** Chocolate
- **Odor:** Faint characteristic
- **Solubility:** Insoluble in water, sparingly soluble in cold alcohol.
- **Melting point:** 42°C
- **Storage:** Temp not exceeding 25 °C

Chemical constituents: Wool fat consists chiefly of cholesteryl (Fig. 5.6.9) and iso-cholesteryl alcohols combined with lanoceric, lanopalmitic, carnaubic, myristic, a little oleic, and possibly also palmitic and cerotic acids.

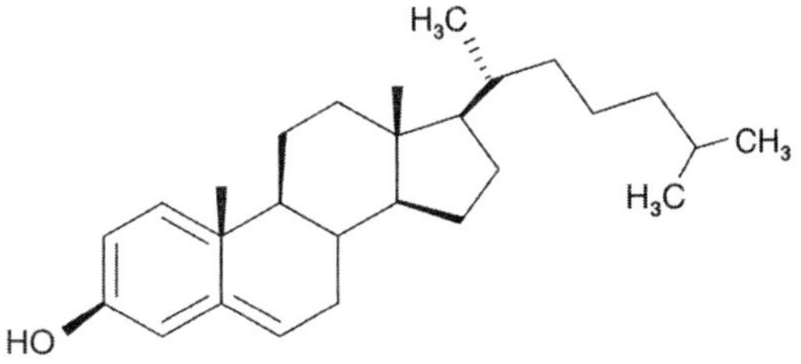

Fig. 5.6.9: Cholesteryl alcohol

Chemical Test

For cholesteryl alcohol: Dissolve 0.1 gm in a mixture of 5 ml of chloroform and 0.5 ml of acetic anhydride; pour gently upon 5 ml of sulphuric acid; a purplish brown ring, passing into green is developed at the surface of contact.

Uses: Wool fat is largely used as an emollient and for promoting the absorption of drugs by the skin.

Adulterants: The most probable adulterants of wool fat are mineral fats (soft paraffin) or animal and vegetable fats and oils.

Lard

Synonyms: Adeps

Biological source: Lard is the purified fat from the abdomen of the hog, *Sus scrofa* Linn., family Suidae.

Botany

- Kingdom   Animalia
- Phylum   Chordata
- Class   Mammalia
- Order   Unigulata
- Family   Suidae
- Genus   *Sus*
- Species   *scrofa*

Part used: Abdomen of hog

Extraction of lard: Lard may be rendered by either of two processes, wet rendering or dry rendering.

Wet rendering: The pig fat is boiled in water or steamed at a high temperature and the lard, which is insoluble in water, is skimmed off of the surface of the mixture, or it is separated in an industrial centrifuge. Wet-rendered lard has a more neutral flavor, a lighter color, and a high smoke point.

Dry rendering: The fat is exposed to high heat in a pan or oven without the presence of water. Dry-rendered lard is somewhat more browned in color and flavor and has relatively lower smoke point.

Properties of Lard

- Color: Soft white
- Odor: Not rancid
- Melting point: Back fat: 30–40°C
                        Leaf fat: 43–48°C
                        Mixed fat: 36–45°C
- Specific gravity: 0.917–0.938
- Iodine value: 45–75
- Acid value: 3.4
- Saponification value: 190–205

Chemical constituents: The lard consists of Saturated fats 38–43%, palmitic acid: 25–28%, stearic acid: 12–14%, myristic acid: 1%, unsaturated fats 56–62%, monounsaturated fats 47–50%, oleic acid: 44–47%, palmitoleic acid: 3%, and linoleic acid: 6–10%.

Chemical Test

Saponification test for triglycerides: Add 25 ml of 10%NaOH to evaporated fat, boil in boiling water bath for 30 min, cool and add excess of Na_2SO_4 solution; soap forms and raise at the top, filter it. To the filtrate, add sulfuric acid, evaporate and collect residue; the residue contains glycerol. Dissolve residue in ethanol. Ethanolic solution used to perform following test:

1. To the ethanolic solution, add few drops of copper sulfate and sodium hydroxide solution clear blue color is observed.
2. To the ethanolic solution add few crystals potassium hydrogen sulfate, heat it; vigorously pungent odor of acrylic aldehydes is produced.

Uses: Used in cooking, emollient, ointment base and protective. Lard oil is used as a antifoaming agent in fermentation and as tablet lubricants, illuminant and to manufacture soap.

Carnauba Wax

Synonyms: Palm wax, tree of life

Biological source: Carnauba is a wax derived from the leaves of the carnauba palm, *Copernicia cerifera* belonging to family Palmae.

Habitat: A plant native to and grown only in the northeastern Brazilian states.

Organoleptic Characters

Color: Hard greenish yellow wax

Odor: No odor

Taste: No taste

Melting point: 50–56°C

Compatibility: Carnauba wax is compatible with most animal, vegetable and mineral waxes and a large variety of natural and synthetic resins.

Extra features: Commercially available in form of flakes.

Chemical constituents: Carnauba wax contains mainly esters of fatty acids (80–85%), fatty alcohols (10–16%), acids (3–6%) and hydrocarbons (1–3%). Specific for carnauba wax is the content of esterified fatty *diols* (about 20%), hydroxylated fatty acids (about 6%) and cinnamic acid (about 10%). Cinnamic acid, an antioxidant, may be hydroxylated or methoxylated.

Chemical Test

Acid value: Weigh accurately 3 g into a 250 ml flask attached to a reflux condenser, add 50 ml of a mixture of isopropyl alcohol and toluene (5:4), and boil gently until the wax is completely dissolved. Remove the flask from the condenser, add about 1 ml of phenolphthalein, and immediately titrate with 0.5 N alcoholic potassium hydroxide to a faint, reddish yellow color. Calculate the acid value as the number of mg of potassium hydroxide required to neutralize the free acids in 1 g of carnauba wax. The acid value so obtained is between 2 and 7.

Saponification value: To the solution from the test for *acid value*, add 15.0 ml of 0.5 N alcoholic potassium hydroxide, reflux for 3 hours, and titrate the excess alkali with 0.5 N hydrochloric acid to a yellow-amber color. Perform a blank determination. The saponification value is between 78 and 95.

Residue on ignition: Heat 2 g in an open porcelain or platinum dish over a flame, it volatilizes without emitting an acrid odor. Ignite the weight of the residue, does not exceed 5 mg. Not more than 0.25% is found.

Uses: Cosmetics, glamour products, pharmaceuticals, ointments, tablet coatings, candles, confections, investment casting, auto, floor and shoe polishes, carbon paper, inks, paper coatings and fruit coatings.

Beeswax

Synonyms: Yellow beeswax, white beeswax, cera flava, cara alba.

Biological source: Beeswax is wax separated from the honey comb of *Apis mellifera* Linn, family Apidae. All bees make wax in epidermal glands to cover their outer layer of cuticle to prevent water loss.

Habitat: West Indies, California, Jamaica, Chili, Egypt, Syria, Morocco.

Preparation of Beeswax

Yellow beeswax: After collecting honey from honey comb, the comb is melted in water so that impurities and residual honey settle down. After straining, wax mixture is allowed to cool, remelted and finally strained to collect yellow beeswax.

White beeswax: It is prepared by process of bleaching by use of chemicals (charcoal, potassium permanganate, chromic acid, ozone, chlorine or treatment with hydrogen

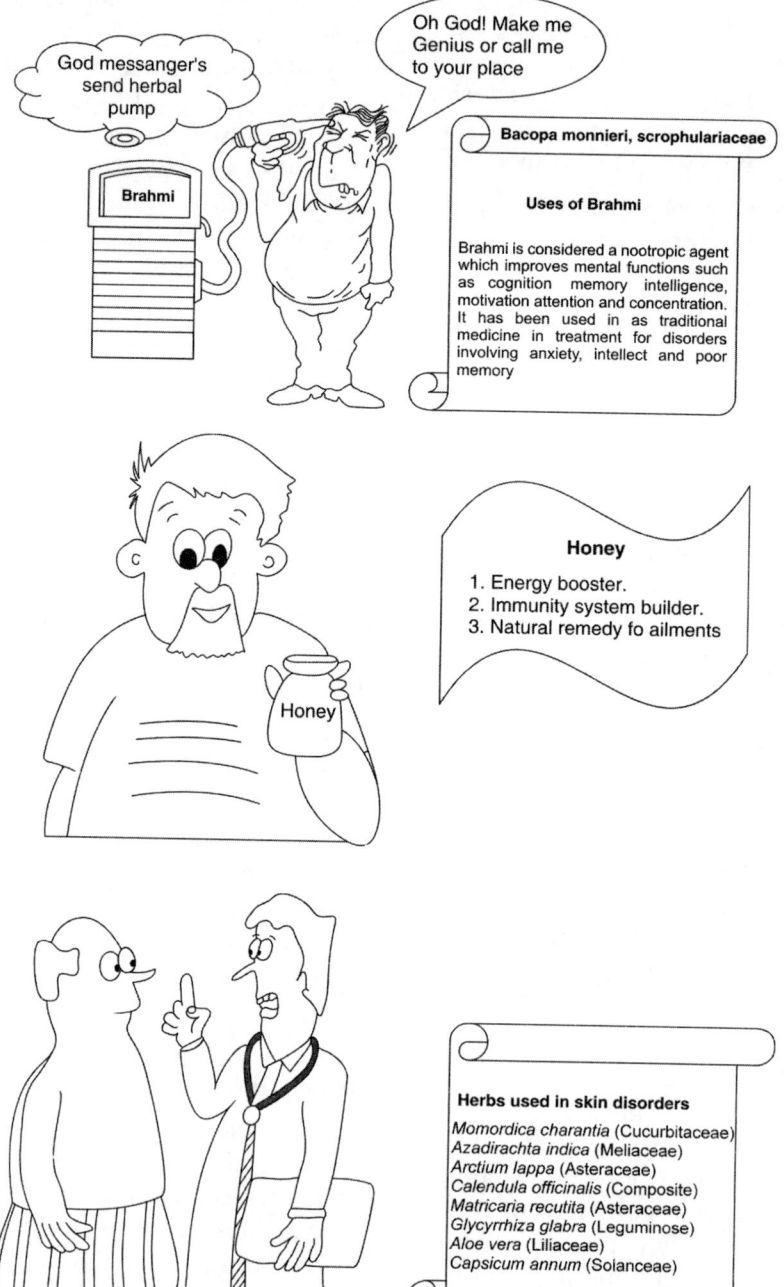

peroxide) or by use of light, air and water. Ribbon, like strips of waxes are formed till bleaching is complete.

Characters of Beeswax

- **Color:** Yellowish to brownish yellow
- **Odor:** Honey-like odor
- **Taste:** Balsamic taste
- **Melting point:** 62–65°C
- **Density:** 0.95–0.96
- **Solubility:** Practically, insoluble in water, slightly soluble in cold alcohol, soluble in hot alcohol, chloroform, benzene and ether.
- **Saponification value:** 3–5

Chemical constituents: The wax contains an ester myricin (78%), free wax acids (14%), moisture and cerolein (aromatic substance). The color of wax is due to presence of pollen pigments and propolis.

Chemical test: Boil 0.5 gm of beeswax with 20 ml of aqueous caustic soda solution for 10 minutes, cool, content is cooled and filtered. The filtrate on treatment with HCl gives clear solution. No turbidity is produced.

Uses: Beeswax is used commercially to make fine *candles, cosmetics* and *pharmaceuticals* including *bone wax*. It is also used as a coating for *cheese*. Beeswax is also an ingredient in *moustache wax,* as well as hair pomades.

Adulterants: Solid paraffin, ceresin, various fats and waxes of vegetable or animal origin with resin and stearic acid.

Drugs from Marine Sources

MARINE DRUGS (Table 6.1)

"It is said that life started in the seas, and many researchers feel that the sea holds the secret to life itself"

Marine biotechnology is the science in which marine organisms are used in full or partially to make or modify products, to improve plants or animals or to develop microorganisms for specific uses. Approximately 70% of the Earth's surface is covered with water. The sea holds an endless source of life. Approximately 85% of water is sea water, which contains sodium chloride and trace minerals. According to researchers only 10% of over 25,000 plants have been investigated for biological activity. The marine environment may contain over 80% of world's plant and animal species. Many bioactive compounds have been extracted from various marine animals, like tunicates, sponges, soft corals, sea hares, nudibranchs, bryozoans, sea slugs and marine organisms.

There are several phyla of marine flora (algae) to be discussed, including:

1. **Phaeophyta** (*benthic brown algae*): Xanthophyll fucoxanthin.
2. **Rhodophyta** (*red algae*): Color comes from red pigments, Xanthophylls.
3. **Chlorophyta** (*green algae*): Predominantly found in fresh water and also in salt water.
4. **Cyanophyta** (*blue green algae*): These contain chlorophyll and other pigments and are microscopic.
5. **Chrysophyta** (*golden brown algae*): Predominantly found in fresh water, and sometimes in seawater.
6. **Dinophyta** (*Pyrrophyta*): These are usually found in the phytoplankton and are microscopic.
7. **Xanthophyta** (*yellow green*): Fresh water, high in carotenoids.
8. **Cryptophyta:** Contain green, blue, and red pigments.
9. **Haptophyta:** A relatively new division of what was formerly thought as chrysophyta.
10. **Bacillariophyta** (*diatoms*): Contain silica cell walls. These cell walls are resistant.

"Poison kills the poison," proverb is the basis finding the biomedical metabolites from living organisms. Their are plenty of metabolites in sea either living or dead form including. Sponges (37%), coelenterates (21%) and microorganisms (18%) are the major sources of biomedical compounds followed by algae (9%), echinoderms (6%), tunicates (6%), molluscs (2%), bryozoans (1%), etc. More than 50% of the 100 isolates from marine sources are potentially exploitable bioactive substances.

Metabolites from Seaweeds (Table 6.3)

Seaweeds are abundant in the intertidal zones and in clear tropical waters. There are a number of seaweeds with economic potential.

Table 6.1: Marine drugs with chemical constituents and uses

S.no.	Botanical name	Chemical constituents	Uses
1.	Ascophyllum nodosum	Alginic acid (a polysaccharide)	Suspending agent, protective colloid, used in cosmetics, shampoos, creams, lotions, and ointments
2.	Alaria esculenta	Vitamins (E, C, B_{12}, B_6, B_3, B, A):, minerals (Zn, F, Cr, Co, Mn, I, Na, Fe, P, Mg, K, Ca), fat, protein, and carbohydrates	Used in cosmetic and hair care products
3.	Laminaria longicruris	Calcium, potassium, iodine, mannitol, and glutamic acid.	Antioxidant activity
4.	Palmaria palmata	Minerals, particularly fluoride, phosphorus, potassium	Used in chowders, salads, etc.
5.	Porphyra umbilicalis	Vitamins A, B, B_2, B_3, B_6, B_{12}, C	Used both in hair and skin treatment products.
6.	Sargassum fluitans	C_{12}–C_{20} saturated fatty acids (arachidonic, oleic, palmitic, myristic, and lauric acids).	Used in the treatment of goiters and have anticoagulant properties
7.	Eisenia bicyclis	Enzyme B-glucuronidase	Anti-inflammatory
8.	Fucus vesiculosus L	Polysaccharides and polyphenols, phlorotannins, polyphenols,	Used internally for obesity, rheumatism, and as a massage for cellulite.
9.	Chlorella vulgaris	Protein, essential amino acids	Good source of chlorophyll used as a blood builder
10.	Spirulina	Protein (55 to 70%), carbohydrates (15 to 25%), lipids (4 to 7%), and minerals (5 to 10%).	It is good source of vitamins and enzymes.
11.	Chondrus crispus	Mucilage, polysaccharides (carrageenans), sulfur compounds, protein, iodine, bromine, iron	Used as a thickener and stabilizer, and to treat and soothe sore throats

Seaweeds are also much higher in protein than land vegetables. They are good sources of iodine and vitamins A, B_2, B_{12}, and C. Seaweeds are rich in compounds pertinent to the cosmetic industry, such as ursolic acid derivates, fucose polymers, and polysaccharides.

- *Polygalactosides* react with the proteins in the outer surface of the skin and hair. Ion–ion interactions form a protective moisturizing complex.
- *Fucose polymers* are very hygroscopic and act as hydrating agents.

Table 6.2: Metabolites from marine cyanobacteria

S.no.	Metabolites/biological source	Activity
1.	Carotenoids and phycobiliprotein pigments from cyanobacteria	Natural food coloring agents, as feed additives, as enhancers of the color of egg yolks, to improve the health and fertility of cattle, as drugs and in the cosmetic industries.
2.	*Lyngbya lagerhaimanii* and *Phormidium tenue*	Anti-HIV activity
3.	*Fusarium chlamydosporum*	Antimicrobial agents
4.	Cyanobacterium *Stigonema* spp	Anti-inflammatory and anti-proliferative properties
5.	Dinoflagellate *Goniodoma pseudogoniaulax*	Antifungal polyether macrolide
6.	*Gambierdiscus toxicus*	Antifungal agents

- *Ursolic acid* and its derivates can form oil-resistant barriers on skin and hair, the same as they do in the waxy coating on apples, pears, cranberry, prunes, and other fruits.

Sea algae are rich in non-essential and essential amino acids (e.g. proline, glycine, and lycine). Elastic fibers in skin are also rich in these amino acids. Therefore, seaweed can play an important role in cosmetics as a moisturizing agent, helping to maintain the skin's elasticity by increasing its hydration.

Metabolites from Sponges (Table 6.4)

Approximately 10,000 sponges have been described in the world and most of them live in marine waters. A range of bioactive metabolites has been found in about 11 sponge genera. Three of these genera (*Haliclona, Petrosia* and *Discodemia*) produce powerful anti-cancer, anti-inflammatory agents.

Metabolites from Fish, Sea Snakes and Marine Mammals

Metabolites extracted from fish, sea snakes and aquatic mammals are scanty. Various fish species are used to extract fish oil, rich in omega-3 fatty acids, which are used in the preparation of various kinds of drugs for the remedies of human beings, such as arthritis and many others. Throughout the world about 500 species of fish are considered

Table 6.3: Metabolites from seaweeds

S.no.	Metabolites/biological source	Activity
1.	Red alga *Sphaerococcus coronopifolius*	Antibacterial activity
2.	Green alga *Ulva lactuca*	Anti-inflammatory activity
3.	*Portieria hornemannii*	Anti-tumor compound
4.	*Ulva fasciata*	Antiviral activity *in vivo*
5.	Brown alga *Stypodium zonale*	Anticancer activity
6.	*Codium iyengarii*	Antibacterial activity

Metabolites of this class occur in diseases such as psoriasis, asthma, arteriosclerosis, heart disease, ulcers and cancer, etc.

Table 6.4: Metabolites from sponges

S.no.	Metabolites/biological source	Activity
1	Cryptotethiacrypta	Potent tumor-inhibiting arabinosyl nucleoside
2.	Dercitus spp. (aminoacridine alkaloid)	Cytotoxic activities
3.	Japanese sponge Theonella spp (Halichondrin-B)	Potential anticancer agent
4.	Theonella spp	In vitro cytotoxity and in vivo antitumor activity
5.	Caminus sphaeroconia	Potent inhibitor of the bacterial type-III secretion system
6.	Xestospongia berguista	Antihistaminic activity
7.	Carribean sponge Batzella spp	Anti-HIV activity
8.	Hyrtios erecta	Anticancer activity

Table 6.5: Metabolites from cnidarians

S.no.	Metabolites/ biological source	Activity
1.	Lobophytum crassum	Antibacterial activity
2.	Pseudopterogorgia (a tricyclic diterpene pentoside)	Anti-inflammatory and analgesic activities
3.	Subergorgia suberosa (sesquiterpenesuberosols A–D)	Anti-inflammatory activity
4.	Clavularia viridis Clavubicyclone	Anticancer activity
5.	Erythropodium caribaeorum (diterpenes)	Antimitotic agents
6.	Pseudopterogorgia elizabethae (pseudopterosins)	Used in cosmetic industries
7.	Eunicea fusca (contains fucoside-A)	Used in cosmetic industries

Table 6.6: Metabolites from bryozoans

S.no.	Metabolites/biological source	Activity
1.	Flustra foliacea (deformylflustrabromine)	Moderate cytotoxicity
2.	Watersipora subtorquata (bryoanthrathiophene)	Antiangiogenic activity
3.	Bugula neritina (Bryostatin)	Anticancer activity
4.	Cribricellina cribreria (β-carboline alkaloid)	Cytotoxic, antibacterial, antifungal and antiviral activities
5.	Flustra foliacea (Indole alkaloids)	Antimicrobial activity

Table 6.7: Metabolites from mollusks

S.no.	Metabolites/biological source	Activity
1	Dolabella auricularia (dolastatin, a cytotoxic peptide)	Antineoplastic substance
2	Hexabranchus sanguineus (ulapualide-A, a sponge-derived macrolide)	Antifungal activity
3	Chromocloris cavae (chromodorolide-A)	In vitro antimicrobial and cytotoxic activities

Table 6.8: Metabolites for tunicates

S.no.	Metabolites/biological source	Activity
1.	Halocynthia aurantium (halocidin)	Antimicrobial peptide
2.	Styela clava clavaspirin	Antibacterial peptide
3.	Didemnum spp (alkaloids)	Antiplasmodial and antitrypanosomal activities
4.	Eudistoma species (eudistomins)	In vitro antiviral activity

toxic. The most spectacular substance of pharmacological importance extracted from fish is tetradotoxin (TTX), the puffer or fugu poison. Other toxins isolated include ciguatoxin from electric rays, which is served as a potent antidote for pesticide poisoning.

Marine Toxins

Marine animals may accumulate and use a variety of toxins from prey organisms and from symbiotic microorganisms for their own purposes. Thus, toxic animals are particularly abundant in the oceans. The toxins vary from small molecules to high molecular weight proteins and display unique chemical and biological features of scientific interest. Marine toxins are naturally occurring chemicals produced by algal or microbial organisms and are concentrated in contaminated seafood. All are heat stable toxins that are not destroyed by normal cooking. The toxins are not detectable by organoleptic means. Except for the scombroid toxins, the toxins accumulate in fish or shellfish through amplification in the food chain. The chemicals that cause Scombroid poisonings are produced by various bacteria on fish that have been thermally abused after harvest. The hazard posed by these toxins is dependant on dose, frequency of exposure, relative toxicity of the chemical and host factors. Many of these substances can serve as useful research tools or molecular models for the design of new drugs and pesticides. Substantial increases in seafood consumption in recent years, together with globalization of the seafood trade, have increased potential exposure to these agents. Marine toxins produce neurological, gastrointestinal, and cardiovascular syndromes, some of which result in high mortality and long-term morbidity.

Algal Toxins

Algae constitute most of the biomass of the oceans. Of ~5000 species of algae, ~40 species, of which most are dinoflagellates (Pyrrhophyta division), produce potent toxins. These algae are a main source of food for shellfish and the larvae of crustaceans. Algae are also an important food source of small herbivorous fish, which may be consumed by larger fish that are, in turn, eaten by humans. Under appropriate environmental conditions, algae can reproduce with extraordinary rapidity, even to the point of discoloring the sea, producing algal blooms that include red tides. Toxin may be so concentrated in waters under these circumstances that it can be aerosolized by surf and cause a transient syndrome of inhalational intoxication in humans.

Paralytic shellfish poisoning: Paralytic shellfish poisoning is a severe disease with rapid onset that may be life. Threatening. The syndrome is exclusively neurological. The illness is caused by saxitoxin and closely related marine toxins. Saxitoxin is a water-soluble, heat-stable tetrahydropurine that is produced by certain dinoflagellates and possibly other algae and bacteria. The mode of action of saxitoxin is blockage of voltage-gated sodium channels in nerve and muscle cell membranes, blocking nerve signal transmission.

Diarrheic shellfish poisoning: Diarrheic shellfish poisoning is a rapid-onset, self-resolving illness with exclusively gastrointestinal symptoms. Symptoms are typically severe, but always self-limiting. The illness is caused by okadaic acid and possibly related toxins produced by certain dinoflagellates. Okadaic acid is a lipophilic polyether that inhibits eukaryotic protein phosphatases and is thought to cause diarrhea by phosphorylation of control proteins that results in sodium release by intestinal mucosal cells.

Amnesic shellfish poisoning: Amnesic shellfish poisoning is a rare illness with symptoms ranging from gastrointestinal disturbance to severe and unusual neurological manifestations. It is caused by domoic acid, a water-soluble, heat-stable amino acid that is produced by certain algal diatoms of *Pseudonitzschia* species.

Ciguatera: Ciguatera is typically a self-limiting illness manifesting combinations of gastrointestinal, neurological, and cardiovascular symptoms. It is the one of the most common forms of seafood intoxication, with an estimated 20,000–50,000 cases occurring annually worldwide. Illness is caused by 2 dinoflagellate toxins. Ciguatoxin and closely related toxins are lipophilic, heat-stable polyethers that open voltage-sensitive sodium channels at the neuromuscular junction, resulting in membrane hyperexcitability, spontaneous repetitive neurotransmitter release, blockage of synaptic transmission, and depletion of synaptic vesicles.

Neurotoxic shellfish poisoning: Neurotoxic shellfish poisoning produces a transient

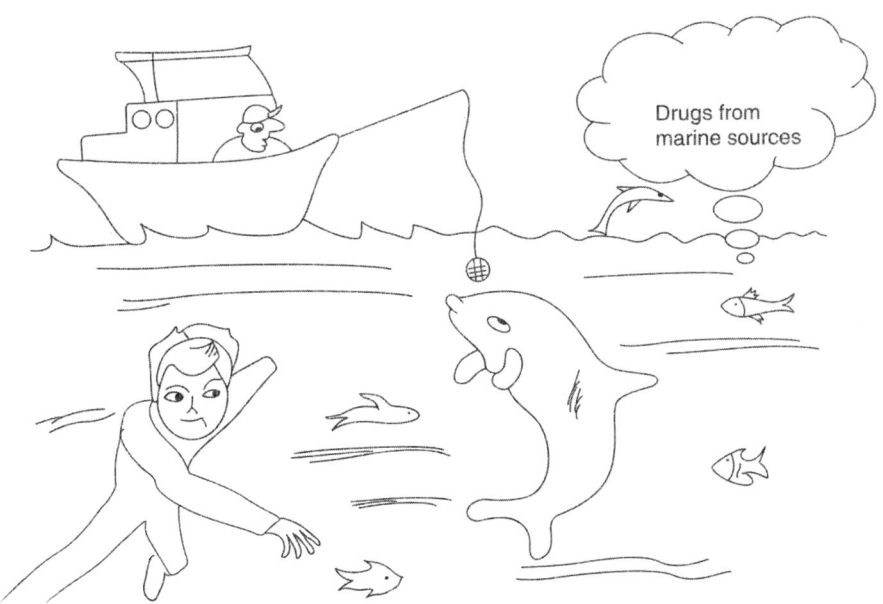

Marine microbes having immense genetic biochemical diversity look likely to become a rich source of novel effective drugs. Marine bacteria constitute ~ 10% of the living biomass carbon of the biosphere

illness characterized by gastrointestinal and neurological symptoms. Illness is caused by members of the brevetoxin family of toxins, which are lipophilic polyethers that, like ciguatera, open voltage-sensitive sodium channels.

Other Toxins

Scombroid fish poisoning (histamine fish poisoning): Scombroid fish poisoning is probably the most common seafood-related intoxication and is mostly caused by consumption of fish with high histamine levels, and symptoms are essentially the same as those associated with histamine toxicity.

Puffer fish poisoning: Puffer fish poisoning is a lethal intoxication resulting from consumption of toxic species of the puffer fish, which is also known as fugu, globefish, or blowfish and which resides in shallow waters of tropical and temperate seas.

7

Drugs from Mineral Origin

Minerals that are essential to life are the source of metals and other inorganic elements involved in the most fundamental processes. These contain metals, such as manganese, copper, zinc, and iron. The human skeleton is composed of calcium and phosphorus and traces of other ions, e.g. magnesium, sulfur, and sodium embedded in an organic matrix. The regulation of body fluid volume and acid–base balance requires the cations, e.g. sodium, potassium, magnesium, and calcium. The principal anion is chloride. Calcium also plays a role in neuromuscular excitability and blood coagulation. Metabolic energy, cellular homeostasis, and most enzyme activities are dependent on phosphorus. The electron-transport chain requires copper and iron. The clement found in body with physiological role but also are not toxic. Examples are rubidium, strontium, titanium, niobium, germanium, and lanthanum. Other elements are toxic when found in greater than trace amounts, and sometimes in trace amounts. These latter elements include arsenic, mercury, lead, cadmium, silver, zirconium, beryllium, and thallium. The interactions of mineral nutrients with carbohydrates, fats, and proteins, minerals with vitamins (qv), and mineral nutrients with toxic elements are areas of active investigation. The amount of each element required in daily dietary intake varies with the individual bioavailability of the mineral nutrient. Bioavailability depends both on body need as determined by absorption and excretion patterns of the element and by general solubility, and on the absence of substances that may cause formation of insoluble products, e.g. calcium phosphate $Ca_3(PO_4)_2$. The essential mineral nutrients are classified either as principal elements or as trace and ultratrace elements.

The list of plant drugs derived from minerals are given below, a few of them have significance as pharmaceutical aids.

SHILAJIT

Synonyms: Vegetable asphalt, bitumen, asphaltum

Origin: Shilajit literally means 'rock overpowering' and is a natural exudate from the rocks of the Himalayas and other mountainous regions of the world. According to *Sushruta*, in the months of May-June, the sap or juice of plants comes out as gummy exudation from the rocks of mountains due to strong heat of sun and *Rasarangini*. *Dwarishtarang* also claim that the Shilajit is an exudation of latex gum-resin, etc. of plants which comes from the rocks of mountains in presence of scorching heat.

Constituents: Shilajit mainly consists of resins, like benzoic acid, hippuric acid, fulvic acid; minerals, like silica, iron, antimony, calcium, copper, lithium, magnesium, manganese, molybdenum, phosphorus, silica, sodium, strontium, and zinc.

Biomedical action: It is a mineral supplement that benefits the kidneys, urinary and reproductive systems. It has diuretic activity, lithotriptic, anti-diabetic, nervine and tonic. It strengthens the whole reproductive system and is a tonic to the sex organs. It also benefits the female reproductive system where there is weakness, infertility, dysmenorrhea.

TALC

Synonyms: Talcum, French talc and soap stone

Origin: The mineral talc is a hydrous magnesium silicate. A massive talcose rock is called steatite, and an impure massive variety is known as soap stone.

Properties: Talc is used commercially because of its fragrance retention, luster, purity, softness, and whiteness. Commercially, important properties of talc are its chemical inertness, high dielectric strength, high thermal conductivity, low electrical conductivity, and oil and grease adsorption. It is insoluble in water, weak acids and weak alkalies.

Composition: Talc is composed of layer of magnesium made of either oxygen or hydroxyl octahedral that lies sandwitched between two layers of silicon oxygen tetrahedron.

Uses: Talc is used in ceramics, paint, paper, and plastics. It is also used as dusting powder, pharmaceutical aid, as a filtration aid and ideal excipient as well as glidant.

ASBESTOS

Synonyms: Amianthus

Origin: Asbestos is a naturally occurring mineral found in underground rock formations. It is recovered by mining and rock crushing. Asbestos is also mined in India, but quantity and quality-wise it is of no relevance to our asbestos cement production. There are two groups of asbestos: serpentine and amphiboles.

- **Serpentine asbestos,** such as chrysotile, has curly shaped fibers that can shear into smaller fibrils. Chrysotile fibers consist of aggregates of long, thin, flexible fibrils that resemble scrolls or cylinders of uniform chemical composition.

- **Amphiboles** crystallise in straight double chains resulting in needle-like structures. They tend to be more brittle.

- **Asbestos fiber,** (composed mainly of magnesium and silica), is a great reinforcing agent. Its tensile strength is greater than steel, it has other rare and highly valued fire retardant, chemical resistant and heat insulating qualities. In fact it is a magic mineral and no other substitute can match its properties.

- Six common forms of asbestos are known as actinolite, amosite, anthophyllite, chrysotile, crocidolite and tremolite.

Description: Asbestos refers to a number of naturally occurring mineral silicates. The macroscopic asbestos fibers are actually bundles of thinner fibers made up of fibrils. Each macroscopic fiber is highly anisotropic and tends to decompose into its thinner constituents under industrial handling.

Properties: Asbestos is neither volatile nor soluble. It can occur in suspension in both air and water. Large fibers are removed from air and water by gravitational settling at a rate which depends on their size. Small fibers can remain suspended for long periods of time. Interaction with natural organic matters may increase precipitation. Designates a group of naturally occurring fibrous serpentine or amphibole minerals that have extraordinary tensile strength, conduct heat poorly and are relatively resistant to chemical attack.

Uses: As insulation, cement, fireproof clothing, and brake linings. However, its use is declining.

KAOLIN

Synonyms: China clay, porcelain clay, bolus alba, terra alba, white bole or argilla

Source: Kaolin is a plastic raw material, particularly consisting of the clay mineral kaolinite. The chemical formula is $Al_2O_3 \cdot 2SiO_2 \cdot 2H_2O$ (39.5% Al_2O_3, 46.5% SiO_2, 14.0% H_2O). It is formed by rock weathering.

Description: Kaolinite ranks among phyllosilicates, which are stratified clay minerals formed by a net of tetrahedral and octahedral layers.

Properties: Kaolinite has very little isomorphic substitution of Al for Si in the tetrahedral layer. Accordingly, it has a low cation exchange capacity. It easily adsorbs water and forms a plastic, paste-like substance. Due to its adsorbent capability and lack of primary toxicity, kaolin is considered a simple and effective means to prevent or ameliorate the adverse effects exerted by many toxic agents.

Composition: Kaolin or china clay is a mixture of different minerals. Kaolin contains 10–95% of the mineral kaolinite and usually consists mainly of kaolinite (85–95%). Kaolinite is made up of tiny sheets of triclinic crystals with pseudohexagonal morphology. It also contains quartz and mica and also, less frequently, feldspar, illite, and montmorillonite.

Uses: Kaolin is used in face powders, liquid powders, powder creams, baby powders, compact rouge, face packs and in some dentifrices. Clinically, *cataplasma kaolini* (kaolin, glycerin, boric acid, methyl salicylate, thymol and peppermint oil) was used in cases of deep-seated inflammation, carbuncles, septic wounds, etc. Kaolin possesses good covering power, good grease-resisting properties and adsorbs perspiration. Kaolin is a safe and dermatologically innocuous material that has a sedative and cooling effect on an inflamed and heated skin.

BENTONITE

Synonyms: Whilknite

Source: Bentonite is a rock formed of highly colloidal and plastic clays composed mainly of montmorillonite, a clay mineral of the Smectite group, and is produced by *in situ* devitrification of volcanic ash. Differences among brands depend on montmorillionite content and percentage of impurities, such as sand. Sodium bentonites are the most popular types in the USA. Other countries often use calcium bentonite, which may have greater or lesser protein removal activity than sodium bentonite

Composition: The principle constituents of bentoninte is montmorillonite. It may also contain feldspar, cristobalite, and crystalline quartz.

Properties: The special properties of bentonite are derived from the crystal structure of the smectite group, which is an octahedral alumina sheet between two tetrahedral silica sheets. It is an ability to form thixotrophic gels with water, an ability to absorb large quantities of water, and a high cation exchange capacity. A hydrated aluminum silicate, bentonite has a negative charge, reacting with positively charged particles, such as proteins. In solution, it behaves like a series of small, absorbent plates.

Use: Bentonite is used in most cement slurries for decreasing slurry weight and increasing slurry volume. In bentonite cement diesel-oil (BCDO) and bentonite diesel-oil (BDO) slurries, bentonite forms a thick, paste-like material that helps prevent lost circulation.

CALAMINE

Synonyms: Prepared calamine

Origin: Calamine is a mixture of zinc oxide (ZnO) with about 0.5% iron(III) oxide (Fe_2O_3). It is a mineral species consisting of zinc carbonate, $ZnCO_3$, and forming an important ore of zinc. It is rhombohedral in crystallization and isomorphous with calcite and chalybite.

Description: The color of the pure mineral is white; more often it is brownish, sometimes green or blue: a bright-yellow variety. The hardness is 5 and specific gravity is 4.4. It is insoluble in water but soluble in hydrochloric acid.

Composition: It contains zinc carbonate (99.9%) colored with iron (III) oxide. The pure material contains 52% of zinc, but this is often partly replaced isomorphously by small amounts of iron and manganese, traces of calcium and magnesium, and sometimes by copper or cadmium.

Uses: It is the main ingredient in calamine lotion and is used as an antipruritic (anti-itching agent) to treat mild pruritic conditions, such as sunburn, eczema, rashes, poison ivy, chickenpox, insect bites and stings. It is also used as a mild antiseptic to prevent infections that can be caused by scratching the affected area, and an astringent to dry weeping or oozing blisters and acne abscesses.

KIESELGUHR

Synonyms: Diatomaceous earth, diatomite, diahydro, kieselguhr, kieselgur and celite.

Origin: It is a naturally occurring, soft siliceous sedimentary rock, that is easily crumbled into a fine white to off-white powder. Diatomaceous earth or kieselguhr is composed of the siliceous shells of fossil diatoms (minute unicellular plants), or of the debris of fossil diatoms.

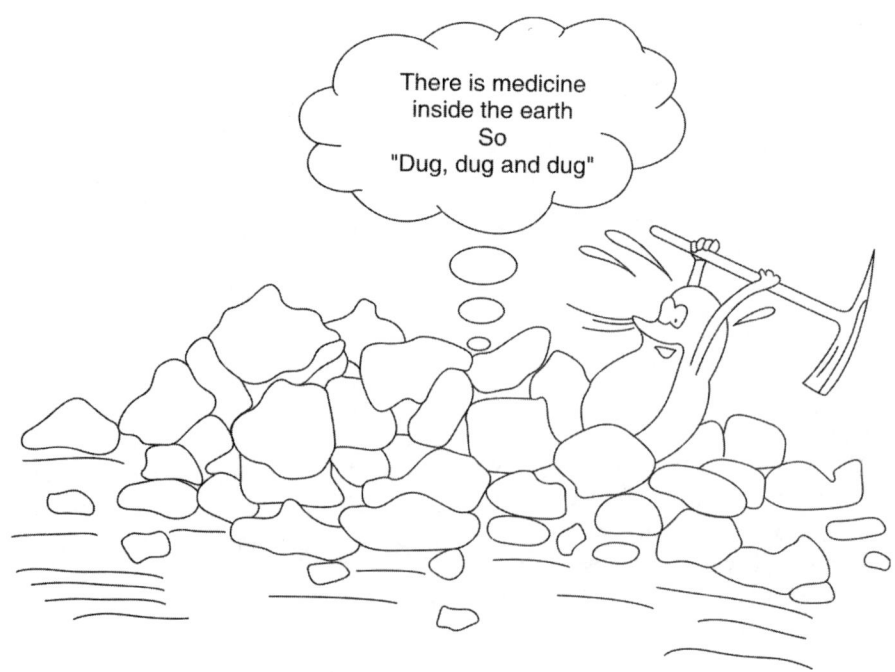

Description: It has a particle size ranging from less than 1 micron to more than 1 millimetre, but typically 10 to 200 microns. This powder has an abrasive feel, similar to pumice powder and is very light, due to its high porosity.

Composition: The typical chemical composition of oven dried diatomaceous earth is 80 to 90% silica, with 2 to 4% alumina (attributed mostly to clay minerals) and 0.5 to 2% iron oxide and consists of fossilized remains of diatoms, a type of hard-shelled algae.

Uses: It is used as a filtration aid, as a mild abrasive, as a mechanical insecticide, as an absorbent for liquids, and as a component of dynamite. As it is also heat-resistant, it can be used as a thermal insulator. Diatomite is also used as an insecticide, due to its physico-sorptive properties.

8

Enzymes and Protein Substances

ENZYMES

An enzyme is usually defined as organic catalyst produced by the living cells but capable of acting outside cells or even *in vitro*. The enzymes may be regarded as proteins which categorically alter the rate of chemical reactions without requiring the aid of an external energy source or being charged themselves. Importantly, an enzyme may be able to catalyze a particular reaction several times effectively. They are proteins, a large group of pharmacologically active molecules that also include monoclonal antibodies, cytokines, growth factors, hemostatic and thrombostatic agents, and vaccines.

Specific Characteristic Features

The various **specific characteristic features** of **enzymes** are as enumerated under:

- Enzymes are reaction specific in that they act exclusively on certain substrates. They give rise to an enzyme substrate complex, which involves not only physical shape but also chemical bonding.
- Enzymes occur as a part of metabolism.
- Enzyme acts at an optimum temperature and a pH, at which it does function most efficaciously. For most human enzymes, these shall be particularly confined to such factors as: pH of cells, body temperature, tissue fluid, and blood.
- Impaired activity of enzymes may be caused due to extremes of pH, temperature, dehydration, UV-radiation, and the presence of heavy metals.
- Certain enzymes need coenzymes (i.e. non-protein molecules, e.g. vitamins) to enable them function properly.

Important **enzymes** exploited commercially that belong to the aforesaid categories are given in Table 8.1:

Table 8.1: Types of enzymes with example

Type of enzymes	Example
Animal enzymes	Lipases, tripsin
Higher-plant enzymes	Amylases, papain, proteases, and soybean lipoxygenase
Microorganisms	*Acetobacter lacti*, *Clostridium aceticum*.
Food and beverage enzymes	Papain, protease

Classification of the **enzymes** based upon their **site of action**:

(a) Endoenzymes (or intracellular enzymes): The enzymes that are solely secreted very much within the cell are termed as endoenzymes. They essentially are involved in the synthesis of different cellular components, food reserves, and also serve as bioenergetic materials. Importantly, as these various processes do occur in the intracellular zones, the enzymes involved are also strategically located in the intracellular region. Examples: Isomerases, phosphorylases, synthetases, etc.

(*b*) **Exoenzymes (or extracellular enzymes):** The enzymes that are exclusively secreted outside the cell are invariably known as exoenzymes or extracellular enzymes. They usually exert a digestive feature in their overall activity and function. Interestingly, they help in the hydrolysis of relatively complex molecules into much simpler compounds for the formation of angiotensin II solely required to maintain and raise the blood pressure.

Examples:
- **Amylases**—hydrolyse **starch** components.
- **Lypases**—hydrolyse **lipids** (i.e. triglycerides); and
- **Proteoses**—hydrolyse **proteins** into **amino acids**.

The International Union of Biochemistry (IUB) initiated standards of enzyme nomenclature which recommend that enzyme names indicate both the substrate acted upon and the type of reaction catalyzed.

Enzymes can be classified by the kind of chemical reaction catalyzed.

1. Addition or removal of water:
    a. Hydrolases—these include esterases, carbohydrases, nucleases, deaminases, amidases, and proteases.
    b. Hydrases, such as fumarase, enolase, aconitase and carbonic anhydrase.
2. Transfer of electrons:
    a. Oxidases
    b. Dehydrogenases
3. Transfer of a radical:
    a. Transglycosidases of monosaccharides
    b. Transphosphorylases and phosphomutases of a phosphate group
    c. Transaminases of amino group
    d. Transmethylases of a methyl group
    e. Transacetylases of an acetyl group
4. Splitting or forming a C–C bond: Desmolases.
5. Changing geometry or structure of a molecule: Isomerases.
6. Joining two molecules through hydrolysis of pyrophosphate bond in ATP or other triphosphate: Ligases.

Enzymes of Pharmaceutical Relevance and Utility

Bromelain

Bromelain is the collective name for closely related proteolytic enzyme is found in tissues of the plant family Bromeliaceae. The crude stem bromelain contains several proteolytically active components together with some non-proteolytic enzymes, inhibitors, and activator several non-proteolytic enzymes have been isolated from crude stem bromelain including a phosphatase, a peroxidase, a cellulase, and other glycosidases.

Physical properties: Bromelain exists as a single polypeptide chain depending on the presence or absence of the N-terminal alanine. Based on the amino acid composition, the molecular weight of bromelain is found to be 22, 828 daltons. Stem bromelain is a glycoprotein with one oligosaccharide moiety per molecule, which is covalently attached to the peptide chain. Stem bromelain is a more basic protein than papain with a pl of 9.45, while fruit bromelain is an acidic protein.

Uses: In medicine, bromelain is effective in the treatment of inflammation and edema in a wide variety of tissues, to cure digestive disorders by means of replacement therapy, and in cardiovascular and circulatory disorders. It is used in the debridement of third degree burns, in the treatment of blunt injuries to the musculoskeletal system. It is also used as a potentiating agent in antibiotic therapy. In laboratory medicine, it is used extensively in blood group serology and in immunology research.

Hyaluronidase

Hyaluronidases are generally glycoproteins. Hyaluronan is a negatively charged high molecular weight linear polysaccharide built from repeating disaccharide units. Hyaluronan is ubiquitously distributed in the extracellular space of higher animals and plays a structural role in cartilage and other tissues.

Uses: Hyaluronidase, in combination with triamcinolone and lidocaine, has been employed to treat recurrences of keloids after laser resection. In scalp-reduction surgery, hyaluronidase has been combined with the local anesthetics to facilitate their diffusion, to enhance the anesthesia, and to ease the dissection. Hyaluronidase is observed duly in the testes and semen. It specifically depolymerizes hyaluronic acid, thereby enhancing the ensuing permeability of the connective tissues by dissolving the various substances that hold body cells together. It also acts to disperse the cells of the corona radiata about the newly ovulated ovum, thus largely facilitating entry of the sperm.

Chymotrypsin

Chymotrypsin is one of the serine proteases. Chymotrypsin is selective for peptide bonds with aromatic or large hydrophobic side chains, such as Tyr, Trp, Phe and Met, which are on the carboxyl side of this bond. It can also catalyze the hydrolysis of ester bond. The main catalytic driving force for chymotrypsin is the set of three amino acids known as catalytic triad. This catalytic pocket is found in the whole serine protease family.

Uses: A pancreatic digestive enzyme that catalyzes the hydrolysis of certain proteins in the small intestine into polypeptides and amino acids.

Collagenase

Collagenases are enzymes that break the peptide bonds in collagen. It is invariably obtained from *Clostridium histolyticum*. Collagenases, members of the matrix metalloproteinase (MMP) family, are involved in the physiological and pathological turnover of connective tissues. Collagenase production is significantly increased at inflammation sites due to the stimulation of proinflammatory cytokines and displays its optimum activity between pH 7 and 8.

Uses: They are an exotoxin (a virulence factor) and help to facilitate the spread of gas gangrene. They normally target the connective tissue in muscle cells and other body organs. Collagenase is mostly used in the form of its 'ointment' for the specific dedebriment of burns, dermal ulcers, and necrotic ulcers.

Deoxyribonuclease [D Nase]

Deoxyribonuclease refers to an enzyme that catalyzes the hydrolysis (depolymerization) of deoxyribonucleic acid (DNA). **Deoxyribonuclease I** (usually called **DNase I**); is an endonuclease coded by the human gene **DNASE1**. DNase usually loses its activity in an aqueous medium. The optimum activity is exhibited between pH 6 and 7.

Uses: It is used to cure of hematomas and localized abscess formation, to minimize the specific viscosity of the pulmonary secretions as its 'aerosol preparations' in inhalers.

Fibrinolysin

Fibrinolysin is an enzyme derived from plasma of bovine origin or extracted from cultures of certain bacteria. It is used locally only and exclusively together with the enzyme desoxyribonuclease. Fibrinolysin and desoxyribonuclease both act as lytic enzymes. The combination is available as ointment containing 1 BU (biological unit) fibrinolysin and 666 BUs desoxyribonuclease per gram.

Uses: Fibrinolysin finds its use in the critical treatment of thrombotic disorders essentially caused due to its fibrinolytic inherent nature.

Muramidase

Lysozymes, also known as muramidase or N-acetylmuramide glycan-hydrolase, are glycoside hydrolases, enzymes that damage bacterial cell walls by catalyzing hydrolysis of 1,4-beta-linkages between N-acetylmuramic acid and N-acetyl-D-glucosamine residues in a peptidoglycan and between N-acetyl-D-glucosamine residues in chitodextrins.

Uses: The enzyme functions by attacking peptidoglycans (found in the cell walls of bacteria, especially Gram-positive bacteria).

Papain

Papain is a proteolytic enzyme that tenderises meat and can act as a clarifying agent in many food industry processes. It is a common ingredient in brewery and meat processing. It is obtained from *Carica papaya* belonging to family *Carcicaceae*. It is soluble in water and glycerine and possesses optimum activity ranging between pH 5 and 6.

Uses: It is used as an anti-inflammatory agent and to relieve symptoms of episiotomy. In industry, it is used as an clarification of beverages, e.g. beer, fruit juices, etc. meat tenderizer, cheese processing as a substitute of rennin, degumming of silk fibers in textile industry and dehairing of animal skins and hides in leather industry.

Pancreatin

Pancreatin (pancreatinum) is usually obtained from the fresh pancreas of the hog or ox. It contains the specific ferments of the pancreas, and represents its external secretion. It is mixture of enzymes, namely: amylase, lipase, and protease. It exhibits its maximum activity in an alkaline medium.

Uses: It is used chiefly as a digestant, for the preparation of predigested or peptonized food products and for conversions of starch into dextrin; proteins into amino acids; and fats into fatty acids and glycerols.

Potency of pancreatin: It has been established that:

1 g of **pancreatin** contains
- 12,000 units of **amylase activity;**
- 15,000 units of **lipase activity;** and
- 10,000 units of **protease activity.**

Pepsin

Pepsin is an enzyme whose precursor form (pepsinogen) is released by the chief cells in the stomach and that degrades food proteins into peptides. It produces its **optimum activity** at a pH of 1.5 to 2. Pepsin on being heated with either pancreatic enzymes or mild alkali aptly loses its biological activity.

Uses: Pepsin is commonly used in the preparation of F(ab')2 fragments from antibodies. It is also used preferable to use only the antigen-binding (Fab) portion of the antibody.

Rennin

Chymosin or rennin is an aspartic acid protease enzyme found in rennet. It is produced by the cow, in the lining of the abomasum (the fourth, final, chamber of its stomach). Rennin is obtained either from the glandular layer of the digesting stomach of the calf, *Bostaurus* (Family: *Bovidae*) or by microbiologically monitored fermentation of *Bacillus cereus, Endothia parasitica,* and *Mucor pusillus.*

Uses: Rennin is a protein-digesting enzyme that curdles milk by transforming caseinogen into insoluble casein. It is also recommended for patients under convalescence and weak in physical status in order to digest milk rather easily. A commercial form of rennin, rennet, is used in manufacturing cheese and preparing junket.

Streptokinase

Streptokinase (SK), a protein secreted by several species of streptococci can bind and activate human plasminogen. It is found to be water-soluble and exhibits optimum activity at pH 7. The various **applications** of **streptokinase** are SK is used as an effective and inexpensive clot-dissolving medication in some cases of myocardial infarction (heart attack) and pulmonary embolism. It is also used as a **fibrinolytic agent** to help in the removal of **bifrin thrombi** from the arteries (i.e. **reperfusion**).

Mechanism of Action: Streptokinase exerts its activity on account of the particular activation of plasminogen into a proteolytic enzyme, e.g. plasmin, that critically carries out the degradation of the fibrin clots, fibrinogen, and certain specific plasma proteins.

L-asparaginase: Asparaginase is an enzyme that catalyzes the hydrolysis of asparagine to aspartic acid. **L-asparaginase** refers to an **enzyme** that serves as an **antineoplastic agent** derived from the organism *Escherichia coli*. It interferes directly with the growth of **cancerous (malignant) cells** that are incapable of synthesizing **L-asparagine** for their necessary metabolism; and, employed in the usual **chemotherapy of very serious lymphocytic leukemia** in preferred sequential combination with other **antineoplastic drugs**.

PROTEIN

Proteins are linear polymers of amino acids connected by amide bonds. They are polymers of 20 different amino acids joined by peptide bonds. They refer as complex nitrogenous compounds that are synthesized by all living organisms. Proteins are found in all living systems ranging from bacteria and viruses through the unicellular and simple eukaryotes to vertebrates and higher mammals, such as humans. Proteins make up over 50% of the dry weight of cells and are present in greater amounts than any other biomolecule.

All cells encode the information content of proteins within genes, or more accurately the order of bases along the DNA strand. Conversion of information or expression into proteins represents the tangible evidence of a living system or life.

$$DNA \rightarrow RNA \rightarrow protein$$

Proteins are joined covalently and non-covalently with other biomolecules including lipids, carbohydrates, nucleic acids, phosphate groups, flavins, heme groups and metal ions. Components, such as hemes or metal ions, are often called prosthetic groups. Complexes formed between lipids and proteins are lipoproteins, those with carbohydrates are called glycoproteins, whilst complexes with metal ions lead to metalloproteins. Amino acids are crucial components of living cells because they are easy to polymerize. α-Amino acids are preferable to β-amino acids because the latter are too flexible to form spontaneously folding polymers. The amino acids of a protein chain are covalently joined by amide bonds, often called peptide bonds, for this reason, proteins are also known as polypeptides. Chemically, the peptide bond is a covalent bond that is formed between a carboxylic acid and an amino group by the loss of a water molecule.

Composition of Proteins

Proteins are composed of a host of vital elements, such as: C, H, O, N, P, S, and Fe, which ultimately make up the greater segment of the animal and plant tissue. In fact, the **amino acids** do represent the basic structure of **proteins**. The backbone is the same for all amino acids and consists of the amino group (NH_2), the alpha carbon and the carboxylic acid group (COOH). Different amino acids are distinguished by their different side chains, R.

The neutral form of an amino acid is shown: in solution at pH 7 the amino and carboxylic acid groups ionize, to NH_3^+ and COO^-. Except for glycine, where R = H, amino acids are chiral (i.e. they have a left–right asymmetry). The form shown is the L-configuration, which is most common. A 'complete protein' contains all the essential amino acids, *viz.* arginine, histidine, isoleucine, lysine, leucine, meltionine, phenylalanine, threonine, tryptophan, and valine.

Sources: The various known and important sources of proteins are, cheese, milk, eggs, meat, fish, and certain vegetables. The proteins are invariably found in both animal and vegetable sources of food. It has been duly observed that there are many **'incomplete proteins'** which are found in vegetables; and they do contain some of the so-called **essential amino acids**. Thus, a **'vegetarian diet'** may judiciously make up for this by combining various vegetable groups which complement each other in their basic amino acid groups. This ultimately provides the body with **'complete protein'**.

Functional Roles for Proteins

Protein is a unique nutrient that performs important and diverse functions in our bodies. Amino acids, which are the basic building blocks of protein, must be present in adequate quantity and quality to provide for new tissue formation during growth and development. This need for protein to make new tissue is also found when new tissues must be formed to heal wounds and fight infections or replace losses resulting from stress, weight loss or injury. Protein is an integral part of all of our tissues, especially our muscles. If adequate amounts of the amino acids, which our body use to make its protein, are not available, growth and repair and maintenance of our muscle tissues cannot be maintained. Proteins have diverse biological functions ranging from DNA replication, forming cytoskeletal structures, transporting oxygen around the bodies of multicellular organisms to converting one molecule into another. Major examples of the biochemical functions of proteins include binding; catalysis; operating as molecular switches; and serving as structural components of cells and organisms.

Binding: Specific recognition of other molecules is central to protein function.

Catalysis: Essentially, every chemical reaction in the living cell is catalyzed, and most of the catalysts are protein enzymes.

Switching: Proteins are flexible molecules and their conformation can change in response to changes in pH or ligand binding. Such changes can be used as molecular switches to control cellular processes.

Structural proteins (Table 8.2): Protein molecules serve as some of the major structural elements of living systems. This function depends on specific association of protein subunits with themselves as well as with other proteins, carbohydrates.

Table 8.2: Structural proteins with their examples

Function	Examples
Enzymes or catalytic proteins	DNA polymerases and trypsin
Transport proteins	Hemoglobin and serum albumin
Contractile proteins	Actin, myosin
Cytoskeletal proteins or structural	Keratin
Defence proteins	Immunoglobulins, venoms and toxins
Effector proteins	Insulin and TSH
Electron transfer proteins	Cytochrome oxidase
Receptors	Acetycholine receptor,
Storage proteins	Ferritin
Repressor proteins	Cro, Jun

Proteins Used as Drugs

Some proteins used normally as therapeutic agents (drugs), have been described briefly in Table 8.3.

Table 8.3: Protein drugs with their description

Protein drugs	Description
Gelatin: Soft-gelatine capsules for vitamin E; **Hard-gelatine capsules** for chloramphenicol and acetamenophen	Gelatin is a protein of uniform molecular constitution derived chiefly by the hydrolysis of collagen. Gelatin is a high grade gelatin in granular form which may be used as a solidifying agent or may be incorporated into culture media for various uses. **Types of gelatin: Absorbable gelatin sponge:** It is a sterile, white, tough, and finely porous spongy, water insoluble, and absorbable substance. It is used as a localized anticoagulant. **Absorbable gelatin film:** Light amber-colored, sterile, nonantigenic thin film invariably produced from a especially prepared gelatin-formaldehyde solution. It is used for mechanical means of protection.
Collagen	Collagens are a class of albuminoids found abundantly in bones, skin, tendon, cartilage and similar animal tissues. Collagen protein is distinctive because it contains high levels of the non-essential amino acids. It contains the specific amino acids — glycine, proline, hydroxyproline and arginine. These particular amino acids are necessary for proper function, growth and repair of the muscle tissues in the body. In essence, collagen protein is the cement that holds everything together. Not only does it hold components of our skeletal – muscular system together, it is also the primary mortar between the bricks of all of our smooth muscle tissues, such as our blood vessels, digestive tract, heart, gallbladder, kidneys and bladder.
Casein	Casein is the principal protein found in cow's milk. It is responsible for the white, opaque appearance of milk in which it is combined with calcium and phosphorus as clusters of casein molecules, called micelles. The principal use of casein products has been as an ingredient in foods to enhance their physical (so-called functional) properties, such as whipping and foaming, water binding and thickening, emulsification and texture, and to improve their nutrition. Casein actually represents the phosphoprotein with a composition of 0.85% P and 0.75% S.
Lectins	Lectins are sugar-binding proteins that are highly specific for their sugar moieties. They play a role in biological recognition phenomena involving cells and proteins. They are mainly used; for determining blood groups; and for carrying out erythrocytic polyagglutination investigative studies; for performing histochemical studies related to either normal and pathological status; for establishing structural elucidation studies of the carbohydrate bearing molecules; and it is used as an tools for studying cell-surface properties in cancer research.
Thaumatin	Thaumatin is a low-calorie (virtually calorie-free) protein sweetener and flavour modifier. The substance is often used primarily for its flavor-modifying properties and not exclusively as a sweetener. It is mostly composed of *five* distinct forms *viz.* thaumatins I, II, III, b, and c. All of them are almost 100,000 times sweeter than sucrose, and do have molecular weights around 22,000. Sweetness of thaumatin builds very slowly. Perception lasts a long time, leaving a liquorice-like aftertaste at high usage levels. Thaumatin is highly water-soluble, stable to heating, and stable under acidic conditions. It is also used largely in such products as chewing gums, breath freshners, as it has enormous usage as a potential low-calorie sweetner.

Aromatherapy

Aromatherapy is both a preventative and an active treatment during illness or disease. It is sometimes used in combination with massage and other therapeutic techniques as part of a holistic treatment approach on the external use of essential aromatic plant oils to maintain and promote physical, physiological, and spiritual wellbeing. Aromatherapy is the art and science of utilizing naturally extracted aromatic essences from plants to balance harmonies and promote the health of body, mind and spirit. It seeks to explore the physiological and psychological and spiritual realm of the individual's response to aromatic extracts to reduce stress and enhance the individual's healing process.

It involves external application of essential oils via full-body massage, added to a warm bath, inhalation, topical application, steam, and used to moisten a compress that is applied to the affected part of the body.

Aromatherapy is a form of alternative medicine makes use of essential oils that is believed to benefit both the mind and body and other aromatic compounds from plants for the purpose of physical wellbeing. Aromatherapists use essential oils to help people to relax from stress and enjoy the sensory experiences of massage, warm water, and pleasant smells. Aromatherapy makes use of essential oil which differs herbal products in chemical constituents due to its extraction technique (distillation). Distillation process extracts out the lighter phytomolecules monoterpenes, sesquiterpenes and esters; aromatic compounds: non-terpene hydrocarbons; some organic sulfides, etc. The aromatic substance from a flower stimulates the olfactory bulb and neurons. The desired emotional response (e.g. relaxation) is activated from the limbic system of the brain. The absorption rate of most essential oils is immediate in skin as they are lipophilic. Essential oils are considered the inner core of all plants and roots as it contains the hormones from which they are extracted. It is nature's antibiotics due to its ability to limit the growth of micro-organisms. Most aromatherapists believe that aromatherapy should be used as an adjunct not as a substitute for mainstream medical or psychiatric care. The history of aromatherapy is described in Table 9.1.

Physical and Psychological Benefits of Aromatherapy

Some common medicinal properties of volatile oil used in aromatherapy include sedative, antiseptic, antimicrobial, expectorant, diuretic, astringent and analgesic. It is used to treat symptoms including mood disorders, gastrointestinal discomfort, skin conditions, menstrual pain and irregularities, stress-related conditions, and wounds.

There are several different techniques for the use of essential oils in aromatherapy:

Massage: Massage is an integral part of the aromatherapy process. It allows a soothing and therapeutic application of essential oils

Table 9.1: History of aromatherapy

S.no.	Aromatherapy pioneer	Milestone
1.	Egyptian's wrote papyrus manuscript (2800 BC)	They explained details of medical herbs, and essential oils
2.	Chinese wrote yellow emperor's book of internal medicine (2000 BC)	They explained use of herbs including opium and ginger
3.	Jeues decalared the book of exodus in the bible (1240 BC)	They emphasized use of cinnamon, myrrh, olive oil and cassia along with different aromatic herbs
4.	Gattefre (1928) French chemist	He devised the term aromatherapy, and described therapeutics possibilities of essential oils
5.	French man, Jews Valnet (1964)	He explained uses of aromatic oils to treat patients with psychiatric and medical disorders

to heal and rejuvenate the body. For use in massage, essential oils are mixed with a vegetable carrier oil, usually wheatgerm, avocado, olive, safflower, grapeseed, or soya bean oil. A ratio is 2.5–5% essential oil to 95–97.5% carrier oil. Massage can work as a stimulant as well as a relaxant. Blending essential oils and massaging them into your body work on the olfactory nerves as well as the limbic system.

Full-body baths: Full body baths are the most beneficial and are very pleasant. They have been used as specific therapeutic aids in the treatment of disorders and for their beautifying effect. In this technique, the essential oil is added to a tubful of warm (but not hot) water as the water is running. The dosage of essential oil is usually 5–10 drops per bath.

Hand or foot baths: Foot baths are especially helpful in treating tired, aching feet, cases of ingrown toe nails, foot fungus problems such as athlete's foot or ringworm, injuries or sprains. These are often recommended to treat arthritis or skin disorders of the hands or feet as well as sore muscles. The hands or feet are soaked for 10–15 minutes in a basin of warm water to which 5–7 drops of essential oil have been added.

Inhalations: Inhalation of essential oils is rapid and deeply affects the physical and emotional bodies. This technique is used to treat sinus problems or such nasal allergies as hay fever. Two to five drops of essential oil are added to the steaming water, and the person leans over the container and inhales the fragrant vapors for five to ten minutes.

Diffusion: Aromatherapy could help us enhance our health and thus enable us to better enjoy our life. Diffusion is recommended for treating emotional upsets. This technique requires the use of a special nebulizer to disperse microscopic droplets of essential oil into the air, or a clay diffuser that allows the oil to evaporate into the air when it is warmed by a small votive candle or electric bulb.

Compresses: An aromatherapy compress is a cloth soaked in water and essential oils. Make a compress solution by adding six drops of essential oil with two cups of distilled water. Place a clean cotton cloth in the aromatic water. Soak the cloth. Squeeze excess liquid and apply the compress to the affected area. Wrap the compress around the injury or ailing area with plastic wrap. Keep the compress in place until it cools or warms to body temperature. Reapply, if needed.

Aromatic salves: Salves are made by melting together vegetable oil and beeswax in a double boiler over medium heat, and adding the desired combination of essential oils.

Internal use: Some essential oils such as oil of peppermint and cinnamon can be used to make teas or mouthwashes, or mixed with a glass of honey and water.

The properties of essential oils are described in Table 9.2.

Extraction of Essential Oil

There are four ways of extraction of essential oil:
1. Expression
2. Steam distillation
3. Extraction by volatile solvents
4. Adsorption in purified fat (enfleurage)

1. Expression: The plant material is crushed and the juice is screened to remove the large particles. The screened juice is centrifuged at a high speed when nearly half of the essential oils is extracted. The other half of the oil is generally not extracted and such residue is used for isolation of the inferior quality of oil by distillation.

Example: Citrus, lemon and grass oils.

2. Steam distillation: Distillation can be performed on mixtures in which two compounds are not miscible. This process is called co-distillation. When one compound of water, the process is steam distillation. This is most widely used method, the plant material is macerated and then steam distilled when the essential oils is distillate, it is extracted by the use of pure organic volatile solvents like light petroleum. However, the method should be used with a great care, since some essential oils are decomposed during distillation and some (esters) are hydrolysed to non or less fragment compounds.

Example: Clove, cumin.

3. Extraction by means of volatile solvents: As described above, some essential oils are sensitive to heat and hence decomposed during distillation, in such cases the plant material is directly treated with light petrol at 50°C and the solvent is then removed by distillation under reduced pressure.

Example: Jasmine, tuberose and hyacinth.

4. Enfluerage: It is also known as essential oil extraction with cold fat. The principle is that fat possesses high power of absorption when brought in contact with fragrant, flowers, readily absorb the perfumes emitted. The fat taken in glass plates is warmed to about 50°C, then its surface is covered with the petals and it is allowed to be kept as such for several days until the fat is saturated with the essential oils for which the old petals may be replaced by the fresh ones. The petals are then removed and the fat is digested with ethyl alcohol fill the essential oils present in fat are dissolved in ethyl alcohol. And if some fat is also dissolved during digestion, it is removed by cooling to about 20°C. The extract having ethyl alcohol and essential oils is distilled under reduced pressure to remove the solvent. But recently, the activated coconut charcoal is used in place of fat owing to the greater stability and more surface as compared to fat.

Example: Tuberose and jasmine

Isolation and Separation of Essential Oils

Isolation

Essential oils are isolated mainly four types of distillation techniques from plant material:
1. Water distillation
2. Water and steam distillation
3. Direct steam distillation
4. Distillation per se.

1. Water distillation: The material is completely immersed in water and is boiled by applying heat either by direct heat or steam jacket. The

Table 9.2: Properties of essential oils for use in aromatherapy

S. no.	Essential oil	Properties
1.	Jasmine (*Jasminum officinale*)	Antidepressant, soothing and moisturizing
2.	Ginger (*Zingiber officinale*)	Stimulant, in digestive problems and poor memory
3.	Rose (*Rosa centifolia*)	Antidepressant, moisturizing and in aging skin
4.	Basil (*Ocimum basilicum*)	In mental strain, poor memory and nervous fatigue
5.	Cinnamon (*Cinnamomum zeylanicum*)	Digestive disorders
6.	Fennel (*Foeniculum vulgare*)	Stomach-related problems
7.	Peppermint (*Mentha piperanta*)	Relieving nasal, sinus and chest congestion
8.	Sandalwood (*Santalum album*)	Perfumery, excellent blending properties and antidepressant
9.	Orange (*Citrus aurantium*)	Sedative can treat anxiety and depression, for constipation and mouth ulcers
10.	Cardamom (*Elettaria cardamomum*)	Aphrodisiac, stimulant and in digestive disorders.
11.	Lemon (*Citrus limonia*)	Antidepressant
12.	Myrrh (*Commiphora molmol*)	Antinflammatory, antiwrinkles and in treatment of mouth ulcers
13.	Neroli (Citrus auranthium)	In treatment of nervous tension and anxiety
14.	Coriander (*Coriandrum sativum*)	Stimulant and carminative
15.	Camphor (*Cinnamomum camphora*)	Relieve nasal congestion and cough, analgesic effect relieving massage blends for sore muscles and arthritic pain
16.	Benzion (*Styrax benzoin*)	In anxiety, energy imbalance, loneliness and sadness.
17.	Nutmeg (*Myristica fragrans*)	Local stimulant to the gastrointestinal tract
18.	Palmarosa (*Cymbopogon martini*)	Treat fevers, infectious diseases, rheumatism and nerve pain
19.	Sage (*Salvia officinalis*)	Stimulant, tonic and carminative

plant material and boiling water are in direct contact in this method. It is also referred as hydrodistillation. Its major disadvantage is that complete isolation of oils is not possible. Hydrodistillation is used only in cases where the plant material by its nature cannot be processed by water and steam distillation or by direct steam distillation.

2. Water and steam distillation: The plant material is lodged on a perforated grid or screen inserted above the bottom of still. The still is filled with water up to sufficient level and the water is heated. This method has many advantages over the hydrodistillation method.

3. Direct steam distillation: The plant material is supported on a grid and saturated steam is injected through the charge by the means of open or perforated coils placed below the grid. This method not only produces the best yield and the purest oil but also enables the operators to attain the end sought most economically and with simple apparatus.

4. Distillation per se: The large quantities of volatile oil are produced without much human labor. It is a fact that the high temperature of steam destroys the unstable perfume components. Since high pressure steam causes considerable decomposition. As such without use of any water or steam is employed in cases of the separation of volatile fractions of turpentine. It becomes possible as well as the resins are mains in the form of molten liquid and support the separation of less volatile fraction.

Separation

i. Chemical methods:

1. Volatile oil treated with NaCl in chloroform. The products are separated and decomposed and collected.
2. Terpenoid alcohol and volatile oil are separated with reaction with pthalic anhydride to form diesters.
3. Terpenoid aldehyde and ketone are separated by reaction with carbonyl reagent, $NaHCO_3$ and 2–4 drops of dinitrophenyl hydrazine and grignard reagent through which are isolated terpenoids, ketones and aldehydes.

i. Physical distillation:

1. Fractional distillation
2. Chromatography

1. *Fractional distillation:* During such type of distillation, mono-terpenoid hydrocarbon and trioxygenated derivatives and residue contain sesquiterpenes which are unextracted.

2. *Chromatography:* Adsorption chromatography is generally used by using silica gel and alumina used as isolation technique.

EUCALYPTUS

Synonyms: Blue gum tree, stringy bark tree

Botanical name: It is obtained from leaves of *Eucalyptus globulus*, belonging to family Myrtaceae.

Habitat: Australia, North and South Africa, India, Southern Europe and Spain.

Characteristics: Colorless to pale yellow with a strong, fresh, camphorous odor and woody undertone.

Oil properties: Eucalyptus has a clear, sharp, fresh and very distinctive smell. It is pale yellow in color and watery in viscosity.

Extraction: Eucalyptus oil is extracted from Steam distillation of fresh or partially dried leaves and young twigs.

Chemical composition: The main chemical components of eucalyptus are: Camphene, citronellal, fenchene, phellandrene and cineole.

Precautions: Eucalyptus oil should be used with care and people with high blood pressure and epilepsy should avoid it. Excessive use of the oil may cause headaches.

Therapeutic properties: Eucalyptus has a cooling and deodorizing effect on the body, helping with fevers, migraine and malaria. The therapeutic properties of eucalyptus oil include: analgesic, antirheumatic, antineuralgic, antispasmodic, antiseptic, balsamic, decongestant, deodorant, diuretic, expectorant, insecticide, rubefacient and stimulant. Eucalyptus oil is useful as warming oil when used for muscular aches and pains, rheumatoid arthritis, sprains and poor circulation. In skin care, it can be used for burns, blisters, herpes, cuts, wounds, skin infections and insect bites. Eucalyptus oil can boost the immune system, and is helpful especially in cases of chickenpox, colds, flu and measles. It is used in burners and vaporizers, blended massage or in the bath and gargles.

GERANIUM

Synonyms: Alum root, spotted cranesbill, wild cranesbill, storksbill, alum bloom, wild geranium.

Botanical name: It is obtained from dried rhizomes and leaves of *Geranium maculatum*, belonging to family Geraniaceae.

Habitat: Flourishes in low grounds and woods from Newfoundland to Manitoba, south to Georgia, Missouri and in Europe.

Oil properties: The oil is mostly colorless but can have a slight light green color to it, and has a watery viscosity. The geranium oil we sell is extracted from the plant *Pelargonium odorantissimum*.

Extraction: The leaves and stalks are used for extraction, and the oil is obtained through steam distillation.

Chemical composition: The essential oil is composed of various chemical constituents and includes the following: geraniol, geranic, citronellol, citronellyl formate, linalol (linalool), euganol, myrtenol, terpineol, citral, methone and sabinene, tannic and gallic acid, also starch, sugar, gum, pectin and coloring matter.

Precautions: Geranium oil is not indicated to cause any side effect, since it is non-toxic, non-irritant and generally non-sensitizing, yet can cause sensitivity in some people and due to the fact that it balances the hormonal system, it might not be a good idea to use in pregnancy.

Therapeutic properties: The therapeutic properties of geranium oil include the following: As an astringent, hemostatic, diuretic, antiseptic, antidepressant, tonic, antibiotic, antispasmodic and anti-infectious. Geranium oil can be used to help in the treatment of the following: Acne, bruises, burns, cuts, dermatitis, eczema, hemorrhoids, lice, mosquito repellant, ringworm, ulcers, breast engorgement, edema, poor circulation, sore throat, tonsillitis, menopausal problems, stress and neuralgia.

JASMINE

Synonyms: Jasmin, jessamine and common jasmine.

Botanical name: Jasmine essential oil is extracted from *Jasminum officinale*, belonging to family Oleaceae.

Extraction: In manufacturing, jasmine oil is produced as a 'concrete' by solvent extraction, and an absolute is obtained from the concrete by separation with alcohol, and an essential oil is produced off the absolute by steam distillation.

Chemical composition: The main chemical components of jasmine oil are: Benzyl, nerol, terpineol, linalyl acetate, methyl anthranilate, jasmone and farnesol.

Oil properties: Jasmine essential oil has a sweet, exotic and rich floral smell and the oil is deep orange-brown in color.

Precautions: Jasmine oil is non-toxic, non-irritant and generally non-sensitizing, although some people do have an allergic reaction to the oil. Jasmine oil is used to ease labor as well as an emmenagogue. It should not be used during pregnancy. It can impede concentration, so should be used with care.

Therapeutic properties: The therapeutic properties of jasmine oil include: antidepressant, aphrodisiac, antispasmodic, antiseptic, stimulant and emollient. It soothes the nerves and produces a feeling of confidence, optimism and euphoria. It revitalizes and restores energy. Jasmine oil facilitates delivery in childbirth; it hastens the birth by strengthening the contractions and at the same time relieves the pain. Jasmine oil helps with sexual problems, such as impotence, premature ejaculation and frigidity. In the respiratory system, it also soothes irritating coughs and helps with hoarseness and laryngitis. It helps with muscle pain, sprains, and stiff limbs. Jasmine tones dry, greasy, irritated and sensitive skin, increases elasticity and is often used to assist with stretch marks and scarring.

ROSE

Synonyms: Bulgarian and Turkish rose, Otto of rose and attar of rose.

Botanical name: Rose oil is extracted from *Rosa damascena* from the Rosaceae family.

Aromatherapy

Habitat: Northern Persia, on the Caspian, or Faristan on the Gulf of Persia.

Oil properties: Rose has a deep, rosy, fresh aroma, the color ranges from clear to a pale yellow or greenish tint and the viscosity is watery to crystalline, when warm or cold, respectively.

Extraction: Rose oil is extracted from the fresh flowers, picked before 8 am in the morning, by steam distillation and the yield is 0.02–0.05%. The aroma can be damaged, if the heat is too high at distillation.

Chemical composition: The main chemical components of Rose otto oil are: Citronellol, geraniol, nerol, farnesol, geranic and eugenol.

Precautions: The rose oil is non-toxic, non-irritant and non-sensitizing but should not be used during pregnancy.

Therapeutic properties: The rose oil soothes the mind and helps with depression, grief, nervous tension and stress and is helpful for poor circulation and heart palpitations. The therapeutic properties of rose oil are: Anti-infectious, antidepressant, antiseptic, antispasmodic, aphrodisiac, astringent, bactericidal, diuretic, emmenagogue, hepatic, laxative, sedative, splenetic and general tonic. Rose otto oil can be used for irregular menstruation, leukorrhea, menorrhagia and uterine disorders. On the skin, it can be used for broken capillaries, dry skin, eczema, herpes, mature and sensitive skin, wrinkles, and rose water can be used for conjunctivitis.

SANDALWOOD

Synonyms: East Indian sandalwood, santal, saunders and sandalwood Mysore.

Botanical name: Sandalwood oil is extracted from *Santalum album* from the Santalaceae family.

Oil properties: The oil has a woody, exotic smell, subtle and lingering. The color of the oil is pale yellow to pale gold.

Extraction: Sandalwood oil is extracted from the chipped heartwood and roots by steam distillation and yields 4–6.5%.

Chemical composition: The main chemical components are: Santalol, furfurol and santalene.

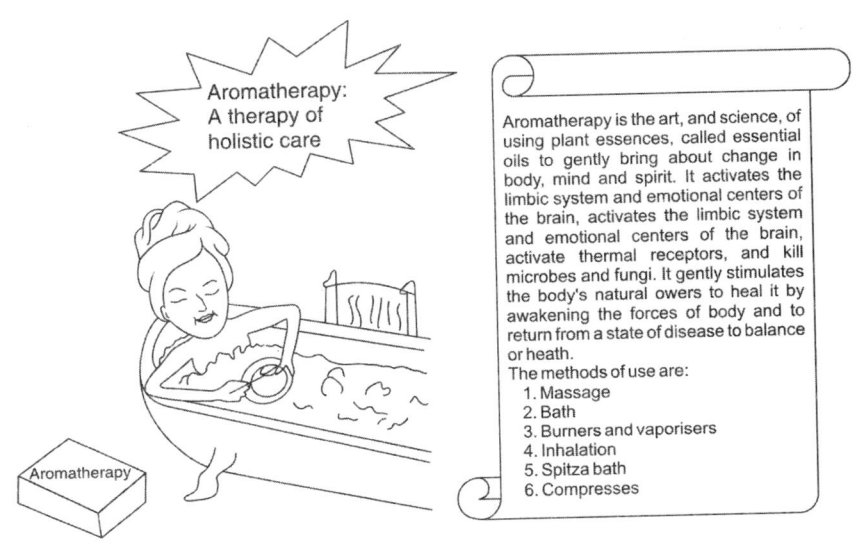

Aromatherapy: A therapy of holistic care

Aromatherapy

Aromatherapy is the art, and science, of using plant essences, called essential oils to gently bring about change in body, mind and spirit. It activates the limbic system and emotional centers of the brain, activates the limbic system and emotional centers of the brain, activate thermal receptors, and kill microbes and fungi. It gently stimulates the body's natural owers to heal it by awakening the forces of body and to return from a state of disease to balance or heath.
The methods of use are:
1. Massage
2. Bath
3. Burners and vaporisers
4. Inhalation
5. Spitza bath
6. Compresses

Precautions: Generally, sandalwood oil is non-toxic, non-irritant and non-sensitizing.

Therapeutic properties: This relaxing oil could be useful for tension, depression, nervous exhaustion, chronic illness and anxiety. Sandalwood oil could be useful for chest infections, sore throats and dry coughs that accompany bronchitis and lung infections. It is used as antiseptic, diuretic, aphrodisiac, astringent, carminative, emollient, expectorant, sedative and tonic.

PEPPERMINT

Botanical name: *Mentha piperita*

Common method of extraction: Steam distillation.

Characteristic

Color: Clear with a yellow tinge.

Consistency: Thin, perfumery

Note: Top, strength of initial aroma: Strong.

Description: Mint leaves are dried spearmint leaves of the species *Mentha spicata*. The dark green leaves have a pleasant warm, fresh, aromatic, sweet flavor with a cool aftertaste.

Possible uses: Asthma, colic, exhaustion, fever, flatulence, headache, nausea, scabies, sinusitis, vertigo.

10 Flavoring Agents, Sweeteners and Bitter Plant Substances

FLAVORING AGENTS

Generally, the term "flavor" is the sensory impression of food that implies an overall integrated perception of all of the contributing senses (smell, taste, sight, feeling, and sound) at the time of food consumption. According to British standards, flavor is a combination of taste and odor which may be influenced by sensation of pain, heat, cold and tactile sensation.

Flavor is very important due to reason that it is substance added for the acceptability of foods, confectionery, medicines and drinks. The flavor of a food is the combined effects of taste, smell and mouthfeel (Table 10.1).

Flavor detection depends on the properties of stimulating molecules:
- Physicochemical properties (i.e. volatility, lipid and water solubility).
- Receptive properties of different receptors present in nose and oral cavity.
- Olfactory, gustatory, trigeminal chemosensory modalities.

Table 10.1: Senses with their responses of flavors

Stimulus	Senses	Response
Food	Sight	Appearance
	Odor	Flavor
	Taste	
	Hearing	Texture
	Touch	

Food flavors are of two types:
1. **Desirable flavor,** e.g. orange juice, potato chip, roast beef
2. **Undesirable flavor** (off flavor), e.g. oxidized, stable, rancid, warmed-over.

Characteristics of ideal flavor:
- It should be harmless, technologically compatible, readily and uniformly miscible, and stable.
- It should be strictly comply with all the legislative requirements prevailing in the country.
- It should be capable of measured in accurate dosage, handled by food processing section.
- It should be economic and resistant to storage.

UK Food Law defines a natural flavor as:
A flavoring substance (or flavoring substances) which is (or are) obtained, by physical, enzymatic or microbiological processes, from material of vegetable or animal origin which material is either raw or has been subjected to a process normally used in preparing food for human consumption and to no process other than one normally so used.

The US Code of Federal Regulations describes a "natural flavorant" as:

The essential oil, oleoresin, essence or extractive, protein hydrolysate, distillate, or any product of roasting, heating or enzymolysis, which contains the flavoring constituents derived from a spice, fruit or fruit juice, vegetable or vegetable juice, edible yeast, herb, bark, bud, root, leaf or any other edible portions of a plant, meat, seafood, poultry, eggs, dairy products, or fermentation products thereof, whose primary function in food is flavoring rather than nutritional (Table 10.2).

Table 10.2: Classification of flavor

Flavors	Flavor class	Subdivision	Example
Flavorings are focused on altering or enhancing the flavors of natural food product, such as meats and vegetables, or creating flavor for food products that do not have the desired flavors.			
Food variety	Fruit flavor	Berry type	Raspberry, banana
		Citrus type	Orange, grapes
	Vegetable flavor		Celery, Lettuce
	Spice flavor	Aromatic	Cinnamon, peppermint
		Lachrymogenic	Garlic, onion
		Hot	Ginger, pepper
	Beverage flavors	Unfermented flavors	Juices, milk
		Fermented flavors	Wine, beer, tea drinks
		Compounded flavors	Soft drink
	Meat flavors	Mammal flavors	Lean beef
		Sea food flavors	Fish, clams
	Fat flavors		Olive oil, coconut fat, butter fat
	Stench flavors		Cheese
	Cooked flavors	Broth vegetablefruit	Beef bouillonlegume, potatoes marmalade
	Processed flavors	Smoky flavors	Ham
		Boiled, fried flavors	Processed meat products
		Roasted, toasted, baked flavors	Coffee, snack foods, processed cereals
Flavors are organic compounds belonging to different chemical classes; alcohol, aldehydes, amines, esters, lactones, trepenes, etc.			

Flavor	Chemical class	Example	Structure
Chemical structure	Heterocyclic compounds	Furan, pyridine, pyrazines	(furan, pyridine, pyrazine structures)
	Nitrogen containing compounds	Trimethylamine	$H_3C-N(CH_3)-CH_3$
	Hydrocarbon	Limonene, α and β pinene	Limonene

(Contd.)

Table 10.2: Classification of flavor (*Contd.*)

Flavor	Chemical class	Example	Structure
			α-Pinene, β-Pinene
	Aldehyde	Vanillin, citral	Vanillin, a(geranial), b(neral)
	Alcohol	Geraniol, eugenol	Geraniol, Eugenol
	Esters	Ethyl acetate	Ethyl acetate
	Acid	Acetic, butyric acid	Acetic acid, Butyric acid
	Ketone	Diacetyl, b-ionone	Diacetyl

(*Contd.*)

Table 10.2: Classification of flavor *(Contd.)*

Flavor	Chemical class	Example	Structure
	Lactones	γ-nonlactone	b-ionone γ-nonlactone

According to origin

Flavor	Description	Example
Entirely natural	Produced naturally by chemical and biochemical (enzymatic) processes. Active in plants or animals during their growth and ripening of vegetable and fruit, meat maturation.	Strawberry flavor
	Herb: They are soft stemmed plant materials which generate aroma when crushed or ground.	Rosemary, curry leaves
	Spices: Aromatic plant materials used in the flavoring or seasoning of the food material.	Coriander, pepper, chilli, etc.
Nature identical chemicals	Chemical components entirely made by man but found in nature	Vanilla, strawberry, mango, banana
Synthetic flavors	Blend of natural and synthetic flavor compounds	
Artificial flavors	These components are entirely made by man and not found in nature	Ethyl vanillin

Flavor changes during food storage:

Flavors are changed during food storage, there are four ways:

- Due to nature of flavor compounds: Evaporation chemical reaction; oxidation (i.e. alcohols, aldehyde), cleavage, polymerization, interaction with other compounds (i.e. lipid oxidation).
- Due to continuing aroma biogenesis: Evolution of the flavor due to aroma compounds production during fruit maturation (green banana flavor, mature banana flavor).
- Due to tissue disruption or enzyme reaction: During processing (cutting, crushing); release of aroma precursors and this induces enzyme reactions (i.e. garlic, onion, cabbage, cauliflower, brussels sprouts, mushrooms.
- Due to processing induced reactions Example: Evolution of Maillard reaction, lipid oxidation.

Objectives of Flavor Chemistry

- To understand the chemical composition of natural flavors and the mechanism of their formation.
- To retard or prevent the development of the off-flavors in foods, reversion flavor in soybean oil, hexenal, 2-pentyl furan (they are resulted from polyunsaturated triglycerides, i.e. linolenate, linoleate).
- To restore the fresh flavor to a processed food.
- To improve the flavor of food by the addition of synthetic flavor.
- To produce new foods with special flavor, such as potato chip flavor.
- To improve flavor by the acceleration of reactions which produce desirable flavor compound (onion flavor: pH 5~7).
- To assist geneticist to breed food raw material with improved flavor compounds or flavor precursors.
- To specify raw material and to control quality of food products.

Flavor Analysis

To analysis flavor which are characterize food flavor, determine concentration of selected aroma compounds, detect presence specific components, evaluate flavor intensity and evaluate flavor compounds partitioning (k). The instrument like gas chromatography (GC), mass chromatography (GCMS), electronic nose as well as trained sensory analyzer also used to analyze the flavor.

Some Important Food Flavors

Camphor

Description: It is a terpenoid ($C_{10}H_{16}O$) which is waxy, white or transparent solid with a strong, aromatic odor.

Biological source: It is obtained from wood of the camphor laurel *Cinnamomum camphora*, belonging to family Lauraceae.

Uses: Flavoring agent, used as ingredient for sweets and widely used for cooking

Clove

Eugenol

Description: Cloves are the immature unopened flower buds of a tropical tree. The compound eugenol is responsible for most of the characteristic aroma of cloves.

Biological source: It is obtained from dried flower bud of *Eugenia caryophyllata* belonging to family Myrtaceae.

Uses: Flavoring agent (sweetly pungent, astringent and strongly aromatic), used in the production of perfumes as well as clove is key ingredient of tea.

Capsaicin

Description: Capsaicin 8-methyl-N-vanillyl-6-nonenamide, it is hydrophobic, colorless, odorless, and crystalline to waxy.

Capsaicin

Biological source: It consists of dried ripe fruits of *Capsicum minimum* and *C. annum* Linn and contains NMT 5% of calices and pedicels, Family Solanaceae.

Uses: Flavoring agent (burning sensation).

Cinnamaldehyde

Cinnamaldehyde

Description: Cinnamaldehyde is the chemical compound that gives cinnamon its flavor and odor.

Biological source: It is obtained from bark of *Cinnamomum zeylanicum* belonging to family Lauraceae.

Uses: Cinnamaldehyde is used in some perfumes of natural, sweet, or fruity scents, as a fungicide and also as a food adulterant. It is used as a flavoring food items like chewing gum, ice cream, candy, and beverages.

Citral

Citral

Description: Citral, or 3,7-dimethyl-2,6-octadienal or lemonal, is a mixture of terpenoids with the molecular formula $C_{10}H_{16}O$.

Biological source: Citral is present in the oils of several plants, including *Lemon myrtle* (90–98%), *Listsea citrata* (90%), *Litsea cubeba* (70–85%), lemongrass (65–85%), lemon tea-tree (70–80%), *Ocimum gratissimum* (66.5%), *Lindera citriodora* (approx. 65%), *Calypranthes parriculata* (approx. 62%).

Uses: Citral is an aroma compound used in perfumery for its citrus effect. Citral is also used as a flavor and for fortifying lemon oil. Citral is used in the synthesis of vitamin A as well as to mask the smell of smoke.

Eucalyptol

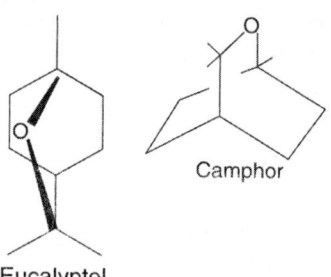

Eucalyptol   Camphor

Description: It is a natural organic compound which is a colorless liquid. It is a cyclic ether and a monoterpenoid.

Biological source: It is the active ingredient of eucalyptus oil obtained from leaf of *Eucalyptus*, species of the plant family Myrtaceae.

Uses: Due to its pleasant spicy aroma and taste, it is used in flavorings, fragrances, and cosmetics. It is also an ingredient in many brands of mouthwash and cough suppressant.

Menthol

Menthol

Description: Menthol is an organic compound made synthetically or obtained from peppermint or other mint oils. It is a waxy, crystalline substance, clear or white in color.

Biological source: It is mainly obtained from *Mentha* species belonging to family Lamiaceae.

Flavoring Agents, Sweeteners and Bitter Plant Substances

Uses: Peppermint has a high menthol content, and is often used as tea and for flavoring ice-cream, confectionery, chewing gum, and toothpaste.

Piperine

Piperine

Description: Piperine is the alkaloid responsible for the pungency of black pepper and long pepper.

Biological source: It is mainly obtained from black pepper (*Piper nigrum*) belonging to family Piperceae.

Uses: It is used as a flavoring agent due to its aromatic characters. Pepper gets its spicy heat mostly from the piperine compound, which is found both in the outer fruit and in the seed.

Vanillin

Vanillin

Description: Vanillin methyl vanillin, or 4-hydroxy-3-methoxybenzaldehyde, is an organic compound with the molecular formula $C_8H_8O_3$.

Biological source: Natural vanillin is extracted from the seed pods of *Vanilla planifolia* belonging to family Orchidaceae.

Uses: As a flavoring, usually in sweet foods, ice-creams, confection and baked goods. Vanillin is also used in the fragrance industry, in perfumes, and intermediate in the production of pharmaceuticals

Zingiberene

Zingiberene

Description: Zingiberene is a monocyclic sesquiterpene that is the predominant constituent of the oil of ginger.

Biological source: It is obtained from rhizomes of *Zingiber officinale* belonging to family Zingiberaceae.

Uses: It is also used as an adjunct to many tonic and stimulating remedies.

SWEETENING AGENTS

Sweeteners/sugars are either simple carbohydrates or complex carbohydrates. Simple carbohydrates are quickly absorbed into the bloodstream, causing the pancreas to crank out insulin to whisk away the excess, resulting very quickly in low blood sugar/fatigue. Sugar (sucrose) imparts a sweet taste that is quick, clean, and short lived. Sugar is also an important functional ingredient for preparing attractive foods. It provides the support for bulkiness, texture, preservation, flavor, and color. However, sugar is a nutritive sweetener. It is easily metabolized, yielding energy of 4 kcal/g (16.7 kJ/g).

The worldwide demand for high potency sweeteners is increasing and, with blending of different sweeteners becoming a standard practice, the demand for the search of alternative natural sweeteners is also increasing. Due to many adverse effects of artificial sweeteners, for example, aspartame, sucralose, acesulphame K and the natural sweetener sucrose found in sugar cane and bee's honey, the search for natural sweeteners derived from plants has been intensified.

Characteristics of Sweeteners

The ideal sweetener should be water-soluble and stable in both acidic and basic conditions and over a wide range of temperatures. Length of stability and consequently the shelf-life of the final product are also important. The final food product should taste much like the traditional one. A sweetener must be compatible with a wide range of food ingredients because sweetness is one component of complex flavor systems. The sweetener must be non-toxic and metabolized normally or excreted unchanged. To be successful, a sweetener should be competitively priced with sucrose and other comparable sweeteners. It should be easily produced, stored, transported and safe.

- The sweetener should have a taste profile like sugar, highly sweet, odorless, colorless, stable to cooking foods, non-carcinogenic, non-caloric, tooth friendly and cheap to market the product.
- A good alternative sweetener should have other qualities clean sweet taste, quick onset, no lingering aftertaste, compatibility with other food ingredients, high water solubility, high dissolution rate, and ease of handling.
- It should also be non-hygroscopic, synergistic with other sweeteners, economical (same or cheaper than sugar based on sweetness equivalence), and have a high degree of consumer acceptance, e.g. no perceived toxicity.

Classification of Sweeteners

- Non-nutritive sweeteners.
- Nutritive sweeteners.

Non-nutritive sweeteners: Non-nutritive sweeteners are essentially kilojoule-free and, therefore, have no effect on blood glucose levels. Generally, these are high intensity sweeteners and contribute only sweetness to the foods to which they are added. These include aspartame, acesulphame K, saccharin, sucralose, cyclamate, neotame and thaumatin.

Nutritive sweeteners: Nutritive sweeteners are usually different types of carbohydrate. Therefore, they are not kilojoule-free and have different effects on blood glucose levels. They impart sweet taste and calories. Products containing nutritive sweeteners may sometimes be labeled as 'carbohydrate modified'. They impart sweetness, viscosity, bulk; desirable texture and mouth feel to beverages. They have water binding properties as well as they decrease freezing point of solution and as a food source in fermentation (Table 10.3).

Alternative sweeteners (a) provide and expand food and beverage choices to control caloric, carbohydrate, or specific sugar intake; (b) assist in weight maintenance or reduction; (c) aid in the management of diabetes; (d) assist in the control of dental caries; (e) enhance the usability of pharmaceuticals and cosmetics; (f) provide sweetness in times of sugar shortage; and (g) assist in the cost effective use of limited resources.

PLANT BITTERS (Table 10.4)

The plants containing bitters (bitter substances) are exclusively used due to their intensively bitter tastes, which reflectively induce stimulation on the salivary gland and the secretion of gastric juice. The bitter taste recognizes at the very moment of excitation. The taste buds are situated at the root of the

Table 10.3: Type of sweeteners with examples

Type of sweeteners	Example	Description
Non-nutritive sweeteners	Aspartame	Aspartame is caloric dipeptide, it yields ~4 kcal/g (16.7 kJ/g), high sweetness potency (200X), negligible caloric contribution
	Neotame	N-[N-(3,3-dimethylbutyl)-L-aaspartyl]- L-phenylalanine 1-methyl ester. It is ~8000 times sweeter than sucrose or ~40 times sweeter than its analcgue, aspartame
	Acesulfame-K	Acesulfame-K 6-methyl-1, 2, 3-oxathiazin-4(3H)-one 2, 2-dioxide, is a white crystalline powder having a long 6 years or more shelf-life. It is a sweetener that resembles saccharin in structure and taste profile
	Saccharin	Saccharin3-oxo-2,3-dihydro-1,2-benzisothiazole 1,1-dioxide (o-sulfobenzimide or o-benzosulfimide), imparts a sweetness (300X) that is pleasant at the onset, lingering, bitter aftertaste
	Cyclamate	Sodium cyclamate, the sodium salt of cyclamic acid. Cyclamate is ~30 times more potent than sugar. Its aftertaste is minor compared to saccharin and acesulfame-K
	Sucralose	Sucralose is a trichloro-galactosucrose. Chemically it is 1,6-dichloro-1,6-dideoxy-b-Dfructofuranosyl-4-chloro-4-deoxy-a-D-galactopyranoside. The sweetness potency of sucralose is found to be 600X
	Stevioside	Stevioside is a naturally occurring sweetener (~200X) extracted from a South American plant, *Stevia rebaudiana* Bertoni.
	Glycyrrhizin	Glycyrrhizin, also known as glycyrrhizic acid, is a glycoside isolated from the roots of licorice, Glycyrrhiza glabra. The sweetness potency of glycyrrhizin is ~33X.

Table 10.4: Properties of bitters

S. no.	Properties	Description
1.	Bitters act as appetizers	Bitters act directly on appetite centers in the hypothalamus and indirectly through increased stomach motility.
2.	Bitters increase secretion of digestive juices	Bitters expedite the process of digestion by boosting the stomach and pancreatic enzyme secretions
3.	Bitters offer protection to the gut tissues	The bitters decrease the harmful effects of the digestive juices and dietary toxins by enhancing the already rapid rate of mucosal regeneration in the stomach and duodenum
4.	Bitters enhance bile flow	The use of bitters leads to a greater production of biliary elements and dilutes the bile as well by increasing the bicarbonate content. They are effective in curing all allergic, metabolic and immunological conditions where the diagnosis points to the digestion
5.	Bitters improve pancreatic functions	Bitters control fluctuations in blood sugar levels permanently and temporarily as well as control late-onset diabetes
6.	Bitters act as tonics	Bitter remedies were mainly resorted to in old age or in a convalescent state in order to be able to improve the quality of nourishment to the body

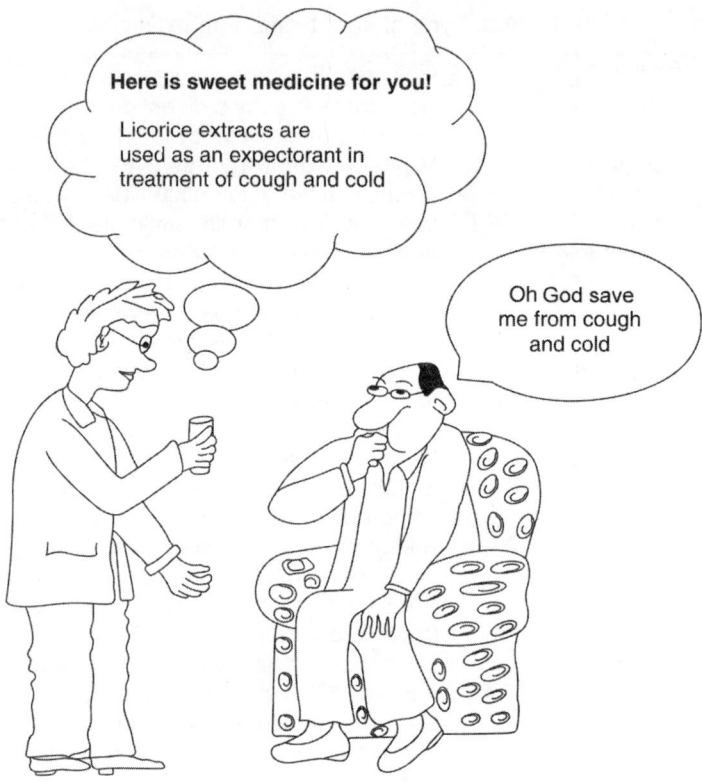

tongue, and keep the bitter taste some time afterwards (after-taste). These are then sending the signal to the brain, which by reflex then affects the swelling of the secerning mucous membranes.

The bitters have, therefore, positive influence on the digestive processes, then it lead to an improvement on appetite as well as an amelioration of the food intake.

The bitter substances are mostly of terpenoid structure, especially the sesquiterpene lactones, monoterpene iridoids and the secoiridoids, example: *Cnicus benedictus* (blessed thistle), and *Ginkgo biloba* (ginkgo). Iridoids are responsible for the chief bitter constituents of the plant family Gentianaceae, *Cichorium intybus* (chicory), *Valeriana officinalis* (valerian) and Quassia bark. Many alkaloids also contribute to the bitter taste as in the protoberberine isoquinoline alkaloids of golden seal (*Hydrastis canadensis*), and Berberis, the morphine alkaloids, the quinoline alkaloids of quinine and angostura and the purine alkaloids. In addition, miscellaneous compounds, like ketones and amino acids are responsible for the bitterness, as found in hops.

11

Plant Anatomy

Plant anatomy (Anatomy—dissection) is the study of internal structure and organization of plants, especially of their parts by means of dissection and microscopic examination. In general, plant anatomy refers to study of internal morphology, pertaining to different tissues.

The simple type of plant body is unicellular. In such forms, the single cell performs all the vital functions of life. It grows, prepares food, undergoes metabolism, reproduces and completes its span of life. The progressive evolution in plants has resulted in increasing complexity of structures. In higher plants, root, stem, leaves and flowers carry out different functions. Due to these divisions of labor, the cells of the plant are differentiated to form different tissues.

The body of a vascular plant is composed of dermal tissue, ground tissue and vascular tissue.

Dermal Tissue (Skin)

Dermal tissue is protective in function. Basing on its origin, it is classified into two types: Epidermis and periderm.

Epidermis: This is the primary surface tissue of the entire plant. Epidermal cells are compactly and continuously arranged. Epidermis provides mechanical protection, allows gaseous exchange through stomata, restricts transpiration with cuticle, and is also involved in storage, photosynthesis, secretion, absorption and perception to stimuli.

Periderm: This is formed during secondary growth replacing primary epidermis.

Ground Tissue

This is inner to dermal tissue and is composed of simple tissues, like parenchyma.

Vascular Tissue

Vascular tissue consists of conducting elements, like xylem and phloem. Vascular tissue may be scattered in ground tissue or regularly arranged forming a ring.

TISSUES AND TISSUE SYSTEMS

Morphologically, a tissue is a group of cells, which are similar in origin, form and function. Physiologically, a tissue is composed of dissimilar cells that perform a common function. The cells form various kinds of tissues. Two or more types of tissues form tissue systems. Tissues can be classified into two types (Fig. 11.1):

- Meristematic tissue, and
- Permanent tissue

Meristematic Tissue (Fig. 11.2)

A meristematic tissue (meristos = divisible) is a group of identical cells that are in a continuous state of division and are self-perpetuating. Some cells in the meristem retain their meristematic activity. Remaining cells stop dividing and acquire certain changes to become permanent tissues of the plant. This

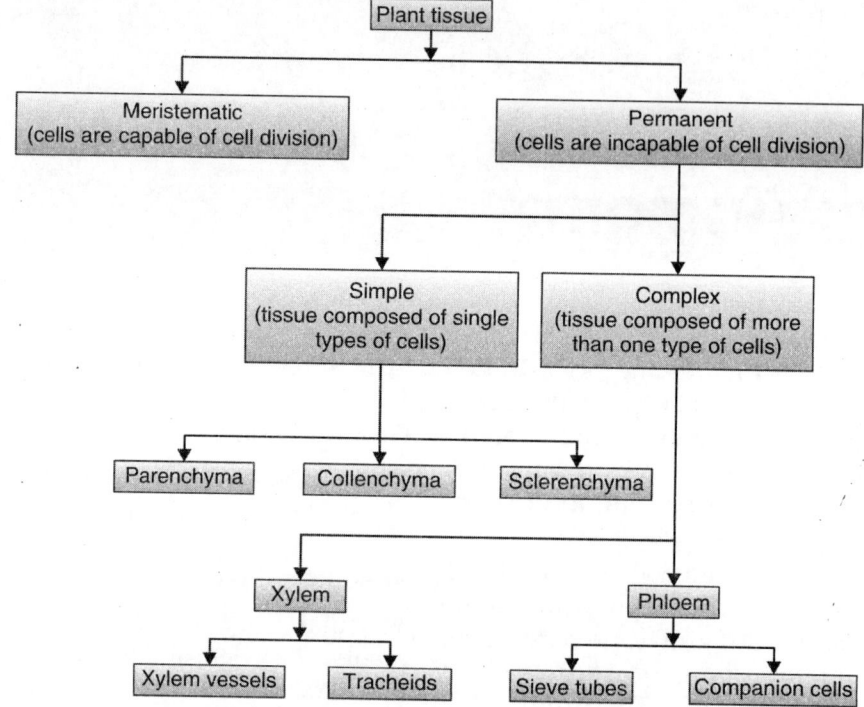

Fig. 11.1: Classification of plant tissues

change from meristematic to permanent tissue is called differentiation.

Characteristics of Meristematic Cells

Meristematic cells are isodiametric, compactly arranged with dense cytoplasm, large nucleus, and small vacuoles or without vacuoles. Their cell walls are thin, elastic and made up of cellulose. The meristematic cells may be round, oval, polygonal or rectangular in shape. They are closely arranged without intercellular spaces.

Classification of Meristem

The meristem is divided into three types – apical meristem, intercalary meristem and lateral meristem.

1. Apical meristem: Apical meristem is completely undifferentiated meristematic tissue found at the tips of roots, stem and

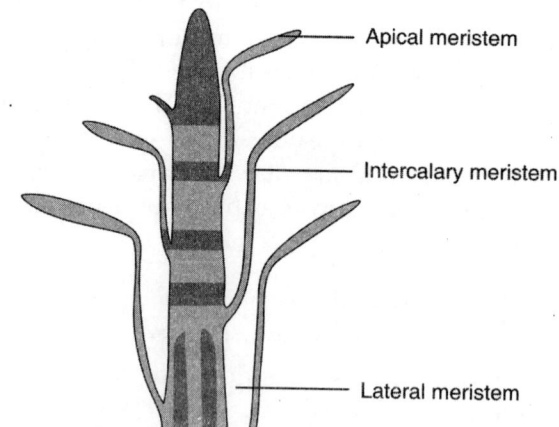

Fig. 11.2: Longitudinal section (LS) of shoot showing positions of meristems

branches, which bring about primary growth of the plants, hence also called as primary meristems. It is divided into three zones:

- Protoderm lies around the outside of the stem and gives rise to epidermal tissues.

- Procambium develops into primary xylem and primary phloem.
- Ground meristem develops into the pith and also gives rise to cortex and pith.

Intercalary meristem: It is derived from the apical meristem, present in nodal region and is responsible for the elongation of internodes. It is prominently found in monocotyledons, e.g. grasses.

Lateral meristem: The meristem is known as lateral meristem because they are involved in lateral growth, is present along the longitudinal axis of stem and root is called lateral meristem, e.g. vascular cambium and cork cambium (phellogen).

Permanent Tissue

Permanent tissues are derived from meristematic tissues (apical meristems). They have lost the power of dividing, having attained their definite form and size. They can be classified into simple and complex tissues on the basis of constituent cells (Fig. 11.3).

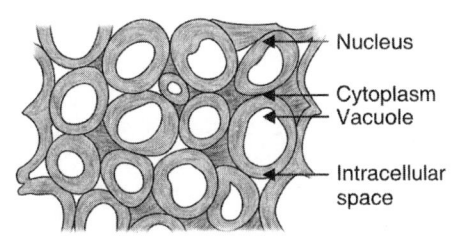

Parenchyma tissue

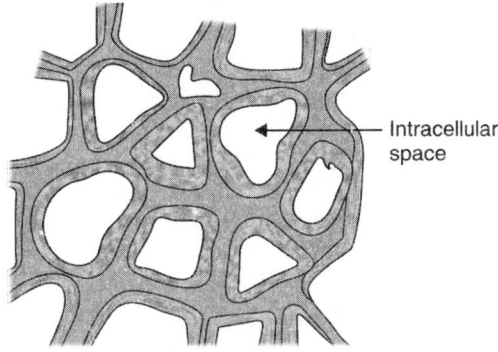

Aerenchyma

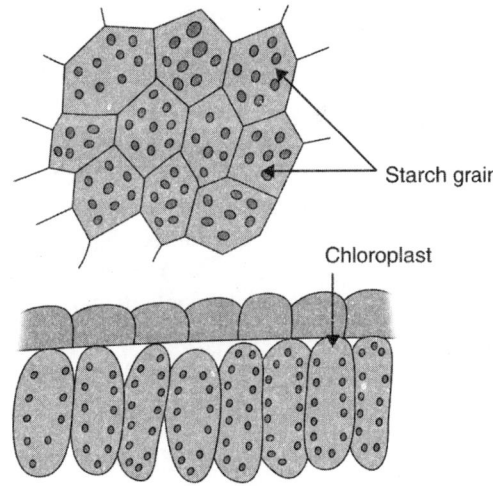

Palisade parenchyma

Fig. 11.4: Types of parenchyma tissues

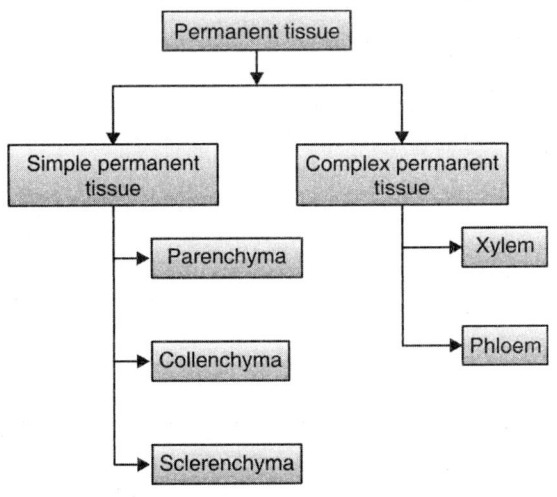

Fig. 11.3: Classification of permanent tissues

Simple Tissue (Table 11.1)

A tissue with the cells of similar structure and function is called simple tissue. It is of three types—parenchyma, collenchyma and sclerenchyma (Figs 11.4 to 11.6).

Table 11.1: Simple tissues

Type of simple tissue	Nature	Occurrence	Function
Parenchyma (Fig. 11.4)	Parenchyma is living cells, which are isodiametric, i.e. equally expanded on all sides. They may be oval, round, polygonal or elongated. The cell walls are thin and made of cellulose. Cytoplasm is dense with a single large vacuole. Intercellular spaces may be present. It may contain chlorophyll. Parenchyma which contains chlorophyll is called chlorenchyma.	Found in the cortex of root, ground tissue in stems and mesophyll of leaves	• Store and assimilates food, e.g. stem and root tubers. • Gives mechanical strength by maintaining turoidity • Store, waste products like tanin, gum, crystals and resins. • It help the plant to float in water, e.g. Nymphaea and Hydrilla due to air filled parenchyma tissue is called aerenchyma. • Its important function is photosynthesis due to chlorophyll.
Collenchyma (Fig. 11.5)	Collenchyma is a living tissue generally occurs in the dicot stems in two or more layers below the epidermis. The cells are elongated and are circular, oval or polygonal in cross-section. Cell wall is unevenly thickened with cellulose at the corners against the intercellular spaces. Besides cellulose, the cell wall contains high amounts of hemicellulose and pectin. Vacuoles are small. Intercellular spaces are generally absent. If it contains chlorophyll it is known as chlorenchyma	Found under the skin, i.e. below the epidermis in dicot stems	Provides mechanical support to the stem and assists in rapid elongation of the stem. Collenchyma may contain chloroplasts and carry out photosynthesis. **Angular collenchyma:** The cell walls of collenchyma are thickened at their angles. This type is called angular collenchyma, e.g. Hypodermis of Datura and Nicotiana. **Lacunate collenchyma:** The cell wall thickening materials are deposited on the walls bordering the intercellular spaces. This type is called lacunate collenchyma, e.g. hypodermis of Ipomoea. **Lamellar collenchyma:** The tangential walls of collenchyma are thickened and the radial walls are devoid of thickening. This type of collenchyma is called lamellar collenchyma, e.g. hypodermis of Helianthus.

(Contd.)

Table 11.1: Simple tissues (*Contd.*)

Type of simple tissue	Nature	Occurrence	Function
Sclerenchyma (Fig. 11.6)	Sclerenchyma is a dead tissue. The cells have lignified secondary walls. They lack protoplasts. The cells are long, narrow, thick and lignified, usually pointed at both ends. The cell wall is evenly thickened with lignin and sometimes is so thick that the cell cavity or lumen is absent. Nucleus is absent and hence the tissue is made up of dead cells. They have simple, often oblique pits in the walls. On the basis of origin, structure and function, sclerenchyma is divided into two types—sclereids and fibers. Sclereids are dead cells. They are found in bark, pith, cortex, hard endocarp and fleshy portions of some fruits. They vary greatly in shape and thickness. The cell wall is very thick due to lignification. Lumen is very much reduced. The pits may be simple or branched. Usually sclereids are isodiametric, but in some plants they are elongated. Fiber cells are dead cells. They are very long and narrow with pointed ends. In transverse section, the fibers are polygonal with narrow lumen. The secondary wall is evenly thickened with lignin. It possesses simple pits.	Found abundantly in stems of plants like hemp, jute and coconut, their length varying from 1 to 550 mm	Gives mechanical support to the plant by giving rigidity, flexibility and elasticity to the plant body. Sclereids are responsible for the rigidity of the seed-coat. Fibers are supporting tissues. They provide mechanical strength to the plants and protect them from the strong winds. The fibers that are found in the seed coat of some seeds are called surface fibers, e.g. cotton.

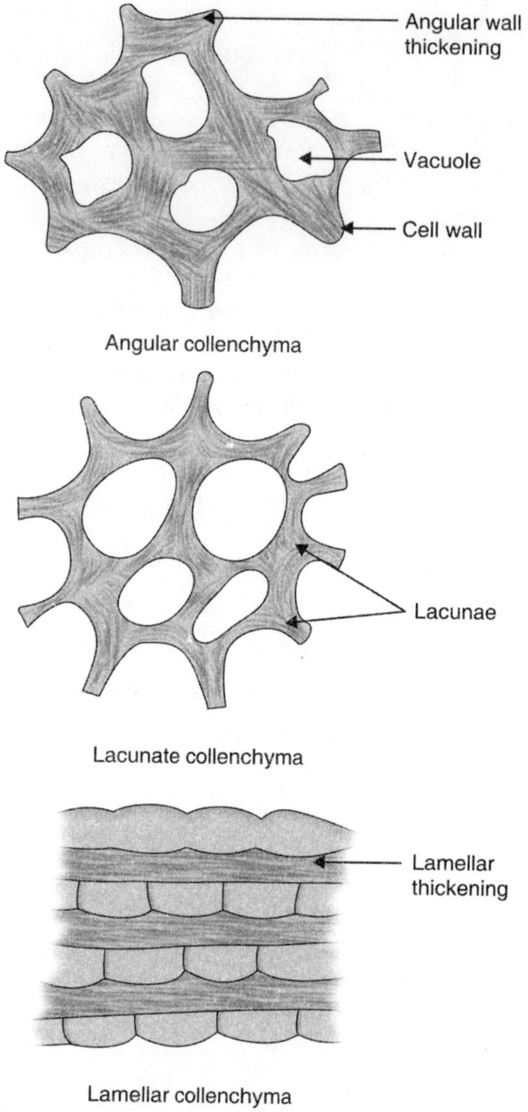

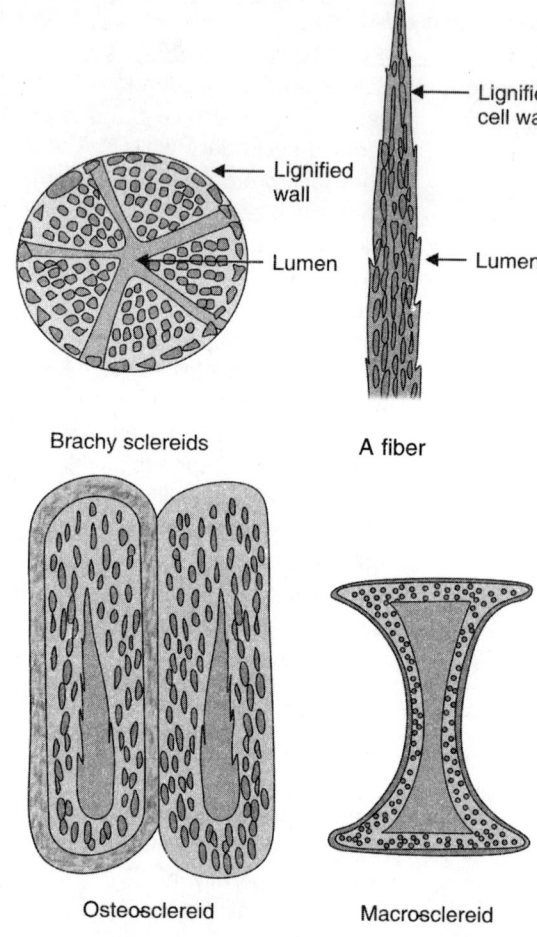

Fig. 11.5: Types of collenchyma tissues

Fig. 11.6: Types of sclerenchyam tissues

Complex Tissues

Complex tissues are made up of more than one type of cells and they work together as a unit. They transport water, salt and prepared food material to various parts of the plant body. They are of two types:
1. Xylem and
2. Phloem

1. Xylem

Nature: Xylem (Greek word 'xylos'= wood) is derived from procambium, is called primary xylem and the xylem, which is derived from vascular cambium, is called secondary xylem. Xylem elements formed earlier are known as protoxylem, whereas the later formed xylem elements are known as metaxylem. Xylem is made up of four kinds of cells—tracheids, vessels or tracheae, xylem fibers and xylem parenchyma (Fig. 11.7).

Plant Anatomy

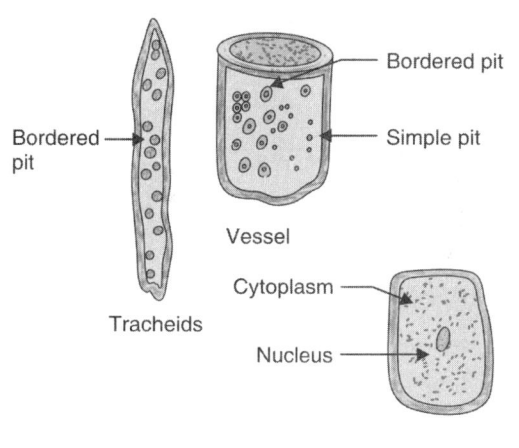

Fig. 11.7: Kinds of xylem cells

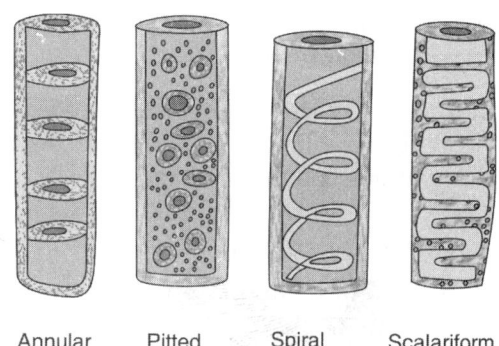

Fig. 11.8: Types of seconary wall thickenings in tracheids

Occurrence: Found in the root, stem and leaves. They occur along with phloem to form the vascular bundle.

Function: Conduct water and minerals upwards from the roots to the stem and leaves. Cells that are lignified to give mechanical strength to the plant.

a. Tracheids

Nature: Tracheids are elongated with blunt ends. Their lumen is broader than that of fibers. Their secondary wall is lignified. In cross-section, the tracheids appear polygonal and thick-walled. The pits are simple or bordered. There are different types of cell wall thickening due to deposition of secondary wall substances (Fig. 11.8).

Types: Annular (ring-like), spiral (spring-like), scalariform (ladder-like), reticulate (net-like) and pitted (uniformly thick except at pits).

Function:
- The chief function is conduction of water and mineral salts takes place through the bordered pits, e.g. gymnosperms and pteridophytes.
- They also provide mechanical support to the plants.

b. Vessels or Tracheae

Nature: Vessels are perforated at the end walls. Their lumen is wider than that of tracheids. The perforated plates at the end wall separate the vessels. They occur parallel to the long axis of the plant body.

Simple perforation plate: A single pore is formed at the perforation plate due to dissolution of entire end wall, e.g. mangifera.

Multiple perforation plate: If perforation plate has many pores, then it is called multiple perforation plate, e.g. liriodendron.

Types of secondary wall thickenings of vessels: Annular, spiral, scalariform, reticulate, or pitted.

Function:
- The main function of vessel is conduction of water and minerals, e.g. water conducting elements in angiosperms, but they are absent in pteridophytes and gymnosperms.
- It also offers mechanical strength to the plant.

c. Xylem Fibers (libriform fibers)

Xylem fibers are dead cells and have lignified walls with narrow lumen. The fibers of sclerenchyma associated with the xylem are known as xylem fibers.

Function: Provide additional mechanical support to the plant body, present both in primary and secondary xylem.

d. Xylem Parenchyma

Xylem parenchyma is the only living tissue amongst the constituents of xylem. The parenchyma cells associated with the xylem are known as xylem parenchyma. The cell wall is thin and made up of cellulose.

Function: The xylem parenchyma cells store food reserves in the form of starch and fat as well as they also assist in conduction of water.

2. Phloem (Fig. 11.9)

Nature: Phloem is also a complex tissue. It conducts food materials to various parts of the plant. The phloem elements which are formed from the procambium of apical meristem are called **primary phloem**. The phloem elements which are produced by the vascular cambium are called **secondary phloem**.

Occurrence: Phloem is found in all parts of the plant, like roots, stem and leaves. It occurs together with the xylem to form the vascular bundle.

Function: The function of the phloem is to conduct prepared food from the leaves to the growing parts of the plant and the storage organs.

Types: Phloem is composed of four kinds of cells: sieve elements, companion cells, phloem parenchyma and phloem fibers.

a. Sieve Elements

Sieve elements are the conducting elements of the phloem. They have thick primary walls. Their end walls are transverse or oblique. The

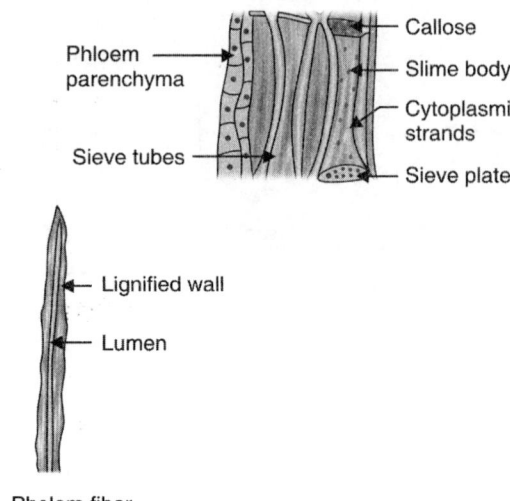

Fig. 11.9: Phloem tissue

end wall contains a number of pores and it looks like a sieve. So it is called a sieve plate.

Types: Sieve cells and sieve tubes.

Sieve cells: They occur in pteridophytes and gymnosperms, Sieve cells have sieve areas on their lateral walls only and are not arranged one above the other in linear rows. They are not associated with companion cells.

Sieve tubes: They occur in angiosperms. They are arranged one above the other in linear rows and have sieve plates on their end walls. They are associated with the companion cells.

b. Companion Cells

The thin-walled, elongated, specialized parenchyma cells, which are associated with the sieve elements, are called companion cells. They are connected to the sieve tubes through pits found in the lateral walls.

Function: They assist the sieve tubes in the conduction of food materials.

c. Phloem Parenchyma

The living parenchyma cells associated with the phloem are called phloem parenchyma.

They store starch and fats. They also contain resins and tannins in some plants.

Occurrence: They are present in pteridophytes, gymnosperms and dicots, absent in monocots.

d. Phloem Fibers

The fibers of sclerenchyma associated with phloem are called phloem fibers or bast fibers. They are narrow, vertically elongated cells with very thick walls and a small lumen (the cell cavity).

Function: They provide strength and support to cells.

THE TISSUE SYSTEM

A group of tissues performing a similar function irrespective of its position in the plant body is called a tissue system. In 1875, Sachs recognized three tissue systems in the plants. They are epidermal tissue system, vascular tissue system and fundamental tissue system.

Epidermal Tissue System

Epidermal tissue system (Fig. 11.10) is the outermost covering of plants. It consists of epidermis, stomata and epidermal outgrowths. Epidermis is generally composed of single layer of parenchymatous cells compactly arranged without intercellular spaces. The outer wall of epidermis is usually covered by cuticle.

Stoma is a minute pore surrounded by two guard cells. The stomata occur mainly in the epidermis of leaves. In some plants, such as sugarcane, the guard cells are bounded by some special cells. They are distinct from other epidermal cells. These cells are called subsidiary or accessory cells. Trichomes and root hairs are some epidermal outgrowths. The unicellular or multicellular appendages that originate from the epidermal cells are called trichomes. Trichomes may be branched

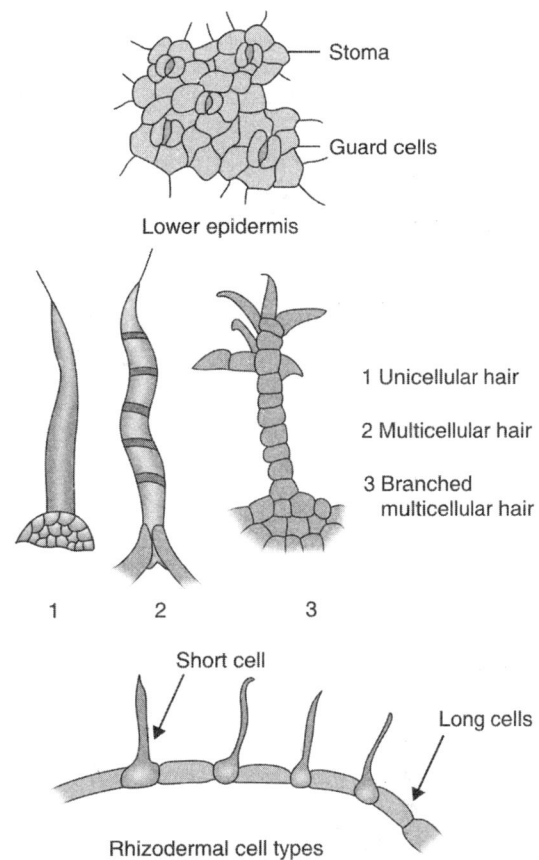

Fig. 11.10: Epidermal tissue system

or unbranched. Rhizodermis has two types of epidermal cells—long cells and short cells. The short cells are called trichoblasts. Root hairs are produced from these trichoblasts.

Functions

- This tissue system in the shoot checks excessive loss of water due to the presence of cuticle.
- Epidermis protects the underlying tissues.
- Stomata involve in transpiration and gaseous exchange.
- Trichomes are also helpful in the dispersal of seeds and fruits.
- Root hairs absorb water and mineral salts from the soil.

Vascular Tissue System

The vascular tissue system consists of xylem and phloem. The elements of xylem and phloem are always organized in groups. They are called vascular bundles (Fig. 11.11).

Open vascular bundle: The vascular bundle in dicot stem consists of cambial tissue in between xylem and phloem.

Closed vascular bundle: In monocot stem, cambium is absent in the vascular bundle.

Conjoint vascular bundle: Xylem and phloem are arranged at the same radius and form a vascular bundle together is known as conjoint vascular bundle.

Depending upon the mutual relationship of xylem and phloem, conjoint vascular bundles are divided into three types collateral, bicollateral and concentric.

Collateral vascular bundle: If xylem and phloem in a vascular bundle are arranged along the same radius with phloem towards the outside

Bicollateral vascular bunde: If phloem occurs on both the outer and inner sides of xylem, most typically seen in Cucurbitaceae.

Concentric vascular bundle: The bundle in which either phloem surrounds the xylem or xylem surrounds the phloem completely.

Exarch: This arrangement of xylem in roots in which protoxylem vessels are present towards the periphery and the metaxylem vessels towards the center.

Endarch: In stem, protoxylem vessels are towards the center, while metaxylem towards the periphery.

Ground or Fundamental Tissue System

The ground or fundamental tissue system constitutes the main body of the plants. It includes all the tissues except epidermis and vascular bundles.

Monocot stem: The ground tissue system is a continuous mass of parenchymatous tissue in which vascular bundles are found scattered.

Dicot stem: The ground tissue system is differentiated into three main zones—cortex, pericycle and pith. The cortex occurs between the epidermis and pericycle. Cortex may be a few to many layers in thickness.

Leaves: The ground tissue consists of chlorenchyma tissues. This region is called mesophyll. The innermost layer of the cortex is called endodermis made up of barrel-shaped parenchyma cells.

Pericycle made up of parenchyma cells occurs between the endodermis and the vascular bundles. Lateral roots originate from the pericycle. Thus their origin is endogenous.

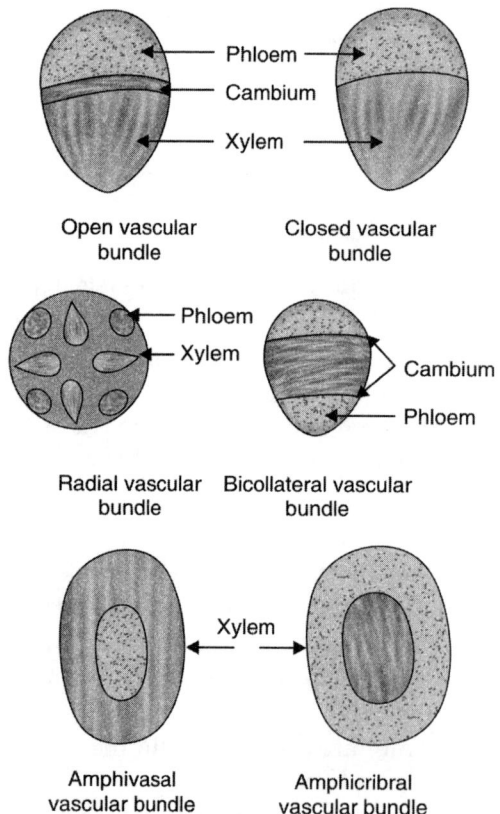

Fig. 11.11: Types of vascular bundles

The central part of the ground tissue is known as pith or medulla made up of thin-walled parenchyma cells which may be with or without intercellular spaces stores starch, fatty substances, tannins, phenols, calcium oxalate crystals, etc.

ANATOMY OF MONOCOT AND DICOT STEMS

Monocot Stem

Primary structure of monocot stem—Maize stem (Fig. 11.12). Internal structure of monocot stem reveals epidermis, hypodermis, ground tissue and vascular bundles.

Epidermis

It is the single outermost layer of the stem, made up of single layer of tightly packed parenchymatous cells. The continuity of this layer may be broken here and thereby the presence of a few stomata.

Hypodermis

Below the epidermis constitute the hypodermis. It consists of sclerenchymatous cells. It gives mechanical strength to the plant.

Ground Tissue

The entire mass of parenchymatous cells lying inner to the hypodermis forms the ground tissue. The cells of the ground tissue are smaller in size, polygonal in shape and compactly arranged but in center cells are loosely arranged, rounded in shape and bigger in size. The vascular bundles lie embedded in this tissue. The ground tissue stores food and performs gaseous exchange.

Vascular Bundles

The vascular bundles are conjoint, collateral, endarch and closed. Vascular bundles are numerous, small and closely arranged in the peripheral portion.

Phloem

The phloem in the monocot stem consists of sieve tubes and companion cells. Phloem parenchyma and phloem fibers are absent.

Xylem

Xylem vessels are arranged in the form of the letter 'Y'. The two metaxylem vessels are located at the upper two arms and one or two protoxylem vessels at the base.

Dicot Stem

Primary structure of dicot stem (Fig. 11.13)—sunflower stem.

Internal structure of dicotyledonous stem reveals epidermis, cortex and stele.

Epidermis

It is protective in function and forms the outermost layer of the stem. It is a single layer of parenchymatous rectangular cells. The cells are compactly arranged without intercellular spaces. The outer walls of the epidermal cells have a layer called cuticle. The cuticle checks the transpiration. The cuticle is made up of a waxy substance known as cutin. Stomata may be present here and there. Epidermal cells are living. Chloroplasts are usually absent. A large number of multicellular hairs occur on the epidermis.

Cortex

Cortex lies below the epidermis. The cortex is differentiated into three zones. Below the epidermis, there are a few layers of collenchyma cells. This zone is called hypodermis. It gives mechanical strength to the stem. These cells are living and thickened at the corners. Inner to the hypodermis, a few layers of chlorenchyma cells are present with conspicuous intercellular spaces. This region performs photosynthesis. Some resin ducts

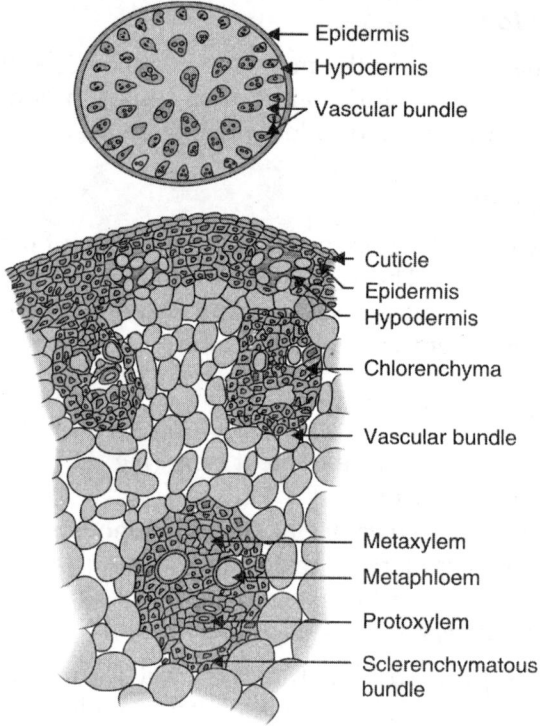

Fig. 11.12: Transverse section of maize stem

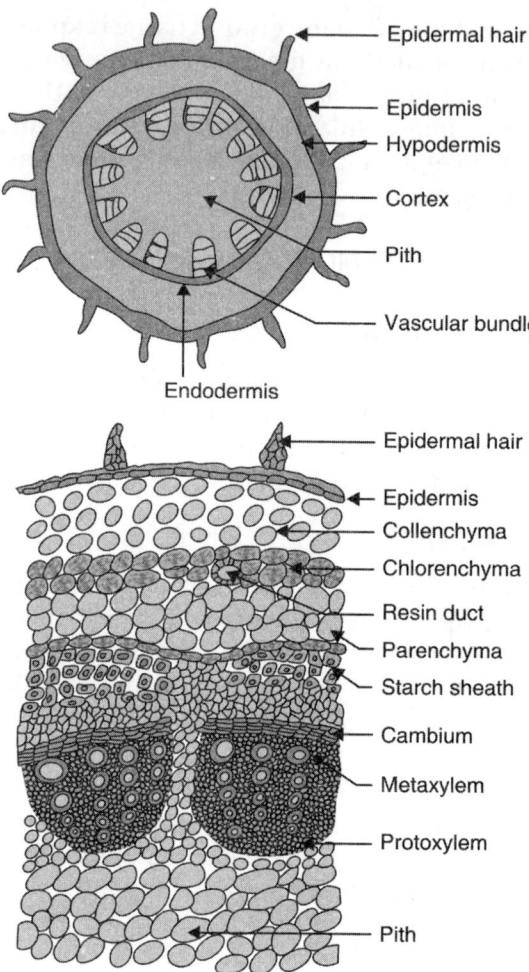

Fig. 11.13: Transverse section of dicot stem

also occur here. The third zone is made up of parenchyma cells. These cells store food materials. The innermost layer of the cortex is called endodermis. The cells of this layer are barrel-shaped and arranged compactly without intercellular spaces. Since starch grains are abundant in these cells, this layer is also known as starch sheath. This layer is morphologically homologous to the endodermis found in the root. In most of the dicot stems, endodermis with casparian strips is not developed.

Stele

The central part of the stem inner to the endodermis is known as stele. It consists of pericycle, vascular bundles and pith. In dicot stem, vascular bundles are arranged in a ring around the pith. This type of stele is called eustele.

Pericycle

Pericycle is the layers of cells that occur between the endodermis and vascular bundles. In the stem of sunflower (Helianthus), a few layers of sclerenchyma cells occur in patches outside the phloem in each vascular bundle. This patch of sclerenchyma cells is called bundle cap or hard bast. The bundle caps and the parenchyma cells between them constitute the pericycle in the stem of sunflower.

Vascular Bundles

The vascular bundles consist of xylem, phloem and cambium. Xylem and phloem in the stem occur together and form the vascular bundles. These vascular bundles are wedge-shaped. They are arranged in the form of a ring. Each vascular bundle is conjoint, collateral, open and endarch.

Phloem

Primary phloem lies towards the periphery. It consists of protophloem and metaphloem. Phloem consists of sieve tubes, companion cells and phloem parenchyma. Phloem fibers are absent in the primary phloem. Phloem conducts organic food materials from the leaves to other parts of the plant body.

Cambium

Cambium consists of brick-shaped and thin-walled meristematic cells. It is two to three layers in thickness. These cells are capable of forming new cells during secondary growth.

Xylem

Xylem consists of xylem fibers, xylem parenchyma, vessels and tracheids. Vessels are thick-walled and arranged in a few rows. Xylem conducts water and minerals from the root to the other parts of the plant body.

Pith

The large central portion of the stem is called pith. It is composed of parenchyma cells with intercellular spaces. The pith is also known as medulla. The pith extends between the vascular bundles. These extensions of the pith between the vascular bundles are called primary pith rays or primary medullary rays. Function of the pith is storage of food.

Anatomical differences between dicot stem and monocot stem (Table 11.2).

ANATOMY OF DICOT AND MONOCOT LEAVES

Leaves are very important vegetative organs because they are mainly concerned with photosynthesis and transpiration. Like stem

Table 11.2: Difference between dicot and monocot stems

Dicot stem	Monocot stem
Hypodermis is made up of collenchymatous cells.	Hypodermis is made up of sclerenchymatous cells.
Ground tissue is differentiated into cortex, endodermis, pericycle and pith.	Ground tissue is not differentiated, but it is a continuous mass of parenchyma.
Starch sheath is present.	Starch sheath is absent.
Pith is present.	Pith is absent.
Pericycle is present	Pericycle is absent.
Medullary rays are present.	Medullary rays are absent
Vascular bundles are open.	Vascular bundles are closed.
Vascular bundles are arranged in a ring.	Vascular bundles are scattered in the ground tissue.
Bundle cap is present.	Bundle sheath is present.
Protoxylem lacuna is absent.	Protoxylem lacuna is present.
Phloem parenchyma is present.	Phloem parenchyma is absent.

and roots, leaves also have the three tissue systems—dermal, ground and vascular. The dermal tissue system consists of an upper epidermis and lower epidermis. Stomata occur in both the epidermis but more frequently in the lower epidermis. The ground tissue system that lies between the epidermal layers of leaf is known as mesophyll tissue. Often it is differentiated into palisade parenchyma on the adaxial (upper) side and spongy parenchyma on the abaxial (lower) side.

A leaf showing this differentiation in mesophyll is designated as dorsiventral. It is common in dicot leaves. If mesophyll is not differentiated like this in a leaf (i.e. made of only spongy or palisade parenchyma) as in monocots, it is called isobilateral. The mesophyll tissue, especially spongy parenchyma cells, enclose a lot of airspaces. The presence of airspaces is a special feature of spongy cells. They facilitate the gaseous exchange between the internal photosynthetic tissue (mesophyll) and the external atmosphere through the stomata. The vascular tissue system is composed of vascular bundles. They are collateral and closed. The vascular tissue forms the skeleton of the leaf and they are known as veins. The veins supply water and minerals to the photosynthetic tissue. Thus the morphological and anatomical features of the leaf help in its physiological functions.

Dicot Leaf

Anatomy of a dicot leaf—Sunflower leaf (Fig. 11.14). Internal structure of dicotyledonous leaves reveals epidermis, mesophyll and vascular tissues.

Epidermis

A dicotyledonous leaf is generally dorsiventral. It has upper and lower epidermises. The epidermis is usually made up of a single layer of cells that are closely packed. The cuticle on the upper epidermis is thicker than that of lower epidermis. The minute openings found on the epidermis are called stomata. Stomata are more in number on the lower epidermis than on the upper epidermis. A stoma is surrounded by a pair of bean-shaped cells called guard cells. Each stoma opens into an air chamber. These guard cells contain chloroplasts, whereas other epidermal cells do not contain chloroplasts. The main function of the epidermis is to give protection to the inner tissue called mesophyll. The cuticle helps to check transpiration. Stomata are used for transpiration and gas exchange.

Mesophyll

The entire tissue between the upper and lower epidermises is called the mesophyll (Gk *meso* = in the middle; *phyllome* = leaf). There are two regions in the mesophyll. They are palisade parenchyma and spongy parenchyma.

Palisade parenchyma cells are seen beneath the upper epidermis. It consists of vertically elongated cylindrical cells in one or more layers. These cells are compactly arranged without intercellular spaces. Palisade parenchyma cells contain more chloroplasts than the spongy parenchyma cells. The function of palisade parenchyma is photosynthesis. Spongy parenchyma lies below the palisade parenchyma. Spongy cells are irregularly shaped. These cells are very loosely arranged with numerous airspaces. As compared to palisade cells, the spongy cells contain lesser number of chloroplasts. Spongy cells facilitate the exchange of gases with the help of air spaces. The air space that is found next to the stoma is called respiratory cavity or substomatal cavity.

Vascular Tissues

Vascular tissues are present in the veins of leaf. Vascular bundles are conjoint, collateral and closed. Xylem is present towards the

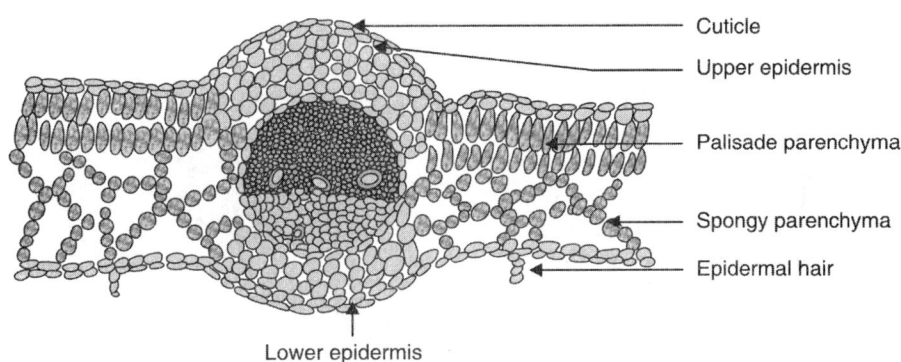

Fig. 11.14: Transverse section of sunflower leaf

upper epidermis, while the phloem towards the lower epidermis. Vascular bundles are surrounded by a compact layer of parenchymatous cells called bundle sheath or border parenchyma. Xylem consists of metaxylem vessels and protoxylem vessels. Protoxylem vessels are present towards the upper epidermis. Phloem consists of sieve tubes, companion cells and phloem parenchyma. Phloem fibers are absent. Xylem consists of vessels and xylem parenchyma. Tracheids and xylem fibers are absent.

ANATOMY OF MONOCOT AND DICOT ROOTS

The embryo develops into an adult plant with roots, stem and leaves due to the activity of the apical meristem. A mature plant has three kinds of tissue systems—the dermal, the fundamental and the vascular systems. The dermal system includes the epidermis, which is the primary outer protective covering of the plant body. The periderm is another protective tissue that supplants the epidermis in the roots and stems that undergo secondary growth. The fundamental tissue system includes tissues that form the ground substance of the plant in which other permanent tissues are found embedded. Parenchyma, collenchyma and sclerenchyma are the main ground tissues. The vascular system contains the two conducting tissues, the phloem and xylem. In different parts of the plants, the various tissues are distributed in characteristic patterns. This is best understood by studying their internal structure by cutting sections (transverse or longitudinal or both) of the part to be studied.

Monocot Root

Primary structure of monocotyledonous root—maize root (Fig. 11.15).

The internal structure of the monocot roots shows the following tissue systems from the periphery to the center. They are epiblema or rhizodermis, cortex and stele.

Rhizodermis or Epiblema

It is the outermost layer of the root. It consists of a single row of thin-walled parenchymatous cells without any intercellular space. Stomata and cuticle are absent in the rhizodermis. Root hairs that are found in the rhizodermis are always unicellular. They absorb water and mineral salts from the soil. Root hairs are generally short lived. The main function of rhizodermis is protection of the inner tissues.

Cortex

The cortex is homogenous, i.e. the cortex is made up of only one type of tissue called parenchyma. It consists of many layers of thin-walled parenchyma cells with lot of intercellular spaces. The function of cortical cells is storage. Cortical cells are generally oval or rounded in shape. Chloroplasts are absent in the cortical cells, but they store starch. The cells are living and possess leucoplasts. The inner most layer of the cortex is endodermis. It is composed of single layer of barrel-shaped parenchymatous cells. This forms a complete ring around the stele. There is a band-like structure made of suberin present in the radial and transverse walls of the endodermal cells. They are called Casparian strips named after Casparay who first noted the strips. The endodermal cells, which are opposite to the protoxylem elements, are thin-walled without Casparian strips. These cells are called passage cells. Their function is to transport water and dissolved salts from the cortex to the xylem. Water cannot pass through other endodermal cells due to Casparian strips. The main function of Casparian strips in the endodermal cells is to prevent the re-entry of water into the cortex once water entered the xylem tissue.

Stele

All the tissues inside the endodermis comprise the stele. This includes pericycle, vascular system and pith.

Pericycle: Pericycle is the outermost layer of the stele and lies inner to the endodermis. It consists of a single layer of parenchymatous cells.

Vascular system: Vascular tissues are seen in radial arrangement. The number of protoxylem groups is many. This arrangement of xylem is called polyarch. Xylem is in exarch condition. The tissue, which is present between the xylem and the phloem, is called conjunctive tissue. In maize, the conjunctive tissue is made up of sclerenchymatous tissue.

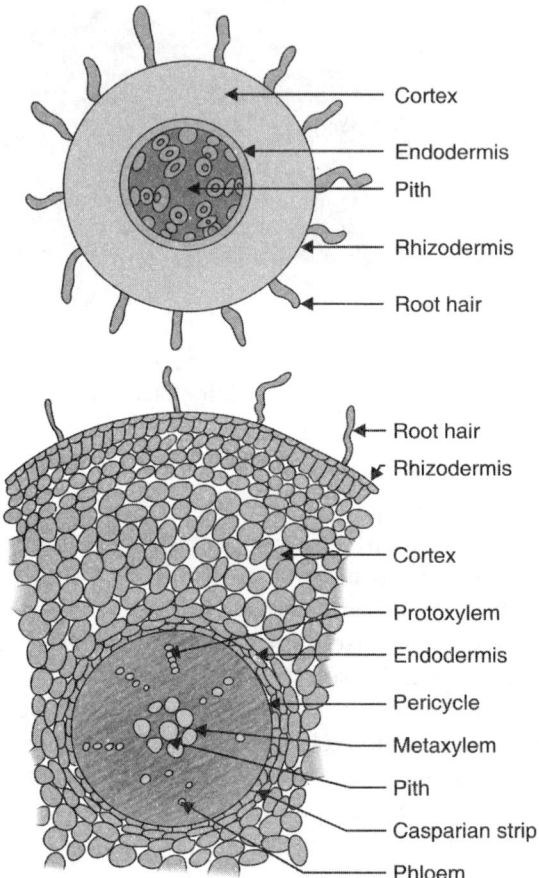

Fig. 11.15: Transverse section of maize root

Pith: The central portion is occupied by a large pith. It consists of thin-walled parenchyma cells with intercellular spaces. These cells are filled with abundant starch grains.

Dicot Root

Primary structure of dicotyledonous root—bean root (Fig. 11.16).

The transverse section of the dicot root (bean) shows the following plan of arrangement of tissues from the periphery to the center.

Rhizodermis or Epiblema

The outermost layer of the root is known as rhizodermis. It is made up of a single layer of parenchyma cells which are arranged compactly without intercellular spaces. It is devoid of stomata and cuticle. Root hair is always single celled. It absorbs water and mineral salts from the soil. The chief function of rhizodermis is protection.

Cortex

Cortex consists of only parenchyma cells. These cells are loosely arranged with intercellular spaces to make gaseous exchange easier. These cells may store food reserves. The cells are oval or rounded in shape. Sometimes they are polygonal due to mutual pressure. Though chloroplasts are absent in the cortical cells, starch grains are stored in them. The cells also possess leucoplasts. The inner most layer of the cortex is endodermis. Endodermis is made up of single layer of barrel-shaped parenchymatous cells. Stele is completely surrounded by the endodermis. The radial and the inner tangential walls of endodermal cells are thickened with suberin. This thickening was first noted by Casparay. So these thickenings are called Casparian strips. But these Casparian strips are absent in the endodermal cells which are located opposite to the protoxylem elements. These thin-walled cells without Casparian strips are called passage cells through which water and mineral salts are conducted from the cortex to the xylem elements. Water cannot pass through other endodermal cells due to the presence of Casparian thickenings.

Stele

All the tissues present inside endodermis comprise the stele. It includes pericycle and vascular system.

Pericycle: Pericycle is generally a single layer of parenchymatous cells found inner to

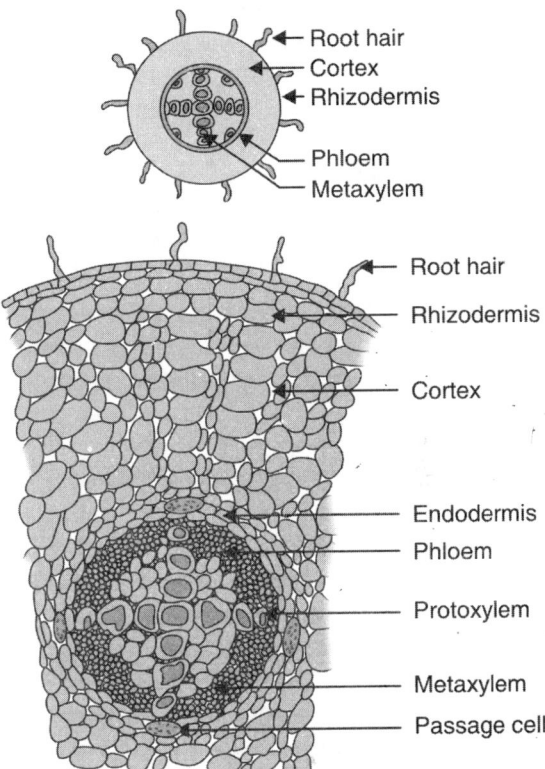

Fig. 11.16: Transverse section of bean root

the endodermis. It is the outermost 'layer of the stele. Lateral roots originate from the pericycle. Thus, the lateral roots are endogenous in origin.

Vascular system: Vascular tissues are in radial arrangement. The tissue by which xylem and phloem are separated is called conjunctive tissue. In bean, the conjunctive tissue is composed of parenchymatous tissue. Xylem is in exarch condition. The number of protoxylem points is four and so the xylem is called tetrarch. Each phloem patch consists of sieve tubes, companion cells and phloem parenchyma. Metaxylem vessels are generally polygonal in shape. But in monocot roots, they are circular.

12 Cosmeceuticals

According to the FDC Act of 1938, a cosmetic is defined as an article intended to be rubbed, poured, sprinkled, or sprayed on, introduced into, or otherwise applied to the human body or any part there of for cleansing, beautifying, promoting attractiveness, or altering the appearance without affecting structure or function. It is noteworthy that in this definition the cosmetic is not allowed to have any activity (i.e. without affecting structure or function). Among the products included in this definition are skin moisturizers, perfumes, lipsticks, fingernail polishes, eye, and facial makeup preparations, shampoos, permanent waves, hair colors, toothpastes, and deodorants, as well as any material intended for use as a component of a cosmetic product. These cosmeceuticals, serving as a bridge between personal care products and pharmaceuticals, have been developed specifically for their medicinal and cosmetic benefits.

Cosmeceuticals are a marketer's playground, which makes it possible to incorporate into skin care products an unlimited number of active substances, derived from a great variety of natural and synthetic sources. Cosmeceuticals (or alternatively, cosmaceuticals) are topical cosmetic pharmaceutical hybrids intended to enhance the beauty through ingredients that provide additional health-related function or benefit. They are applied topically as cosmetics, but contain ingredients that influence the skin's biological function. The variety of ingredients which have been incorporated in cosmeceuticals is staggering, including vitamins, antioxidants, minerals, herbs, hormones, anti-inflammatory, mood influencing fragrances (aromatherapy), and even such exotica as placenta, amniotic fluid.

Natural extracts, from animal, botanical, or mineral origin, have been used as "active ingredients" of drugs or cosmetics for as long as human history. Oils, butter, honey, beeswax, lead, and lemon juice were common ingredients of the beauty recipes. A nutritional cosmetic, which is probably better known in the industry as nutricosmetics, encompasses the concept that orally ingestible dietary products may support healthier and thus more beautiful skin. This is not totally unlike the term nutraceutical; however, this latter term typically refers to foods and dietary supplements that support better overall health. Similarly, the term cosmeceutical refers to products generally designed for topical application and which contain active ingredients with benefits for improved skin health (Fig. 12.1).

Cosmeceuticals could be characterized as follows:
- The product has pharmaceutical activity and can be used on normal or near-normal skin.
- The product should have a defined benefit for minor skin disorders (cosmetic indication).
- As the skin disorder is mild, the product should have a very low-risk profile.

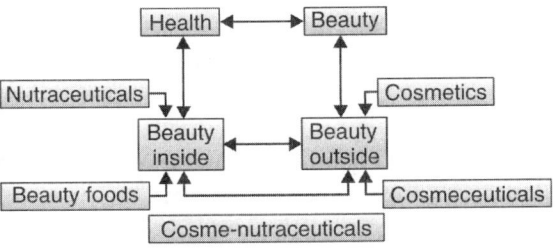

Fig. 12.1 Digrammatic corelation between nutraceuticals, beauty foods and cosmeceuticals

The use of natural ingredients in cosmetic products has a very long history. Since ancient times, women have turned to the goodness of nature to help increase their own beauty. Production of bioactive compounds from biological materials and their use in nutrition, cosmetics, and pharmacy is the need of hour. Bioactive ingredients represent compounds that have numerous specific pharmacological and technological values, such as natural antioxidants, natural preservatives, natural coloring agents, anti-microbiological active compounds, and others. During processing and storing, food, cosmetics, and pharmaceutical products are exposed to environmental factors, such as atmospheric composition, light, and temperature. These factors promote their spoilage. The following changes caused by oxidation may occur during cosmetic formulation storage: Fragrance profile change, vitamin and active ingredient decomposition, color change, and development of rancidity. A major cause of this quality deterioration is the autoxidation of unsaturated lipids initiated by free radicals. Antioxidants are crucial additives in cosmetic preparations for increasing their shelf life. Additionally, they can also be useful bioactive cosmetic ingredients to protect the skin against free radical formation induced by UV radiation and chemical environmental stress. Natural extracts with antioxidant properties recently have gained popularity because many studies show that natural ingredients are better and safer than synthetic ones. The interest in natural antioxidants is further heightened by the suggestions that many of these compounds, such as plant phenolics, often possess anti-oxidant, antimicrobial, anti-inflammatory, chemopreventive, anticarcinogenic, anti-atherogenic, and antitumor activity.

STRUCTURE OF THE SKIN

Macroscopic Characteristics

The skin is the largest, most extensive organ of our body. In fact, the average adult has about 170–200 cm^2 of skin with a weight that varies between 15 kg and 17 kg (obviously varying according to the subject's height and dimensions). The thickness of the epidermis, the outermost layer of the skin, can be from 0.5 mm in the thinnest areas (e.g. the eyelids) to 4–6 mm at its thickest points (as on the palm of the hand and the sole of the foot). This thickness parameter becomes especially important when a substance is applied to the skin, be it a pharmaceutical or cosmetic product. In fact, once in contact with the skin, any substance can penetrate the cutaneous barrier in a way directly proportional to the skin's thickness at that point. The skin tissue houses within its structure other important constituents: hairs, nails, etc. (the skin's annexes). The whole of the skin is covered with hairs. In some areas, the hairs are more developed and more colored, as on the scalp, in the pubic region, and in the armpit. In other areas, they are finer and much paler. These characteristics vary above all according to sex but also with individual biology. Tiny, invisible openings are found over the entire skin surface. These are the outlets of the eccrine sudoriparous glands, which, together with the apocrine sudoriparous glands and the sebaceous glands.

Microscopic Characteristics (Fig. 12.2)

Epidermis: The most external layer in contact with the environment.

Dermis: Below the epidermis, it is the structural component of the skin and the underlying organs.

Hypodermis: Immediately below the dermis, composed of a layer of adipose cells and representing a "cushion" of fat between the skin and the organs underneath.

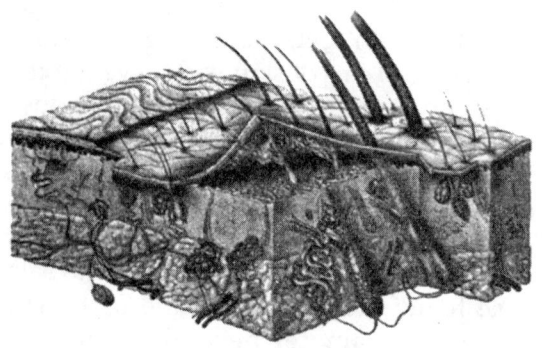

Fig. 12.2: Diagram of a skin section

The Epidermis

The epidermis is composed of different types of cells that overlap, not randomly but in a well-defined manner. There are four different cell types:

1. Keratinocytes
2. Melanocytes
3. Langerhans' cells
4. Merkel cells

The Keratinocytes

The "keratinocytes" are the predominant cell type and owe their name to the characteristic protein they produce in the course of their life, "keratin." This protein is responsible for specific, important skin functions.

The Melanocytes

Interposed between the keratinocytes of the basal layer, there are "melanocytes" that synthesize "melanin," the pigment responsible for skin color. The number of melanocytes can vary according to body area and are usually present as a ratio of the number of keratinocytes.

Biochemistry of melanin: Melanin is the pigment contained in the structures called melanosomes produced by the melanocytes. It is transferred to the surrounding epidermal keratinocytes, which maintain functional contact forming an epidermal melanin unit.

Langerhans' Cells

These cells are situated above the basal layer and, like the melanocytes, have a dendritic appearance. The Langerhans' cells unite against exogenous antigens and "present" them to both skin and lymph node T lymphocytes. They are also involved in immune surveillance against viral and tumor antigens.

Merkel Cells

These cells are found mainly in certain areas of the body: the fingertips, the oral mucosa, the lips, and the hair follicles. Merkel cells are considered as "tactile receptors," that is they are the structures responsible for our sense of touch.

The Dermis

The dermis is positioned below the epidermis and is the tissue that supports the skin and its annexes (hair, nails, etc.). Its thickness varies from area to area, being thinnest on the eyelids and thickest on the back. The dermis tends to become progressively thinner with age. This layer is formed by cells, fibers, and ground substance is richly innervated and vascularized. The most abundant cells are the *fibroblasts*. These cells are the production site of the other dermal components: both the fibers of the dermis and the ground substance are synthesized within the fibroblasts. In addition to fibroblasts, *mastocytes* (mast cells), *lymphocytes*, and *histiocytes* are present.

The Hypodermis

The hypodermis is situated below the dermis and is composed of "adipocytes" grouped into "lobes" separated by an area of connective tissue. The thickness of the hypodermis varies considerably according to the body site, nutritional state, and sex of the individual. Adipose cells are characterized by the remarkable quantity of lipids they contain. These lipids are grouped into a single globule in the cytoplasm, so large that the nucleus is forced to occupy a peripheral position. In fact, the distribution of subcutaneous fat is a strictly hormone-dependant secondary sexual characteristic. The number of adipose cells changes in the first phases of child development, at first increasing and then remaining stable. During puberty in women, there is an increase in subcutaneous fat predominantly in the area of the buttocks, hips, thighs and breasts. In men, on the other hand, the increase in lipid content is in the area of the torso and abdomen.

The Hair System

The entire surface of the skin is supplied with hairs, but on the head the hairs are longer and more pigmented. There are three types of hair:
1. Vellus hair
2. Terminal hair
3. Lanugo hair

Anatomy and Histology of Hair

Hairs develop from the hair follicles (Fig. 12.3), which are true organs formed by the invagination of the epidermis during the fetal development. These organs are divided into three main parts:
1. The infundibulum is the portion from the opening on the skin surface to the mouth of the sebaceous gland duct.
2. The isthmus is the section between the sebaceous gland duct and the point of intersection with the hair erector muscle.
3. The inferior portion extends from the erector muscle to the bulb of the hair follicle.

The *hair root* is a generic term that includes the entire inferior portion and the isthmus. The *bulb* is the enlarged terminal part of the hair follicle in the root. The root produces the hair *shaft*, which is defined as the hair structure visible above the skin surface. Below the bulb, the dermis re-enters the hair

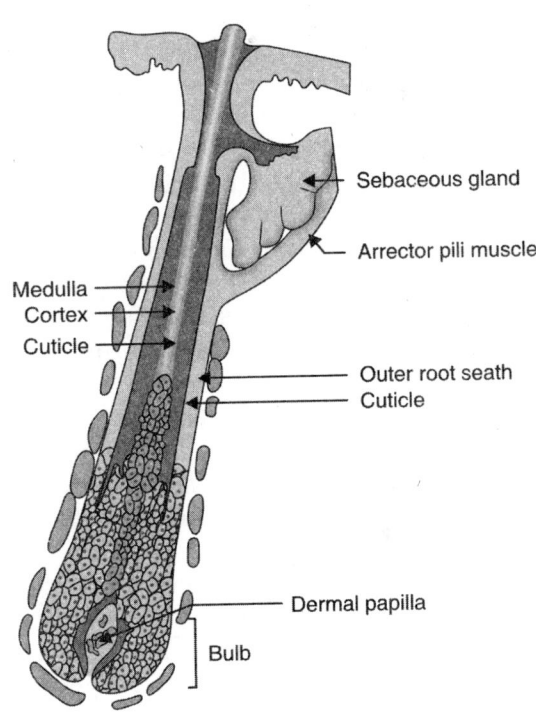

Fig. 12.3: Diagram of a hair follicle

follicle, producing the *dermal papillae*, as the hair follicle is formed by introtlexions of the epidermis; this re-establishes the junction with the dermis. In this way, the hair follicle is surrounded by the basal membrane. In this region, it is particularly thick and assumes the name *vitreous membrane,* because together with the basal membrane it forms a kind of connective sheath that surrounds the whole follicle. The part on the hair follicle between the bulb and the isthmus is known as the *keratogenous zone.* The maturation of the cells that produce the hair shaft occurs in this area.

The most important part of the hair follicle is the bulb. In the basal layer, immediately above the papillae, cells continuously divide and begin their ascent. Slowly as this process proceeds, the cells subdivide in the layers that make up the follicle. In fact, if a hair is cut perpendicularly to the follicle, one can easily see how, independently of the zones and structure described earlier, each of these is formed by the union of layers and from inwards towards the outside of the follicle we can recognize the following layers: the *medulla, cortex,* and *cuticle.* These three layers form the hair shaft. The cuticle is followed by the *cuticle of the internal epithelial sheath, Huxley's layer,* and *Henle's layer.* Beyond these layers, the *external epithelial sheath* begins and this, too, is composed of cell layers becoming increasingly thinner from the epidermal surface to the bulb. In the germinative layer, or *hair matrix,* the keratinocytes are in contact with melanocytes, which are present only in this region. Here the melanocytes produce the pigment that will give rise to our hair coloring. The connective sheath also envelops the sebaceous gland and the hair erector muscle. The latter structure, important in furry animals in controlling the angle of the hair and so regulating heat exchange, is all but useless in man-nevertheless, this thin muscle is able to raise the hair. The follicles are set obliquely to the skin's surface and the erector muscle, by contracting and nipping both the follicle and the epidermis, are able to raise the hair. This is the phenomenon of *horripilation,* commonly called goose flesh, which occurs during shivering due to cold or fear.

ORIGIN OF BOTANICAL EXTRACTS

Botanical extracts have been used for centuries and are present in today's products either for their own properties or as substitute of animal materials. There are plant powders for hair coloring (Henne), scrubs (apricot kernel, corn), or masks (oat flour); plant extracts ("as is" or purified); and biotechnology extracts obtained through fermentation, cloning, soilless culture (aquaculture, artificial media, etc.), which are developed from microorganisms, plant organs, total plants, or through the use of specific enzymes.

Antioxidants

Free radicals have been shown to play a major role in sun damage as well as in aging or in pollution (tobacco, stress). They act by degrading the skin structural fibers (collagen, elastin), cell membranes, DNA, or by creating inflammatory reactions. Free radical actions can be blocked by *Vegetable oils rich in tocopherols and tocotrienols.* α-Tocopherol contributes directly to cell membrane structure by stabilizing it and allowing (Table 12.2).

CHARACTERIZATION OF COSMETIC CARE PRODUCTS

Physical Characterization

Appearance

Assessment and description of appearance are one of the easiest, most practical, and nevertheless powerful tests. It may be performed macroscopically, describing color, clearness, transparency, turbidity, and state

Table 12.1: Botanicals and their uses

Use	Botanical
Acne	Hops, lavender, papaya, asparagus, blackberry leaf
Antibacterial	Grapefruit, lavender, rosemary, quassia, bayberry, sandalwood
Antidandruff	Quassia, lemon grass, orange peel, rosemary, chamomile
Antioxidants	Ginkgo, tumeric
Antiseptics	Lavender, lemon, grapefruit, hops, chamomile, rosemary, onion, garlic, black walnut, eucalyptus, myrrh, cinnamon
Astringents	Vinca minor, lemon, raspberry, rose, rosemary, sandalwood,
Cleansers	Papaya, lemon, pineapple
Deodorants	Rosemary, cardamon, coriander, orange peel
Eczema	Sarsaparilla, thyme
Emollients	Aloe vera, fenugreek, orange flowers
Eye	Chamomile, cucumber, fennel hair cosmetics
Dark hair	Black or neutral henna, jaborandi, raspberry
For treatment of dry hair	Orange flowers, chamomile, quince seed, fenugreek, basil,
Hair, to add sheen	Lemon Peel, Rosemary, chamomile
For hair, split ends	Fenugreek, lavender, basil, rosemary, sage.
Rubefacients	Capsicum, cinchona
Soothing	Cucumber, red poppy, licorice
Sunburn	Aloe vera, calendula, lemon, Lavender, capsicum
Skin, dry	Aloe vera, fennel, orange peel, ginseng, capsicum, licorice.
Skin, oily	Caraway, cucumber, lemon grass, rose, grapefruit.

of matter. In addition, microscopic investigation is recommended; taking microphotographs is useful for documentation.

Rheology

Rheological properties (viscosity, consistency) are important characteristics of most types of cosmetic care products because they have an impact on preparation, packaging, storage, application, and delivery of actives. Thus these properties should be assessed for characterization and quality control of the product. Most disperse systems and thus cosmetic care products show non-Newtonian flow behavior, namely pseudoplastic, plastic, or dilatant behavior. A wide variety of techniques and methods have been developed to measure viscosity properties. These procedures can be classified as either absolute or relative. The absolute either directly or indirectly measures specific components of shear stress and shear rate to define an appropriate rheological function. Methods used for absolute viscosity measurements are flow through a tube, rotational methods, or surface viscosity methods. Methods used for relative viscosity measurements are those using orifice viscometers, falling balls, or plungers. Such instruments, although they do not measure stress or shear rate, offer valuable quality-control tests for relative comparison between different materials. Apparatus based on rotational or even oscillating principles to assess viscoelastic properties are state of the art.

pH

Measurement of pH value (concentration of hydrogen ions) in aqueous vehicles (solutions, suspensions, o/w emulsions, gels) is a valuable control mean. First of all, if possible, a pH value in the physiological range is generally targeted, ideally similar to that of the skin or the specific application site, to prevent irritation. Many reactions and processes depend on pH, e.g. efficacy of antimicrobial preservatives, stability and degradation of substances, and solubility.

Table 12.2: Botanical extracts

Biological source	Chemical constituents	Uses
Rosa canina (fruits), Actinidia, *Malphigia punicifolia*	Ascorbic acid	Ascorbic acid thus plays a role in improving cell resistance due to a better use of lipids. Ascorbic acid is an anti-inflammatory agent that degrades and eliminates histamine. It can be used in after-sun products; It has an immunostimulating activity
Gingko, Eucalyptus sambucus	Flavonoids	Anti-free-radical properties
Sophora japonica, Oenothera biennis, Borage officinalis, and *Ribes nigrum*	Oils rich in PUFA of the n-6 type	They are important in bringing essential fatty acids to the skin contributing to the maintenance or the restoration of epidermal lipids.
Oil and plant butters (rice, wheat, coffee, mango, sorgho, baobab, soya, corn, carob)	Essential fatty acids (EFA)	Maintain skin suppleness and reduce water loss.
Camelia, Argania, Medicago, Spinacia (spinach)	Nonsaponifiable fraction rich in sterols	Antiage products
Sugar cane, Camauba, Ceroxylon, Jojoba, Rose	Plant waxes	They are used to protect lips, hands, or face from dehydration.
Agaricus, *Morus alba*	Ceramides and glycosylceramides	Used for their action on skin or hair to provide hydration or reconstitute epidermal barrier function.
Limnanthes alba or Shambrilla oil	Long-chain fatty acids	As a massage oil
Guarana, tea, coffee, cocoa	Methylxanthines (caffeine, theobromin)	cAMP-phosphodiesterase inhibitors and thus accelerate lipid degradation.
Centella asiatica	Asiatic acid	Anti-inflammatory properties, but they are also α-glucuronidase inhibitors
Amino acids obtained by biotechnology through the action of microorganisms or enzymes on plant extracts are used for stimulation of systems that are active in aging as well as slimming (arginin, glutamin, HGH), hair growth (glutamic acid), or immunity (arginin)		
Centella asiatica	Asiaticosides	Stimulate synthesis of collagen and fibronectin
Eleutherococcus	Saponins	To protect membranes
Ganodema extract	Polysaccharides, triterpenes, and steroids	Are immunostimulating, immunoregulating, prolong all life and to slow down aging
Arctophylos uva-ursi, coactis, and *adenotricha*	Arbutin and methylarbuti	Depigmenting effect

Thus, pH measurement is a "must," and it is easily performed with the available measurement systems.

Homogeneity

In many cases, at a first step, homogeneity may be assessed visibly; precipitation in a solution or distinct phase separation in an emulsion is easily detected. Nontransparent, multiphasic systems are more difficult to check. In these cases, microscopic investigation of representative samples is suggested along with quantitative assays regarding active ingredients (uniformity of content).

Droplet or Particle Size and Distribution

The physical stability of colloidal systems as well as emulsions or suspensions partially depends on the particle size. In particular, preparations containing small particles with identical electrical charge are more resistant to flocculation and sedimentation than systems containing larger or uncharged entities. Similarly, reduced particle size is an indicator of improved kinetic stability of emulsions or suspensions. For that reason, determination of particle size and size distribution is an important characterization method. Various optical methods are available: A minireview is given, and a selection is listed as follows:

1. Perhaps the most commonly used method today is based on laser diffraction, suitable to measure solid particles and also dispersed droplets under special conditions, size range 1 to 600 (mm).
2. Dynamic light scattering, also known as photon correlation spectroscopy, is used for measuring micelles, liposomes, and submicron suspensions (size range 0.003–3 mm).
3. Optical or electron microscopy is a further method of choice.

Chemical Characterization

Besides physical characterization, chemically based investigations are indispensable to assess the quality of a product. It is well known

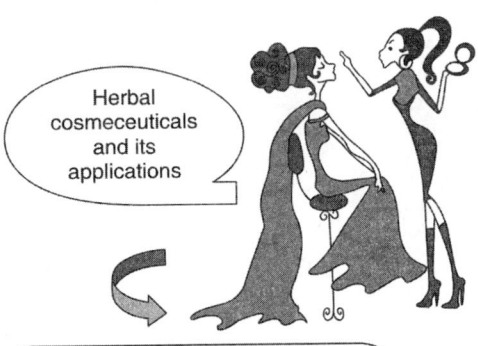

Herbal cosmeceuticals and its applications

Solids: Face powders, masks, compact powders, make-up, etc.
Semi solids: Creams, ointments, iminents, wax base creams, pastes, etc.
Liquids: Lotions, moistures, hair oil, bonditioners, shampoos, cleansing milk, mouthwashes, deodorant, iminents, sprays, etc.

Cosmetic applications in:
1. To enhance the general appearance of face and other body parts
2. To minimize the skin defects to a considerable extent.
3. To maintain or improve the status of skin and hair

that the quality and composition of a vehicle can influence the chemical stability of ingredients. Many reactions, such as ester hydrolysis or other degradations, may be enhanced or sustained by a change in pH, presence of catalytic or stabilizing agents, respectively. Thus, development and optimal selection of the best vehicle are supported by chemical stability investigations.

Biological Characterization

Further important assessment methods are based on biological tests. This is to evaluate and validate the desired targeted effects *in vivo* after application of the product. Examples include hydration of the skin, protection against sun radiation, and protection against skin irritating substances during work. This subject is treated in other chapters of this textbook.

Sensory Assessment

The sensory assessment is a useful tool for product and concept development and for quality control in the cosmetic industry. Although a very subjective and liable method, valuable data are obtained, if sensory assessment is conducted in a systematic way. The consistency of a material can be assessed by using three attributes: smoothness, thinness, and warmth.

Internally, the skin shelters and protects all the physiochemical phenomenon necessary for life, externally it is a barrier against mechanical forces, both physical and chemical, which can be hostile to life.

13

Poisonous Teratogenic and Hallucinogenic Plants

Toxicology is one of the oldest sciences. Plant toxicology has a rich history, a subset of the human experience. History study helps us avoid mistakes, prevent duplication of research, gain new insights, and improve cooperation by sharing a common legacy. The plants included in this chapter are toxic species, which although have little finding in modern medicine.

POISONOUS PLANTS (Table 13.1)

Plants hallucinogens are those which distort the senses and usually produce hallucinations (experiences that depart from reality). Although most hallucinations are visual, they may also involve the senses of hearing, touch, smell, or taste—and occasionally several senses simultaneously are involved. The actual causes of such hallucinations are chemical substances in the plants. These substances are true narcotics. Contrary to popular opinion, not all narcotics are dangerous and addictive. Strictly and etymologically speaking, a narcotic is any substance that has a depressive effect, whether slight or great, on the central nervous system.

Table 13.1: Common toxins with their examples and effects

Common toxins	Examples	Effects
Alkaloids	Solanine, tomatine	20 mg/100 g of potato and 36 mg/100 g of tomatoes are unfit to eat
Enzyme inhibitors	Protease inhibitors	Inhibit trypsin, chymotrypsin, and other protein digesting enzymes
	Saponins	Disrupt red blood cells, cause diarrhea, vomiting and may reduce blood serum cholesterol
	Cyanogenic glycosides dhurrin and amygdalin almonds (bitter almonds), sorghum, choke and pin cherries, and pits of apple, apricot, cherry, plum	12 bitter almonds can kill a child
Plant phenolics	Safrole and coumarin	Quite toxic and have been banned
Tannins	Bananas, grapes, raisins, sorghum, spinach, red wine, beer	Cause of enzymatic browing, bind protein, precipitate protein of epithelium, cause liver damage, inhibit virtually every digestive enzyme
Fats, sugars, proteins, and vitamin antagonists	Rancid or oxidized fat erucic acid (mustard, rapeseed), sugars proteins and vitamin antagonists	Liver degeneration and kidney nephrosis, headache, dizziness, and flushing, rapid heart rate, cramps facial increased blood pressure, and headaches, tumor promoters

Narcotics that induce hallucinations are variously called hallucinogens (hallucination generators), psychotomimetics (psychosis mimickers), psychotaraxics (mind disturbers), and psychedelics (mind manifesters) (Table 13.2).

Table 13.2: List of plant producing systemic poisoning in humans arranged by family and genus

Family	Examples
Berberidaceae	Podophyllum
Euphorbiaceae	Euphorbia, Ricinus and Jatropha
Leguminosae	Cassia, Abrus and Gymnocladus
Ginkgoaceae	Ginko
Apocynaceae	Thevetia, Acokanthera
Liliaceae	Allium, Aloe, Scilla and Urginea
Solanaceae	Atropa, Capsicum, Datura, Hyoscyamus and Nicotiana
Taxaceae	Taxus
Loganiaceae	Strychnos and Gelsemium
Meliaceae	Melia and Swietenia
Umbelliferae	Conium, Oenanthe
Polygonaceae	Rheum
Scrophulariaceae	Digitalis
Rosaceae	Prunus, Malus and Eriobotrya

Chemical Composition

Hallucinogens are limited to a small number of types of chemical compounds. All hallucinogens found in plants are organic compounds—that is, they contain carbon as an essential part of their structure and were formed in the life processes of vegetable organisms. No inorganic plant constituents, such as minerals, are known to have hallucinogenic effects. Hallucinogenic compounds may be divided conveniently into two broad groups:

1. Containing nitrogen in their structure.
2. Not containing nitrogen.

Those with nitrogen are far more common. The most importants of those lacking nitrogen are the active principles of marihuana, terpenophenolic compounds classed as dibenzopyrans and called cannabinols—in particular, tetrahydrocannabinols. The hallucinogenic compounds with nitrogen in their structure are alkaloids or related bases.

Indoles are hallucinogenic alkaloids or related bases, all of them nitrogen-containing compounds. It is the most surprising that of the many thousands of organic compounds that act on various parts of the body very few are hallucinogenic. The indole nucleus of the hallucinogens frequently appears in the form of tryptamine derivatives. It is composed of phenyl and pyrrol segments (Fig. 13.1 and Table 13.3).

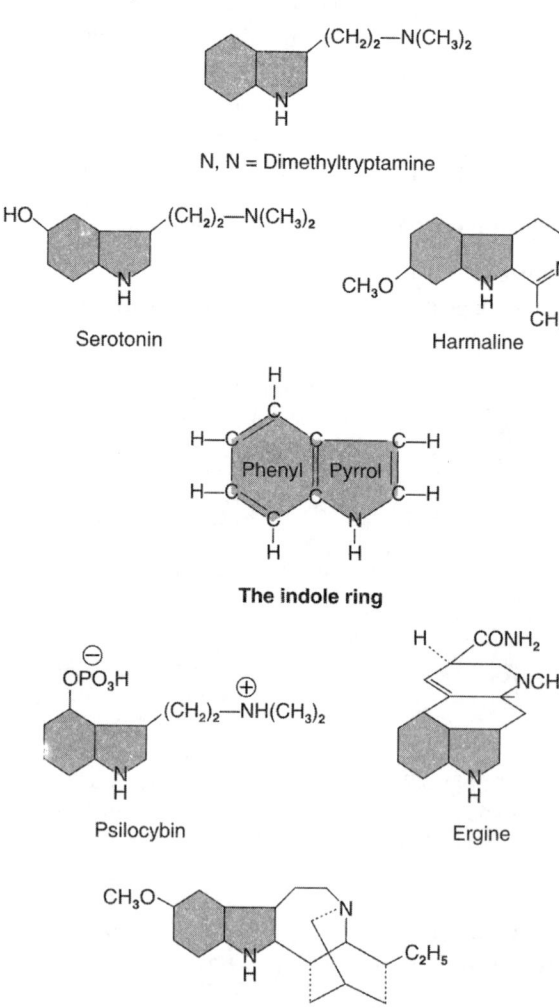

Fig. 13.1: Hallucinogens alkaloids with the indole nucleus

Table 13.3: List of poisonous plants with their description

Poisoning of plants	Examples	Toxic mechanism	Clinical manifestations	Specific therapeutics
Anticholinergic poisons	Atropa datura Hyoscyamus solanum	Competitive antagonism of acetylcholine at the muscarinic subtype of the acetylcholine receptor	1. Dry, warm, and flushed skin 2. Garbled speech 3. Sinus tachycardia 4. Urinary retention 5. Delirium 6. Hallucinations.	It includes sedation with a benzodiazepine or reversal of their clinical syndrome with physostigmine
Calcium oxalate crystals	Brassaia caladium Caryota philodendron	Calcium oxalate crystals penetrate the mucous membranes and induce the release of histamine and other inflammatory mediators.	After biting or chewing 1. Local oropharyngeal pain 2. Local swelling 3. Garbled speech After swallowing 1. Inflammation of the posterior oropharynx 2. Oropharyngeal edema 3. Airway compromise	Demulcents, viscous lidocaine, analgesics or with copious irrigation
Cardioactive steroids/cardiac glycosides	Adonis calotropis Digitalis thevetia	1. Indirectly increase Intracellular Ca^{2+} concentrations in myocardial cells. 2. It enhances cardiac inotropy (contractility) and slows the heart rate.	Abdominal pain and induce vomiting, which serves both as an early sign of toxicity to limit poisoning.	Antigen-binding regions (Fab) of animal-derived antidigoxin antibodies
Convulsant poisons (seizure)	Caulophyllum lobelia Myoporum nicotiana	1. Seizures including antagonism of 2. Gamma-aminobutyric acid (GABA) 3. Imbalance of acetylcholine homeostasis	1. Tonic-clonic convulsions 2. Loss of consciousness as a result of central nervous system dysfunction, urinary or fecal incontinence,	Anticonvulsant benzodiazepine or lorazepam, should be administered parenterally for persistent seizures.

(Contd.)

Table 13.3: List of poisonous plants with their description (Contd.)

Poisoning of plants	Examples	Toxic mechanism	Clinical manifestations	Specific therapeutics
		4. Excitatory amino acid mimicry 5. Sodium channel alteration	3. Tongue biting	
Cyanogenic compounds	Eriobotrya Hydrangea Malus, Prunus	Cyanide inhibits the final step of the mitochondrial electron transport chain, resulting rapidly in cellular energy failure or hypoglycemia	1. Abdominal pain, vomiting 2. Lethargy 3. Sweating 4. Altered mental status, seizures 5. Cardiovascular collapse, and multisystem organ failure.	1. Aggressive supportive care 2. Intravenous fluid therapy 3. Intravenous sodium bicarbonate 4. Antidotal therapy
Gastrointestinal toxins		Irritant toxins indirectly stimulate contraction of the gastrointestinal smooth muscle Hepatotoxins may directly injure the liver cells, commonly through the production of oxidant metabolites	Nausea, vomiting, abdominal cramping, and diarrhea	Vomiting may be mitigated by antiemetic agents such as metoclopramide; occasionally, resistant emesis may require a serotonin antagonist, such as ondansetron.
Mitotic inhibitors	Catharanthus Colchicum Gloriosa Podophyllum	These agents interfere with the polymerization of microtubules, which must polymerize for mitosis to occur, leading to metaphase arrest	Gastrointestinal abnormalities, including vomiting and diarrhea. Nervous system toxicity, including ataxia, headache, seizures, and encephalopathy	Initial management includes aggressive supportive and symptomatic care
Nicotine-like alkaloids	Caulophyllum Conium Gymnocladus Lobelia nicotiana	These agents are direct-acting agonists at the nicotinic subtype of the acetylcholine receptor in the ganglia of both the parasympathetic and sympathetic limbs of the autonomic nervous system	Sympathetic stimulation, including hypertension, tachycardia, and diaphoresis, and parasympathetic stimulation, including salivation and vomiting	Antihypertensive drugs, including nitroprusside or diltiazem. Seizures should respond to intravenous benzodiazepine, such as lorazepam or diazepam.

(Contd.)

Table 13.3: List of poisonous plants with their description (Contd.)

Poisoning of plants	Examples	Toxic mechanism	Clinical manifestations	Specific therapeutics
Pyrrolizidine alkaloids	Echium Heliotropium Senecio	Pyrrolizidine alkaloids are metabolized to pyrroles, which are alkylating agents that injure the endothelium of the hepatic sinusoids or pulmonary vasculature.	Acute hepatotoxicity caused by massive pyrrolizidine alkaloid exposure produces gastrointestinal symptoms, right upper quadrant abdominal pain, hepatosplenomegaly, and jaundice as well as biochemical abnormalities consistent with hepatic necrosis	Standard supportive care, liver transplantation

Pseudohallucinogens

These are poisonous plant compounds that cause what might be called secondary hallucinations or pseudohallucinations. Though not true hallucinogenic agents, they upset normal body functions that they induce a kind of delirium accompanied by what to all practical purposes are hallucinations. Some components of the essential oils—the aromatic elements responsible for the characteristic odors of plants—appear to act in this way. Components of nutmeg oil are an example. Many plants having such components are extremely dangerous to take internally, especially if ingested in doses high enough to induce hallucinations.

Fly agaric mushroom (*Amanita muscaria*) is one of the man's oldest hallucinogens. Fly agaric mushrooms grow in the north temperate regions of both hemispheres. The Eurasian type has a beautiful deep orange to blood-red cap flecked with white scales. The cap of the usual North American type varies from cream to an orange-yellow. There are also chemical differences between the two, for the New World type is devoid of the strongly hallucinogenic effects of its Old World counterpart.

Amanita muscaria typically occurs in association with birches.

The use of this mushroom as an orgiastic and shamanistic inebriant was discovered in Siberia in 1730. These tribes had no other intoxicant until they learned recently of alcohol. These Siberians ingest the mushroom alone, either sun-dried or toasted slowly over a fire, or they may take it in reindeer milk or with the juice of wild plants, such as a species of Vaccinium and a species of Epilobium. When eaten alone, the dried mushrooms are moistened in the mouth and swallowed, or the women may moisten and roll them into pellets for the men to swallow.

Agara (*Galbulimima belgraveana*) is a tall forest tree of Malaysia and Australia. In Papua, natives make a drink by boiling the leaves and bark with the leaves of ereriba. When they imbibe it, they become violently intoxicated, eventually falling into a deep sleep during which they experience visions and fantastic dreams. Some 28 alkaloids have been isolated from this tree, and although they are biologically active, the psychoactive principle is still unknown. Agara is one of four species of Galbulimima and belongs to the Himontandraceae, a rare family related to the Magnolias.

Ereriba, an undetermined species of Homalomena, is a stout herb reported to have narcotic effects when its leaves are taken with the leaves and bark of agara. The active chemical constituent is unknown. Ereriba is a member of the aroid fomily, Araceae. There are some 140 species of Homalomena native to tropical Asia and South America.

Kwashi (*Pancratium trianthum*) is considered to be psychoactive by the Bushmen in Dobe, Botswana. The bulb of this perennial is reputedly rubbed over incisions in the head to induce visual hallucinations. Of the 14 other species of Pancratium, mainly of Asia and Africa, many are known to contain psychoactive principles, mostly alkaloids. Some species are potent cardiac poisons. Pancratium belongs to the amaryllis family Amaryllidaceae.

Galanga or Maraba (*Kaempferia galanga*) is an herb rich in essential oils. Natives in New Guinea eat the rhizome of the plant as an hallucinogen. It is valued locally as a condiment and, like others of the 70 species in the genus, it is used in local folk medicine to bring boils to a head and to hasten the healing of burns and wounds. It is a member of the ginger family, Zingiberoceae. Phytochemical studies have revealed no psychoactive principle.

Marihuana, Hasheesh, or Hemp (species of the genus *Cannabis*), also called Kif, Bhang, or Charas, is one of the oldest cultivated plants. It is also one of the most widely spread weeds, having escaped cultivation, appearing as an adventitious plant everywhere, except in the polar regions and the wet, forested tropics. Cannabis is the source of hemp fiber, an edible fruit, an industrial oil, a medicine, and a narcotic. Despite its great age and its economic importance, the plant is still poorly understood, characterized more by what we do not know about it than by what we know. Cannabis is a rank, weedy annual that is extremely variable and may attain a height of 18 feet. Flourishing best in disturbed, nitrogen-rich soils near human habitations, it has been called a "camp follower," going with man into new areas. It is normally dioecious—that is, the male and female parts are on different plants. The male or staminate plant is usually weaker than the female or pistillate plant. Pistillate flowers grow in the leaf axils. The intoxicating constituents are normally concentrated in a resin in the developing female flowers and adjacent leaves and stems.

Belladonna (*Atropa belladonna*) is well known as a highly poisonous species capable of inducing various kinds of hallucinations. It entered into the folklore and mythology of virtually all European peoples, who feared of its deadly power. It was one of the ingredients of the truly hallucinogenic brews and ointments concocted by the so-called witches of medieval Europe. The attractive shiny berries of the plant still often cause it to be accidentally eaten, with resultant poisoning. The name belladonna ("beautiful lady" in Italian) comes from a curious custom practiced by Italian women of high society during medieval times. They would drop the sap of the plant into the eye to dilate the pupil enormously, inducing a kind of drunken or glassy stare, considered in that period to enhance feminine beauty and sensuality. The main active principle in belladonna is the alkaloid hyoscyamine, but the more psychoactive scopolamine is also present. Atropine has also been found, but whether it is present in the living plant or is formed during extraction is not clear. Belladonna is a commercial source of atropine, an alkaloid with a wide variety of uses in modern medicine, especially as an antispasmodic, an antisecretory, a mydriatic and a cardiac stimulant. The alkaloids occur throughout the plant but are concentrated especially in the leaves and roots. There are four species of Atropa distributed in Europe and from central Asia to the Himalayas. Atropa belongs to the nightshade family, Solanaceae. Belladonna is native to Europe and Asia Minor. Until the 19th century, commercial collection was primarily from wild sources, but since that time cultivation has been initiated in the United States, Europe, and India, where it is an important source of medicinal drugs.

Henbane (*Hyoscyamus niger*) was often included in the witches' brews and other toxic preparations of medieval Europe to cause visual hallucinations and the sensation of flight. An annual or biennial native to Europe, it has long been valued in medicine as a sedative and an anodyne to induce sleep. The principal alkaloid of henbane is hyoscyamine, but the more hallucinogenic scopolamine is also present in significant amounts, along with several other alkaloids in smaller concentrations. Henbane is one of 20 species of Hyoscyamus, members of the nightshade family, Solanaceae. They are native to Europe, northern Africa, and western and central Asia.

Dhatura and Dutra (*Datura metel*) are the common names in India for an important Old

Table 13.4

Specific agents	Major species	Usual effects
Tobacco (*Nicotiana*) (Plant with nicotinic as well as teratogenic alkaloids)	Swine, cattle	Arthrogryposis, spinal curvature, torticollis
Poison hemlock (*Conium*) (Plant with nicotinic as well as teratogenic alkaloids)	Swine, cattle	Arthrogryposis, other skeletal malformations, cleft palate
Lupine, bluebonnet (*Lupinus*) (Plant with nicotinic as well as teratogenic alkaloids)	Cattle, sheep	Arthrogryposis, other skeletal malformations, celft palate
Locoweed (*Astragalus* and *Oxytropis*)	Herbivores, sheep	Arthrogryposis, or contracted tendons
Hybrid sudan or sudan grass (*Sorghum*)	Herbivores	Ankylosis, contracted tendons
Lathyrism (*Lathyrus* spp.)	Herbivores	Various skeletal deformities

Table 13.5

Specific agents	Major species	Usual effects
Potato (*Solanum tuberosum*)	Hamster	Spina bifida, exencephaly
Fescue (festuca with ergot alkaloids produced by the endophytic fungus *Acremonium coenophialum*)	Horses	Dystocia with thick placenta, and oversize, weak foals with overgrown hooves
Mercury	All species, especially cats	Hypoplasia of the cerebellum and other brain defects
Organotins	Wildlife in aquatic ecosystems	Skeletal malformations, defective myelinogenesis
Selenium	Poultry, waterfowl	Hypoplasia of upper and/or lower beak, hindlimbs, wings, and eyes
Halogenated dibenzodioxins and related halogenated aromatics	Laboratory animals predatory water birds	Cystic kidneys, cleft palate. Crossed beaks in cormorants
Vitamin A and derivatives such as isotretinoins	Humans, swine, rabbits, other species	Shortened limbs, altered gait, spinal column abnormalities, cleft palate, malformed ears, craniofacial bone and brain anomalies, microphthalmia
Corticosteroids	Dogs, possibly other species	Cleft palate
Griseofulvin	Cats	Cyclops

(Contd.)

Poisonous Teratogenic and Hallucinogenic Plants

Table 13.5 (Contd.)

Specific agents	Major species	Usual effects
Thalidomide	Human beings, lab rodents	Hypoplasia of the limbs (phocomelia)
Cocaine	Human beings	Severe neurologic impairment
Ethanol	Human beings	Shortened palpebral fissures (eye opening is small relative to the globe) and ocular problems, premaxillary abnormalities resulting in a flattened midface and an indistinct philtrum. Low birth weght, learning impairment, mental retardation, and microencephaly. Hearing impairment and ears rotating posteriorly. Gait abnormalities, scoliosis, shortened digits. Atrioventricular septal defects. Renal disorders. Threshold dose is only 1 ounce of alcohol/day (causes reduced birth weight). Overall, 5.9% of human newborn babies are affected by some degree of fetal alcohol syndrome.

World species of Datura. The narcotic properties of this purple-flowered member of the deadly nightshade family, Solanaceae, have been known and valued in India since prehistory. The plant has a long history in other countries as well. Some writers have credited it with being responsible for the intoxicating smoke associated with the Oracle of Delphi. Early Chinese writings report an hallucinogen that has been identified with this species. And it is undoubtedly the plant that Avicenna, the Arabian physician, mentioned under the name jouzmathel in the 11th century. Its use as an aphrodisiac in the East Indies was recorded in 1578. The plant was held sacred in China, where people believed that when Buddha preached, heaven sprinkled the plant with dew. Nevertheless, the utilization of Datura preparations in Asia entailed much less ritual than in the New World. In many parts of Asia, even today, seeds of Datura are often mixed with food and tobacco for illicit use, especially by thieves for stupefying victims, who may remain seriously intoxicated for several days. *Datura metel* is commonly mixed with cannabis and smoked in Asia to this day. Leaves of a white-flowered form of the plant (considered by some

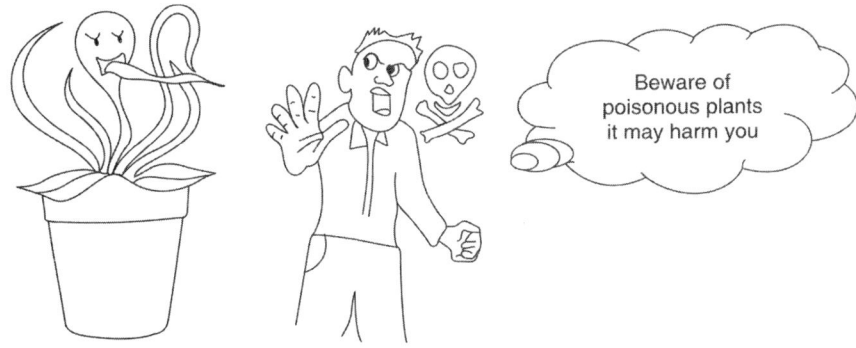

botanists to be a distinct species, *D. fastuosa*) are smoked with cannabis or tobacco in many parts of Africa and Asia. The plant contains highly toxic alkaloids, the principal one being scopolamine. This hallucinogen is present in heaviest concentrations in the leaves and seeds. *Datura ferox*, a related Old World species, not so widespread in Asia, is also valued for its narcotic and medicinal properties.

In addition to the hallucinogenic plants used by primitive peoples, numerous other species containing biodynamic principles are known to exist. Many are common household varieties like catnip, cinnamon, and ginger. No reliable studies have been made of on hallucinogenic properties of such plants. Some of the effects reported to have been caused by them may be imaginary; other reports may be outright hoaxes. Nevertheless, many of these plants do have a chemistry theoretically capable of producing hallucinations. Experimentation continues with plants—common and uncommon—known or suspected to be hallucinogenic, and new ones are continually being discovered.

14
Ayurvedic Pharmacy and Standardization of Ayurvedic Formulation

Ayurveda, literally means (*Ayur:* Life; *Veda:* Science) science of life in Sanskrit, is a way of life which aims at the holistic management of health and diseases widely practiced in Indian subcontinent and its concepts and approaches are considered to have been perfected between 2500 and 500 BC.

According to tradition, the teachings of Ayurveda were recollected by Brahma, the Lord of Creation, as he awoke to begin the task of creating the universe that we inhabit now. This idea suggests that Ayurveda transcends the period of this universe, stretching beyond the concept of time itself, having no beginning and no end. Brahma taught this knowledge to Daks, a Prajapati (the protector of all beings), whom in turn taught it to the As´viný Kumaras (the twin holy physicians), who in turn taught it to Indra (King of the Gods). When disease and illness began to trouble humanity the great *risis* ('sages') of the world assembled in the Himalayan mountains, seeking to learn Ayurveda from Lord Indra.

Ayurveda was preached by sears, like Atreya, Charaka, Sushruta, Madhva, Kashyapa. The *Charaka Samhita* states that the term 'Ayurveda' is derived from two words, *ayus* and *veda*. Many Ayurvedic commentators define *ayus* as 'life', but *Charaka* expands upon this definition, telling us that *ayus* is the '... combination of the body, sense organs, mind and soul', the factor (*dhari*) responsible for preventing decay and death, which sustains (*jývita*) the body over time (*nityaga*), and guides the process of rebirth (*anubandha*). The second part of the word is *veda* and can be translated as 'knowledge' or 'science', but more specifically suggests a deeply profound knowledge that emanates from a divine source.

Ayurveda is known as the 'divine science of life'. As a s´*astra* ('teaching') of the *Vedas*, Ayurveda is allied with the four principal Vedas of ancient India, which similarly issued forth from Lord Brahma at the time of Creation. The Vedas include the *Rigveda*, *Yajurveda*, *Samaveda* and the *Atharvaveda*, and are considered by Hindus to be a sacred knowledge, an eternal and unending truth called the *Sanatana Dharma* (Table 14.1).

Table 14.1: History of Ayurveda

Historical time table of Ayurveda
1500 BCE Vedic religion Rig, Yajur, Sama and Atharva Vedas: 125 herbal medicines mentioned in Atharva Veda
C.600 BCE Rise of heterodox traditions of Jainism, Buddhism. Also growth of what is now called Hinduism
150 B CE–100 CE Charaka Samhita: The earliest complete ayurvedic treatise. Herbs are here classified by action and morphology. Again reformatted by Drdhabala circa 400CE
C.100–500 Susruta Samhita: Detailed surgical text Bhela Samhita:
500 Dhanvantari Nighantu: an early compilation of herbs into certain functional groups based on the property of the herbs
C.600 Astangahrdaya Samhita—by Vagbhata: A collated work on the essence of Ayurveda
C.650–950 Madhava Nida-na (aka Rogavinis´caya): The first text committed solely to pathology

(Contd.)

Table 14.1: History of Ayurveda (Contd.)
Historical timetable of ayurveda
C.875 Siddhayoga by Vrnda. Early ayurvedic text of the same type as Cakradatta
900–1400 Goraksa Samhita: Early hathayoga text where many ayurvedic concepts are fused with tantric yogic practice
1075 Chikitsa samgraha/Cakradatta by Chakrapani professional ayurvedic handbook of the medieval era
1100 Dravyagunasamgraha: The first Nighantu written by Chakrapani
C.1300 Anandakanda: An early alchemical treatise
1374 Madanaphala Nighantu: A further compilation of herbs and minerals
1300–1400 Sarngadhara Samhita: Collected work on ayurvedic formulas and preparations. First record of pulse-taking as a diagnostic method. A pivotal work linking early ayurvedic thought with new tantric alchemical techniques
1449/50 Laksman Otsava: A text describing pulse-taking
1474–1538 Jvaratimirabhaskara of Ca-mun.da. The first mention of Astasthanaparýksa, the eight methods of diagnosis (pulse, tongue, urine, eyes, face, faeces, voice and skin)
1596 Bhavaprakasa Nighantu by Bhavamis´ra: The most important ayurvedic materia medica treatise
C.1600 Ayurvedasutra: A text mixing ayurvedic, yogic and tantric thought. Rasaratnsamuccaya: A pivotal alchemical text compiling much earlier thought and theory
1676 Yogaratnakara: A pivotal work reflecting the assimilative trait of Unani and European influences on Ayurveda
1760 Rajavallabha Nighantu: Progressive material medica
1815 Samgraha Nighantu
1893 Bhaisajya Ratnavalý: Govindadasa's work listing numerous medical preparations and introducing different European diseases
C.1900 Nadýprakas´ana: S´aný kara Sen
1924 Nighantu Ratnakara

The Meaning of '*Dosa*'

'*Dosa*' is described and translated in many different ways; 'constitution', 'functional principle', 'humour'.

- Constitution means one's fixed and lifelong inherited health.
- Functional principle means an invisible catalytic active.
- Humour comes from the Latin '*umere*' meaning moist.

There are three *dosa*s (*tridosa: vata, pitta, kapha*– Fig. 14.1) that are discussed in detail below.

Vata

The *vata dosa* (Table 14.2) is comprised of *akas´a* (ether) and *vayu* (wind). Each *dosa* contains aspects of all the *pancamahabhuta*, but space and wind are predominant in *vata*. *Vata* is cold, light, rough, mobile, subtle, clear, dry and astringent. The primary site of *vata* is the colon. It also resides in the bladder, thighs, ears, bones and the sense of touch. Vata governs bodily functions concerned with movement. The flow of food through the digestive tract and the circulation, the flow of breath and blood, elimination of wastes, expression of speech, it moves the diaphragm, muscles and limbs, regulates the nervous system and it also stimulates the function of the intellect. Vata is especially involved in the movement of electrical activity up and down the nerves and, therefore, has a major function in the nervous system and brain.

Pitta

The *pitta dosa* (Table 14.3) is made up of *tejas* (fire) and *jala* (water). *Pitta* exists as water or oil in the body, thus preserving the tissues from the destructive aspect of fire. It is pungent, hot, penetrating, greasy, oily, sharp, liquid, spreading and sour. Pitta governs bodily functions concerned with heat, metabolism and energy production. It maintains

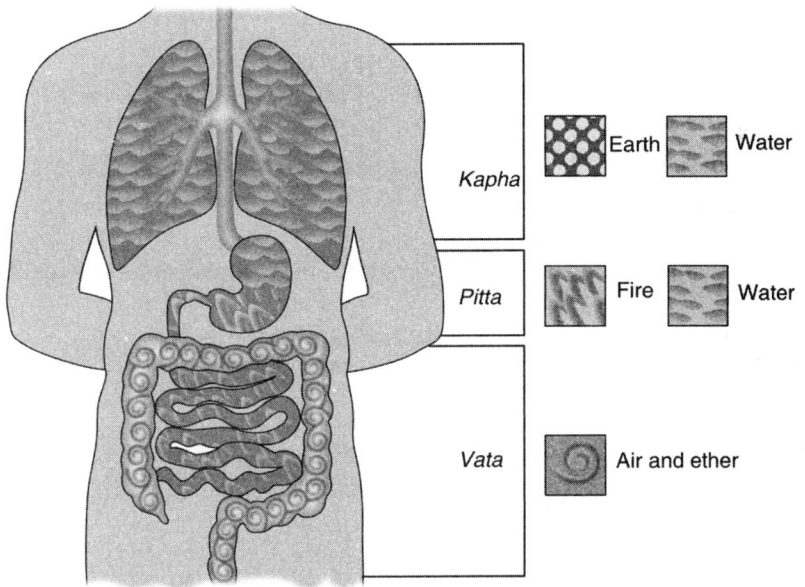

Fig. 14.1: Three seats of dosha: *Vata, pitta* and *kapha*

endocrine function, hormone levels, digestion, body temperature, visual perception, hunger, thirst, and skin quality. Mentally, it plays a role in understanding and in digesting sensory impressions. It resides in the eyes, blood, sweat glands, the small intestine, stomach and lymph. Its primary site is in the small intestine.

Table 14.2: Vata dosa

Body type	Thin body, irregular shape, knobby knees, tall, crooked teeth, thin fingers and cruly hairs.
Activity	Performs activity quickly
Skin type	Dry skin especially in winter
Tendency	Worry, constipation, light and interrupted sleep and irregular hunger and digestion
Qualities	Grasp new information, also quick to forget, enthusiastic and vivacious
Miscellaneous	Walks quickly, talkative and often changes mind

Table 14.3: Pitta dosa

Body type	Balanced, regular athletic body, straight hair, ruddy complexion and prominent eyes.
Activity	Performs activity with medium speed
Aversion	Hot weather
Tendency	Reddish hair and complexion, irritability and anger
Qualities	Good public speakers, great precision, strong intellect and enterprising and sharp in character
Preferences	Cold food and drinks
Miscellaneous	Medium memory and time to grasp new information

Kapha

The *kapha dosa* (Table 14.4) is a combination of the *prithvi* (earth) and *jala* (water) elements. It is slow, heavy, cool, dense, soft, greasy, unctuous, sticky, cloudy, liquid and sweet. *Kapha* literally holds the body together. It is cohesive, gives shape and form, aids growth and development, lubricates and protects, helps smelling and tasting. It relates to phlegm in the body. It resides in the chest, throat, head, pancreas, stomach, lymph, fat, nose and tongue. Its primary site is the stomach. Kapha governs bodily functions concerned with physical structure and fluid balance. Kapha is mainly concerned with fluid balance and the buildup of the gross structure of the body including fat, tissues and muscles.

Table 14.4: Kapha dosa

Body type	Solid, heavier build, big bones, ears and teeth, large eyes and lips and overweight
Activity	Performs activity slowly
Skin type	Oily, smooth
Hair type	Plentiful, thick and wavy
Tendency	Excess mucous, chronic congestion, sinus problems, allergies and lethargy as well as depression
Qualities	Steady personality, sweet and happy by nature
Preferences	Greater strength and endurance
Miscellaneous	Gains weight easily, slow digestion and mild hunger

Qualities of Balance and Imbalance in *Vata*, *Pitta* and *Kapha* (Table 14.5)

The Ayurvedic approach is not to treat symptoms but to treat the underlying imbalances in *Vata*, *Pitta* and *Kapha*. When these imbalances disappear, usually symptoms disappear too.

Ayurvedic medicines are available in the form of powder, tablets, pills, liquid and semi-solid which are classified into the following different categories:

- Arishta and Asava
- Rasa Rasayan
- Lauha
- Bati
- Churna
- Avaleha
- Ghrita
- Parpati
- Taila
- Goggulu

Method of Preparation

1. Arishta and Asava: Asavas and Arishtas are made by soaking the herbs either in powder

Table 14.5: Signs of dosa balance and excess

Dosa	Balanced state	Increased state	Decreased state
Vata	Inspiration, expiration, mental alertness, proper formation of body tissues, desire and enthusiasm, normal elimination enthusiasm sound sleep strong immunity	Weight loss, constipation, weakness, dark complexion, dark discoloration, loneliness, insomnia and depression	Lack of enthusiasm, confusion, no desire to speack and less consciousness
Pitta	Regulation of hormones, strong digestion, sharp intellect, courage, enzyme regulation, eye sight quality and maintains lustrous complexion normal heat and thirst mechanisms	Redness, burning, fever, inflammation, burning urine, impatience and anger, sour taste in mouth	Poor digestion and coldness
Kapha	Muscular strength structure, flexibility and solidity. Vitality and stamina, strong immunity, affection, generosity, stability of mind healthy, normal joints	Excess salivation, obesity, edema, tumors, heaviness, excessive desire to sleep and itching	Dryness, anxiety and cracking joints

form or in the form of decoction (*kasaya*) in a solution of sugar or jugglery, as the case may be, for a specific period of time, during which it undergoes a process of fermentation generation alcohol and facilitates the extraction of the active ingredients contained in the herbs.

2. Rasa Rasayan: Ayurvedic medicines containing mineral drugs as main ingredients are called Rasa Rasayan or Ras-yoga. They are in pill form or in powder form/forest, minerals such as Anrala, Swarna, Rajata, Tamra, etc. and sulfur impurified state are used to convert Bhasma form, called Kajuali then other drugs are added in small quantities, mixed well and grounded to form fine powder.

3. Lauha: Lauha kalpas are preparation of Loha Bhasma as main ingredient with other drugs. The other active ingredients are made to fine powder and mixed with Loha Bhasma.

4. Vati or Gutika: Medicines prepared in the form of tablets or pills are known as Vati or Gutika, these are made of one or more drugs of plant, animal or mineral origin.

5. Churna: Churna is a fine powder form of drugs. All these herbs and other active ingredients are cleaned, dried and powdered together by mechanical means to the fineness of at least 80 mesh.

6. Avaleha madak paak: Avaleha or Lehya is a semi-solid preparation of drugs. These are prepared by the addition of jagger sugar or sugar dandy and boiled with prescribed drug juices decoction, honey, if required, is added when the preparation is cold and mixed well.

7. Ghrita: Ghrita are preparations in which ghee is boiled with prescribed Kasayas (decoction) and Kalkas of drugs according to formulation as per Ayurvedic formulary.

8. Parpati: First Kajjali is prepared with purified mercury and sulfur. Then other drugs as per Ayurvedic Formulae are added and mixed well in grinder. The powder is then heated in iron vessel and melted. This melted material is purified as per Ayurvedic method, cooled and again flakes of medicines are powdered.

9. Taila: Tailas are prepared by boiling prescribed Kasyas (decoction) and Kalkas of drugs in oils according to the formula prescribed in Ayurvedic formulary.

10. Goggulu: Ayurvedic medicines prepared by the exudates, and obtained from the plant *Commiphara mukul*, are known as Goggulu. There are five different varieties of Goggulu in Ayurvedic Shastra but usually two varieties, Mahiskasa and Kanaka are preferred for medicinal preparation. Exudates in small pieces are taken in a piece of cloth and boiled in Gomutara or Dugdha or Triphala Kasayua until the exudates pass into the fluid through the cloth to the maximum. The fluid after filtering is boiled till it forms a mass. After drying, the mass is formed into a paste by adding ghee till it becomes waxy.

Quality Control and Standards

At present, there is no pharmacopoeial standard on each of the active ingredients of Ayurvedic medicine, like allopathic medicine. For standardization and quality control of Ayurvedic drugs, various steps can be followed like physical description, physical tests, pharma-coginized techniques, etc. to ascertain the species of plants and study their pharma-coginostic character for the purpose of identification, detection and analyzing the crude drug. Generally, quality of Ayurvedic products is fully dependent on the quality of raw materials and process of manufacture. The quality control process of some Ayurvedic formulations can be contained from 'Pharmacopoeia Laboratory of India Medicine, near ALTC, Ghaziabad (UP)'. The products are to be manufactured as per Indian System of Medicines of Ministry of Health.

All the steps involved in preparation and standardization should be recorded in the chronological order. As per pharmacopoeia standards, it starts with collection, washing and authentication of Ayurvedic drug samples. The steps of formulating drug into dosage form include grinding, sieving, boiling, filtering and cooling. The botanical identification is performed for Churna, vati, pills, and capsules. This is followed by modest chemical test for chemical constituents and the following parameters, like:

1. Foreign matter.
2. Ash values (total ash, acid-insoluble, water-soluble ash).
3. Extractive values (alcohol and water-soluble).
4. Thin layer chromatography.
5. Shelf life study.
6. Estimation of heavy metals.
7. Microbial load.
8. Pesticide residue, etc.

In case of Avaleha, Syrup, Asava, Arishta, Tala and Ghrita, phytochemical tests are applicable. In these formulations, TLC, HPLC, GLC, GC/MS procedures are helpful to identify the constituents. But in Bhasma, the methods of preparation and Shodhana (purification) as well as Bhasmikarana (incineration) are also standardized. The particle size analysis, and physiochemical characterization of Bhasma are needed.

Ayurvedic medicines are all the medicines intended for internal or external use, for or in the diagnosis, treatment, mitigation or prevention of disease or disorder in human beings or animal. Ayurvedic drugs are obtained from the natural source that is from animal, plants and minerals. Ayurvedic dosages forms are classified into four groups depending upon their physical forms as described in Table 14.6.

Table 14.6: Classification of ayurvedic medicines

S. no.	Type	Dosage form
1	Solid	Pills, Gutika, Vatika
2	Semi-solid	Avleha, Paka, Lepa, Grita
3	Liquid	Asava, Arishta, Arka, Taila, Dravaka
4	Powder	Bhasma, Satva, Mandura, Pisti, Parpati, Lavana, Kshara, Churna

Asava and Arishtas

Asava and Arishta are alcoholic preparations. Former is made with decoctions of herbs in boiling water while later is prepared by directly using fresh herbal juices or decoction to undergo fermentations. These are unique liquid dosage forms that contain self generated alcohol.

Method of Preparation of Asava and Arishta

Procedure: The basic drugs from which the extract is to be prepared are first clean and rinsed with water to get rid of dirt. In the case of fresh plant, they are cleaned, pulverized and pressed for collection of juice.

Asava: If the drug is dry and is to be used in the preparation of asava, it is coarsely crushed and added to the water to which the prescribed quantities of honey, jaggery or sugar are added.

Arishtas (Fig. 14.2): A decoction is obtained by boiling the drugs in the specified volume of water. The water used should be clean, clear and potable. When the extract is obtained, the sugar, jaggery and/or honey are added and completely dissolved. The major components are divided into four types according to their specific role in the process:

1. Main drug.
2. Flavoring agent (herbs): The flavoring

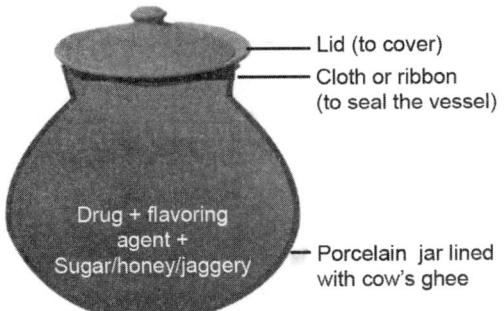

Fig. 14.2: Preparation of arishtas

agents are coarsely powdered and added to the sweetened extract. Too fine a powder of the flavoring agent is undesirable as it causes sedimentation in the prepared medicine and its filtration is difficult.

3. Sugar/jaggery/honey (fermentation initiator).
   - Pure, white cane sugar.
   - Jaggery should be of sweet taste and at least one year old.
   - The honey should be genuine.
4. Earthen pot.

The main purpose of earthen pot is fermen-tation. Internal surfaces of the pot are wiped with the clean cloth and cow's ghee is smeared to surface to prevent oozing out of the contents, the sweetened and flavored drug extract is poured into it up to of the capacity. This unfilled space provides room for the fermenting liquid when it rises up frothing and evolving a large amount of gases. For fermentation, yeast obtained from the flowers which contain the wild species of yeast is used. The sealing of vessel is done by winding around a long ribbon of cloth smeared with clay on one surface. After sealing, the pot is kept in a dark place without disturbance for a month and then filtered and taken for use.

Standardization of Asava/Arishta

It generally involves the following parameters.

1. **Organoleptic parameters:**
   a. Color of sample
   b. Odor of sample
   c. Taste of sample
   d. Determination of pH of sample

2. **Physical parameters:** These parameters are for standardization of drug material:
   a. Determination of foreign organic matter
   b. Determination of ash value
      - Total ash value
      - Acid-insoluble ash
      - Water-soluble ash
      - Sulfated ash
   c. Determination of extractive value:
      - Alcohol-soluble extractive value
      - Water-soluble extractive value
   d. Determination of moisture content
   e. Determination of physical constants:
      - Melting point
      - Boiling point
      - Refractive index
      - Optical rotation
   f. Determination of specific gravity
   g. Determination of solid content
   h. Determination of alcohol content

3. **Chemical parameters:** Chemical parameters involve following parameters in chemical evaluation:
   a. Alkaloids — Drag endroff's test
   b. Glycosides — Molish test
   c. Flavonoids — Shinoda test
   d. Phenolic — Lead acetate test
   e. Tannins — Ferric chloride test

f. Steroids — Salkowski reaction
g. Amino acids — Ninhydrine test
h. Carbohydrates — Fehling's test, Benedict test

4. **Toxicological parameters:** These involve following parameters:
   a. Pesticides residue
   b. Heavy metal
   c. Microbial contamination

Avaleha or Lehya

Avaleha or Lehya is a semi-solid preparation of drugs, prepared with addition of jaggery, sugar or sugar-candy and boiled with prescribed juices or decoction. The Lehya should neither be hard nor a thick fluid. When pulp of the drugs is added and ghee or oil is present in the preparation, this can be rolled between the fingers.

These preparations generally have:
1. Kasaya or other liquids,
2. Jaggery, sugar or sugar-candy,
3. Powders or pulps of certain drugs,
4. Ghee or oil, and
5. Honey.

Method of Preparation

1. Jaggery, sugar or sugar-candy is dissolved in the liquid and strained to remove the foreign particles and boiled over a moderate fire.
2. It should be removed from fire, when pressed between fingers it becomes thready (Tantuvat), or when it sinks in water without getting easily dissolved.
3. Powdered drugs are then added in small quantities and stirred continuously to form a homogenous mixture.
4. Ghee or oil is added and mixed well.
5. Finally, honey is added when the preparation becomes cool and mixed well.

Storage: The Lehya should be kept in glass or porcelain jars. It can also be kept in a metal container which does not react with it. Normally, the Lehya should be used within one year.

Examples: Kalyanaka Guda, Ashvagandhadi Lehya.

Tailas

Tailas are also known as medicated oils forming a group of drugs in ayurvedic system of medicine with the principle is to extract the therapeutic compounds into oil.

Preparation: The method of preparation requires heating of oil with prescribed kashayas (decoction) and Kalkas (powdered drugs) according to formula. They are generally used for Abhyanga (external application).

It consists of:
1. Drava [Any liquid medium as prescribed in the composition]
2. Kalka [Fine paste of the specified drug]
3. Sneha Dravya [Tailas]
4. Gandha Dravya [Perfuming agents]

The medicated Tailas will have the odour, color and taste of the drugs used in the process. If a considerable amount of milk is used in the preparation, the Tailas will become thick and may solidify in cold seasons. Tailas are preserved in good quality of glass, steel or polythene containers. These medicated preparations retain the therapeutic efficacy for 16th months.

Churnas

Churna is defined as a fine powder of drug or drugs in Ayurvedic system of medicine. Drugs mentioned in Patha, are cleaned properly, dried thoroughly, pulverized and then sieved. The Churna is free flowing and retains its potency for one year, if preserved in airtight containers. The Churna consisting of fine powder of herbs in appropriate ratio was subjected to standardization by means of various physical, chemical and microbiological methods.

Powders are solid dosage form of medicament meant for internal and external uses. They are available in crystalline or amorphous form. Powder of a single drug is called simple and that of a compound formulation is called compound powder.

Storage: The packed materials should be stored in cool, dry and dark conditions.

Standardization of Churnas

It generally involves the following parameters:
1. Determination of sieve size
2. Loss on drying/moisture content
3. TLC
4. Total ash
5. Acid-insoluble ash
6. Water-soluble ash
7. Extractive value in water, alcohol and other solvents
8. Phytoconstituents
9. Microbial contaminations
10. Heavy metal limit test for mercury, arsenic, cadmium, and lead
11. Microscopic analysis

Lepas

Lepas are semi-solid preparations intended for external application to the skin or certain mucous membranes for emollient, protective, therapeutic or prophylactic purposes where a degree of occlusion is desired. They usually consist of solutions or dispersions of one or more medicaments in suitable bases.

The base should not produce irritation or sensitization of the skin, nor should it retard wound healing; it should be smooth, inert, odorless, physically and chemically stable and compatible with the skin and with incorporated medicaments. The proportions of the base ingredients should be such that the ointment is not too soft or too hard for convenient use. The consistency should be such that the ointment spreads and softens when stress is applied.

Standardization of Lehyas

- Loss of drying
- Ash values
- Extractive values
- pH
- Thin layer chromatography

Bhasmas

The Bhasmas are the powder of substances obtained by calcinations. The preparation of Bhasmas include following stages:
1. Purva Karma: Sodhana (purification).
2. Pardhana Karma: Marana (incineration/calcination).
3. Paschat Karma: Amritikarna, Lohitikarna.

Sodhana (Purification)

It is prepared from purified minerals, metals, marine and animal products. The following changes are observed: After purification, the materials become free from impurities and become fine as well.

Second Stage (Marana)

The purified drug is mixed with Kasaya of drugs, and it is ground with motar and pestle for specified period of time. The cakes are prepared and their size and thickness depends on heaviness of the drug. The cakes are dried on the sunlight and placed in Sarava (shallow earthen plate) and closed with other plate and sealed with clay smeared cloth and dried. The pit is dug in open space and sealed plates and cow dung are filled in the pit. Fire is put on

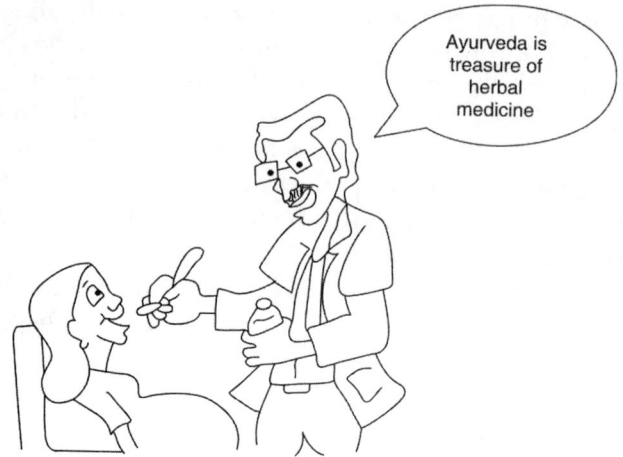

all the sides and when burning is over, allowed to cool. The earthen pot is removed and seal is opened and contents are taken out. The medicine is ground into fine powder in a Khalva (motar and pestle). The process of triturating is repeated as many times for proper fitness and quality.

Standardization of Bhasmas

a. Determination of foreign organic matter
b. Determination of ash value:
   - Total ash value
   - Acid-insoluble ash
   - Water-soluble ash
   - Sulfated ash
c. Determination of extractive value:
   - Alcohol-soluble extractive value
   - Water-soluble extractive value
d. Determination of moisture content
e. Determination of physical constants:
   - Melting point
   - Boiling point
   - Refractive index
   - Optical rotation
f. Determination of specific gravity
g. Determination of solid content
h. Determination of alcohol content

Plant Tissue Culture

INTRODUCTION

Plant tissue culture (PTC) is applied for aseptic culture of cells, tissues, organs and their components under suitable *in vitro* physical and chemical conditions using nutrient media (liquid/semi-solid) for the production of primary and secondary metabolites or for plant regeneration (Fig. 15.1).

Plant cell culture is based on two concepts plasticity and totipotency. The plasticity allows plants to alter their metabolism, growth, and development to best suit their environment. When plant cells and tissues are cultured *in vitro* they generally exhibit a very high degree of plasticity, which allows one type of tissue or organ to be initiated from another type. In this way, the whole plant can be subsequently regenerated. This regeneration of whole organisms depends upon the concept that all plant cells can, given the correct stimuli, express the total genetic potential of the parent plant. This maintenance of genetic potential is called totipotency.

HISTORY OF PLANT TISSUE CULTURE

The science of plant tissue culture takes its roots from the discovery of cell followed by propounding of cell theory. In 1838, Schleiden and Schwann proposed that cell is the basic functional and structural unit of all living organisms. They visualized that every cell is capable of autonomy and, therefore it should be possible for each cell, if given an environment, to regenerate into whole plant.

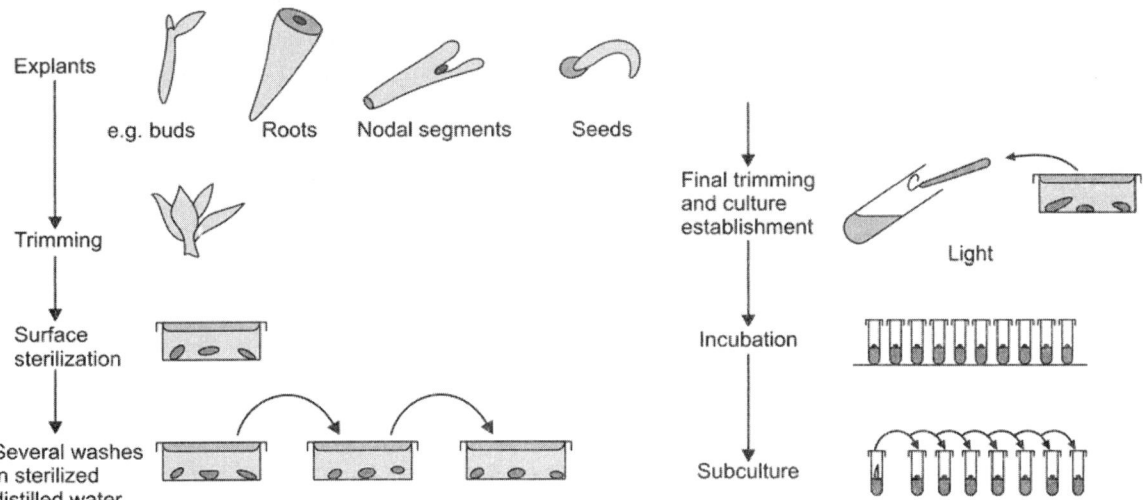

Fig. 15.1: Basic tissue culture production

Based on this premise, in 1902, a German physiologist, Gottlieb Haberlandt, for the first time, attempted to culture isolated single palisade cells from leaves in knop's salt solution enriched with sucrose. The cells remained alive for up to one month, increased in size, accumulated starch but failed to divide. Though he was unsuccessful but laid down the foundation of tissue culture technology for which he is regarded as the father of plant tissue culture. After that some of the landmark discoveries took place in tissue culture which are summarized in Table 15.1.

Table 15.1: Landmark contribution of plant tissue culture by various contributors

Contributors	Milestone
1902	The German botanist Gottlieb Haberlandt regarded as the father of plant tissue culture proposed concept of *in vitro* cell culture.
1904	Hannig cultured embryos from several cruciferous species.
1922	Root and stem tips were successfully cultured by Kolte and Robbins.
1926	Went discovered first plant growth promoting hormone –Indole acetic acid (IAA)
1934	White suggested vitamin B as growth supplement in tissue culture media for tomato root tip.
1939	Gautheret, White and Nobecourt established endless proliferation of callus cultures
1941	Overbeek was first to add coconut milk for cell division in Datura
1946	Ball raised whole plants of Lupinus by shoot tip culture
1954	Muir was first to break callus tissues into single cells
1955	Skoog and Miller discovered kinetin as cell division hormone
1957	Skoog and Miller gave concept of hormonal control (auxin: cytokinin) of organ.
1959	Reinert and Steward regenerated embryos from callus clumps and cell suspension of *Daucus carota*.
1960	Cocking was first to isolate protoplast by enzymatic degradation of cell wall.
1962	Murashige and Skoog developed MS medium with higher salt concentration.
1962	Kanta and Maheshwari developed test tube fertilization technique.
1966	Steward demonstrated totipotency by regenerating carrot plants from single cells.
1970	Smith and Nathans discovered first restriction enzyme from *Haemophilus influenzae* (HindIII)
1970	Baltimore isolated reverse transcriptase from RNA tumor virus
1972	Carlson produced first interspecific hybrid of Nicotiana by protoplast fusion
1972	Berg produced first recombinant DNA, combining SV40 virus and ë virus
1974	Reinhard introduced biotransformation in plant tissue cultures
1977	Chilton *et al.* successfully integrated Ti plasmid DNA from *Agrobacterium tumefaciens* in plants
1978	Melchers *et al.* carried out somatic hybridization of tomato and potato resulting in pomato.
1981	Larkin and Scowcroft introduced the term somaclonal variation
1983	Pelletier *et al.* conducted intergeneric cytoplasmic hybridization in radish and grape
1984	Horsh *et al.* developed transgenic tobacco by transformation with *Agrobacterium*
1987	Klien *et al.* developed biolistic gene transfer method for plant transformation
2005	Rice genome sequenced under International Rice Genome Sequencing project

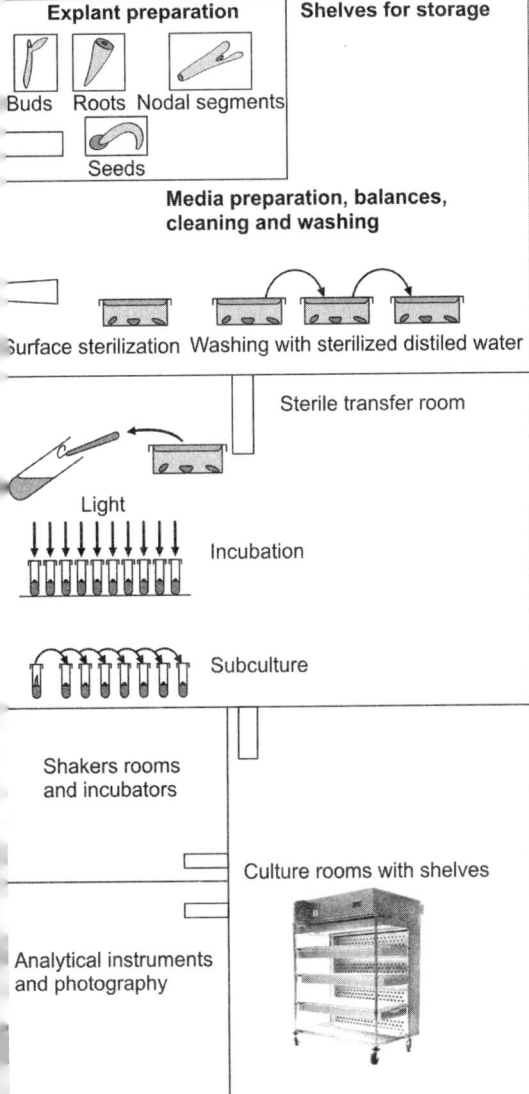

Fig. 15.2 Design of plant tissue culture laboratory

Basic Requirements for Tissue Culture Laboratories

A laboratory, in which tissue culture techniques are performed, usually includes the following facilities (Fig. 15.2):

1. Equipment and apparatus
2. Washing and storage area
3. Media preparation area
4. Sterilization area
5. Environmentally controlled incubators or culture rooms fully equipped with control devices.
6. Observation/data collection area equipped with computers.

Equipment and Apparatus

The variety of equipment essential for tissue culture laboratories are given in Table 15.2.

Washing and Storage Area

Cleanliness is the major consideration while designing the plant tissue culture laboratory. The washing area should contain large sinks, some lead-lined to resist acids and alkalis, draining boards, and racks, and have access to demineralized water, distilled water, and double-distilled water.

Media Preparation Area

The media preparation area should have ample storage space for the chemicals, culture vessels and closures, and glasswares required for media preparation and dispensing. The media preparation requires a balance sensitive to milligram quantities for weighing hormones and vitamins, a less sensitive scale may be used for weighing agar and carbohydrates. The media reagents should be shelved near the balance for convenience. A refrigerator in the media room is necessary for storing stock solutions and chemicals that degrade at room temperature. A combination of hot plate and magnetic stirrer is a time saver for dissolving inorganic reagents. Either a pH meter or pH indicator paper is required for adjusting the final pH of the medium. Sufficient and double-distilled water must be available in the media room. Sterilization equipment is an integral part of media preparation room. Wet-heat sterilization involves either an autoclave or a

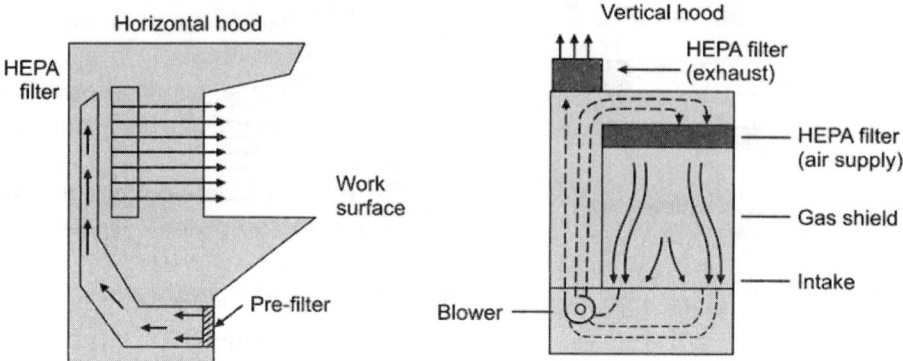

Fig. 15.3: Laminar air flow hood

Table 15.2: Description of equipment used in PTC

Equipment	Description
Spirit burner	For flame sterilization of instruments.
Refrigerator/freezer	To store temperature sensitive chemicals as well as stock solutions.
Balances	To weigh various chemicals needed for preparation of medium.
Hot plate cum magnetic stirrer	To make media and for dissolution of nutrients.
pH meter	To adjust pH of the medium.
Autoclave	Moist heat sterilization is needed for the sterilization of media, water and glasswares.
Hot air oven	For sterilization of the equipment.
Shaker	To maintain cell suspension culture.
Laminar air flow hood	For aseptic transfer of explants to media and for sub-culturing (Fig. 15.3).
BOD incubators	To maintain constant temperature to facilitate callus culture and maintenance.
Centrifuge	To sediment cells and clean protoplasts.
Glasswares and plastic wares	Erlenmeyer's and volumetric flask, petridish, measuring cylinder, pipettes, micropipettes and funnels.

pressure cooker. Some hormones and vitamins are sterilized by ultrafiltration at room temperature. After sterilization of the culture vessels by dry heat and autoclaving the medium, the culture tubes are poured in the transfer chamber.

Aseptic Chamber

The single most important factor in the selection of a suitable working area is the flow of air currents over the sterile area. Such air currents must be avoided because they carry spores of contaminating micro-organisms. An interior room, similar to a photographic darkroom, is an excellent location for aseptic procedures. Because opening, the door creates a draft, post a "No Admittance" sign on the door during the aseptic operations. If precautions are observed in a draft-free room, the open laboratory bench can be used.

General Procedures Involved in Plant Tissue Culture

In vitro culturing of plant tissue involves the following steps:
1. Sterilization of glasswares and equipments
2. Preparation and sterilization of explants
3. Production of callus from the explants
4. Proliferation of cultured callus
5. Sub-culturing of callus
6. Suspension culture

Sterilization of Glasswares and Equipment

Hot-air Oven

Heat sterilization is the most widely used and reliable method of sterilization, involving destruction of enzymes and other essential cell constituents. The process is more effective in hydrated state where under conditions of high humidity, hydrolysis and denaturation occur, thus lower heat input is required.

Dry heat sterilization: It is usually carried out in a hot-air oven: Articles to be sterilized are first wrapped or enclosed in containers of cardboard, paper or aluminum. Then, the materials are arranged to ensure uninterrupted air flow. Oven may be preheated for materials with poor heat conductivity. The temperature is allowed to fall to 40°C, prior to removal of sterilized material.

Moist heat sterilization: Moist heat may be used in three forms to achieve microbial inactivation. Moist heat sterilization involves the use of steam in the range of 121–134°C. Steam under pressure is used to generate high temperature needed for sterilization. Saturated steam (steam in thermal equilibrium with water from which it is derived) acts as an effective sterilizing agent. Steam for sterilization can be either wet saturated steam (containing entrained water droplets) or dry saturated steam (no entrained water droplets). Autoclaves use pressurized steam to destroy micro-organisms, and are the most dependable systems available for the decontamination of laboratory waste and the sterilization of laboratory glassware, media, and reagents. For efficient heat transfer, steam must flush the air out of the autoclave chamber. Before using the autoclave, check the drain screen at the bottom of the chamber and clean, if blocked. If the sieve is blocked with debris, a layer of air may form at the bottom of the autoclave, preventing efficient operation. Autoclaves should be tested periodically with biological indicators like cultures of *Bacillus stearothermophilus* to ensure proper function. This method of sterilization works well for metals and glass items but is not acceptable for rubber, plastics, and equipment that would be damaged by high temperatures.

Table 15.3: Agents used in plant tissue culture

Agents	Used in percentage (%) surface sterilization
Sodium hypochlorite	Laundry bleach is 5.25% sodium hypochlorite.
Ethanol (or isopropyl alcohol)	70% ethanol is used prior to treatment with other compounds
Calcium hypochlorite	Calcium hypochlorite may be less injurious to plant tissues than sodium hypochlorite. The concentration that is generally used is 3.25%.
Mercuric chloride	It is extremely toxic to both plants and humans. It is critical that many rinses be used to remove all traces of the mineral from the plant material.
Hydrogen peroxide	The concentration of hydrogen peroxide used for surface sterilization of plant material is 30%.

Preparation of Explants

Explants: Cell, tissue or organ of a plant that is used to start *in vitro* cultures. The different explants can be used for tissue culture, commonly used are auxiliary buds and meristems.

Sterilization of explants is usually done to remove microbial contaminants. Usually, preferred method is surface sterilization of the explants with an agent such as bleach at a concentration and for a duration that will kill or remove pathogens without injuring the plant cells beyond recovery. Explants or material from which material will be cut can be washed in soapy water and then placed under running water for 1 to 2 hours.

Steps of surface sterilization of the explant are as given in Figs 15.4 to 15.7.

Production of Callus from the Explants

The callus is unorganized, growing mass of cells which is dedifferentiation of explants.

1. The sterilized explants are transferred aseptically onto defined medium.
2. The flask is transferred to BOD incubator for maintenance of the culture.
3. Temperature (25 ± 2°C) and light is needed necessary for callus.
4. Sufficient amount of callus is produced within three to eight days of incubation

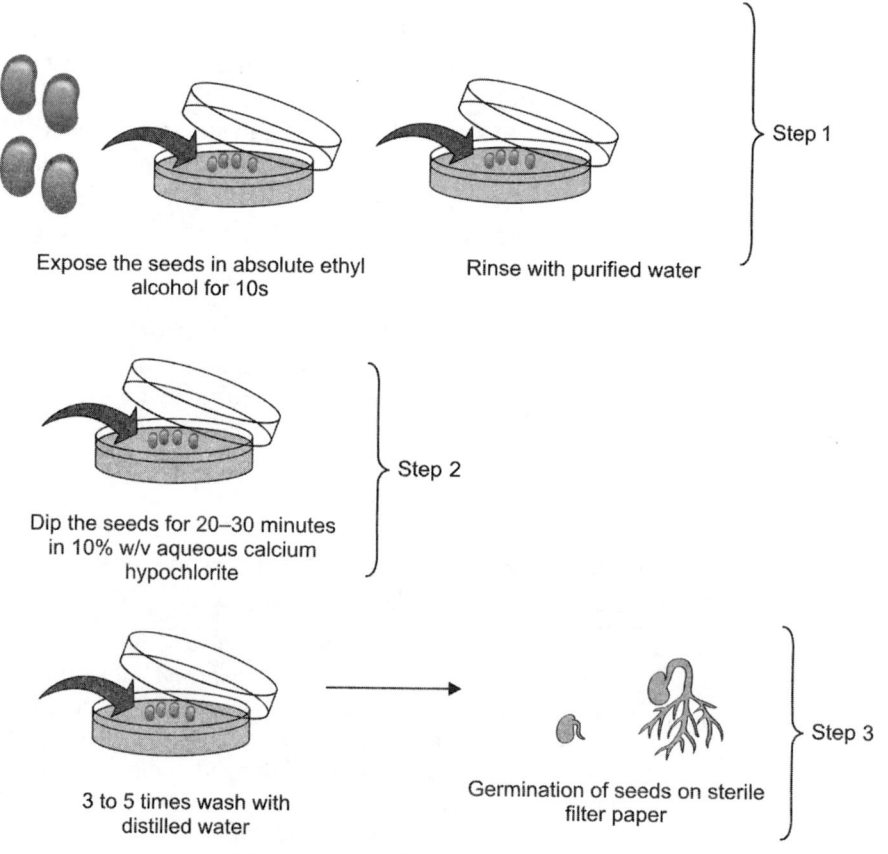

Fig. 15.4: Surface sterilization of seeds

Fruits

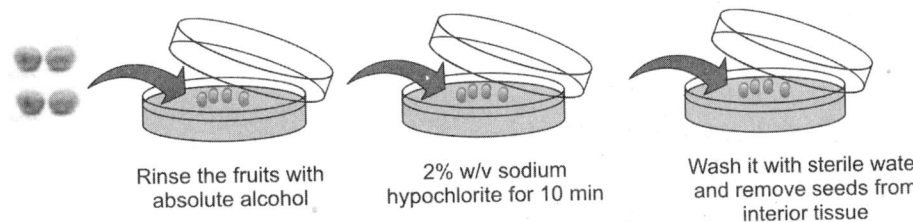

Fig. 15.5: Surface sterilization of fruits

Proliferation of Callus

The culture developed is cut into small pieces and introduced into the fresh medium consisting of the hormones and nutrients, which support growth and proliferation of explants. Proliferation medium is the medium in which more amount of callus is produced.

Stem

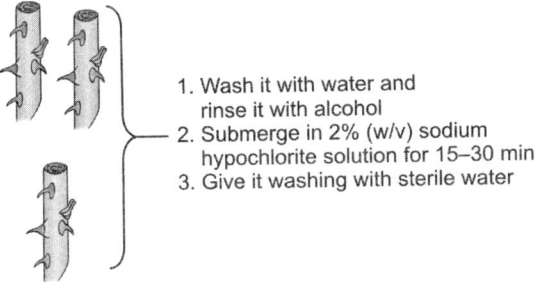

1. Wash it with water and rinse it with alcohol
2. Submerge in 2% (w/v) sodium hypochlorite solution for 15–30 min
3. Give it washing with sterile water

Fig. 15.6: Surface sterilization of stem

Leaves

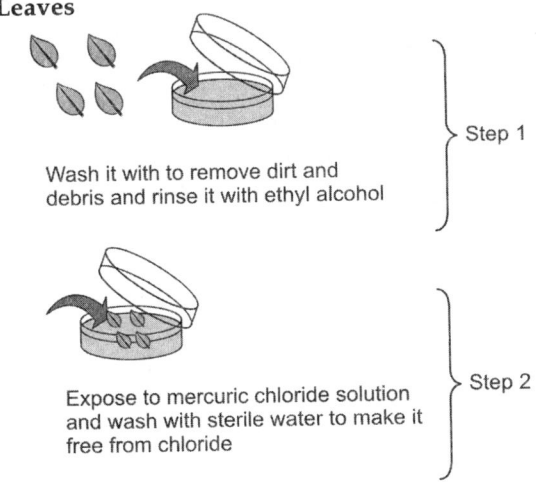

Fig. 15.7: Surface sterilization of leaves

Subculturing of Callus

The periodic transfer of cells to the fresh medium at the interval of 4 to 6 weeks should be done to maintain viability of the cells.

Suspension Culture

Cell suspension culture techniques are very important for plant biotransformation and plant genetic engineering. When friable callus is placed into the appropriate liquid medium and agitated, single cells and/or small clumps of cells are released into the medium and continue to grow and divide, producing a cell-suspension culture. The inoculum used to initiate cell suspension culture should neither be too small to affect cells number nor too large too allow the build up of toxic products or stressed cells to lethal levels.

CULTURE MEDIA

The nutritional requirements of isolated plant cell culture are to be fulfilled for optimal growth of culture. Tissue culture media were first developed from nutrient solutions used for culturing whole plants, e.g. root culture medium of White and callus culture medium of Gautheret. White's medium was based on Uspenski and Uspenska's medium for algae, Gautheret's medium was based on Knop's salt solution. Basic media that are frequently used include Murashige and Skoog (MS) medium, Linsmaier and Skoog (LS) medium, Gamborg (B5) medium and Nitsch and Nitsch (NN) medium.

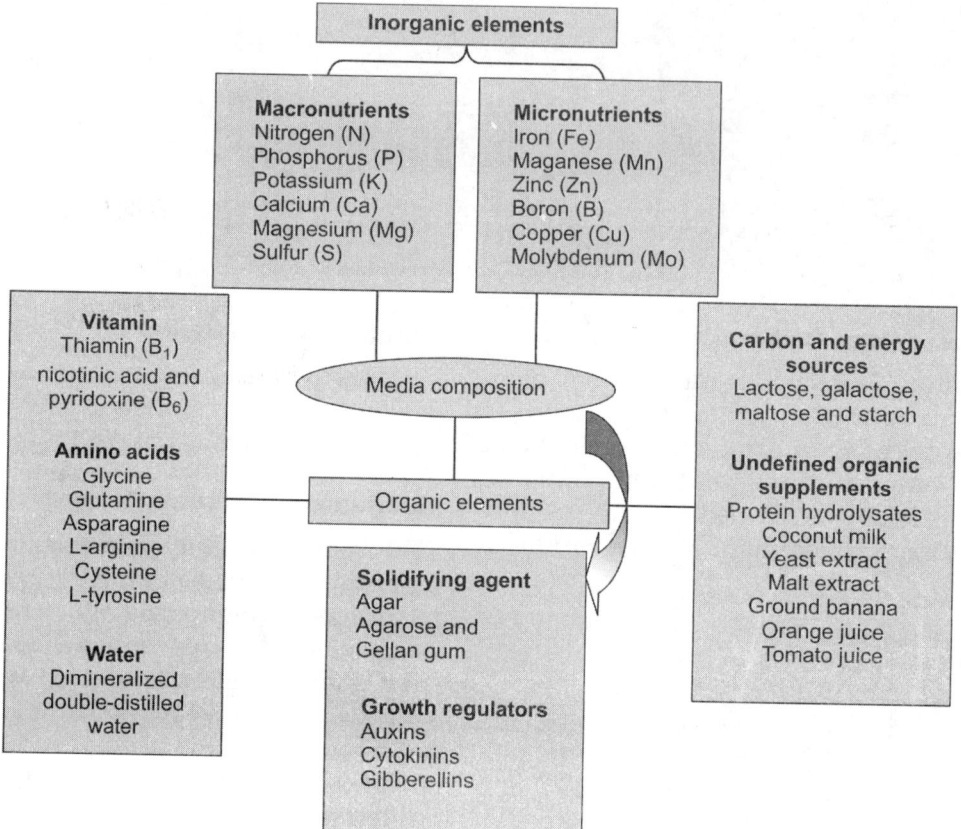

Fig. 15.8 Composition of media used in plant tissue culture

The medium consists of macro- and microelements, sugar, vitamins, amino acids, growth regulators and miscellaneous supplements, like yeast extract and fruit juices.

Media Composition (Fig. 15.8)

Plant tissue and cell culture media are generally made up of macronutrients, micronutrients, vitamins, amino acids or other nitrogen supplements, sugar(s), other undefined organic supplements, solidifying agents or support systems, and growth regulators (Table 15.4).

Media Preparation

The method for preparation of culture media is as follows:

1. To make concentrated stock solutions which can be immediately diluted to preferred concentration before use.
2. Solutions of macronutrients are better to be prepared as stock solutions of 10 times the strength of the final operative medium. Stock solutions can be stored in a refrigerator at 2–4°C.
3. Micronutrients stock solutions are made up at 100 times of the final concentration of the working medium. The micronutrients stock solution can also be stored in a refrigerator or a freezer.
4. Iron stock solution should be 100 times concentrated than the final working medium and stored in a refrigerator.

Table 15.4: Composition of nutrient media

Nutrients	Composition	Functions
Macronutrients		
Nitrogen (N)	25–60 mM	Required for plant cell or tissue growth
Potassium (K)	20–30 mM	
Phosphorus (P)		
Calcium (Ca)		
Magnesium (Mg)	1–3 mM	
Sulfur (S)		
Micronutrients		
Iron (Fe)	1 µM	Micronutrients have role in the functioning of the genetic apparatus and are involved with the activity of growth substances
Manganese (Mn)	20–90 µM	
Zinc (Zn)	5–30 µM	
Boron (B)	25–100 µM	
Copper (Cu)	0.1 µM	
Molybdenum (Mo)	1 µM	
Carbon and energy source		
Sucrose	2–3%	For supplying carbohydrate needs by CO_2 assimilation during photosynthesis
Glucose		
Fructose		
Lactose		
Galactose		
Rafinose		
Maltose		
Starch		
Vitamins		
Thiamin (B_1)	0.1–10 mg/liter	Vitamins are added in small amounts for growth and survival
Nicotinic acid	0.1–5.0 mg/liter	
Pyridoxine (B_6)	0.1–10 mg/liter	
Myoinositol	50–5000 mg/liter	
Amino acids and nitrogen		
L-glutamine	up to 8 mM	Amino acids are added in small amounts for growth
L-asparagine	100 mg/liter	
L-tyrosine	100 mg/liter	
Solidifying and gelling agents		
Agar	0.5 and 1.0%	Plant tissue and organs are most suitably retained above the surface of culture medium by increasing its viscosity with some kind of gelling agent

(Count.)

Table 15.4: Composition of nutrients media (Count.)

Nutrients	Composition	Functions
Support system Perforated cellophane Filter paper bridges Filter paper wicks Polyurethane foam Polyester fleece		
Growth regulators Auxins Cytokinins Gibberellins		Their selection and the concentrations depend on the plant species and the purpose of the culture.

5. Vitamins are prepared as either 100 or 1000 times concentrated stock solutions and stored in a freezer (–20°C) until used, if it is desired to keep them for long otherwise they can be stored in a refrigerator for 2–3 months and should be discarded thereafter.
6. Stock solutions of growth regulators are usually prepared at 100–1000 times the final desired concentration.
7. Concentrations of inorganic and organic components of media are generally expressed in mass values (mg/l and p.p.m.) in tissue culture.

Media Sterilization

Prevention of contamination of tissue culture media is important for the whole process of plant propagation and helps for decreasing the spread of plant parasites. Contamination of media could be controlled by adding antimicrobial agents, acidification or by filtration through microporous filters. To reduce possibilities of contamination, it is recommended that sterilization rooms should have the least number of openings. Media preparation and sterilization are preferred to be performed in separate compartments. Sterilization area should also have walls and floor that withstand moisture, heat and steam. Sterilization of media is routinely achieved by autoclaving at the temperature ranging from 115°–135°C. Advantages of autoclaving are The method is quick and simple, whereas disadvantages are the media pH changes and some components may decompose and so loose their effectiveness. As for example autoclaving mixtures of fructose, glucose and sucrose resulted in a drop in the agar gelling capacity and affecting pH of the culture medium through the formation of furfural derivatives due to sucrose hydrolysis. Filtration through microporus filters (0.22–0.45 M) also used for thermolabile organic constituents such as vitamins, growth regulators and amino acids. Additives of antimicrobial agents are less commonly applied in plant tissue culture media. Limitation for their use was reported and attributed to harm imposed on plants as well.

TYPE OF PLANT TISSUE CULTURE
(Fig. 15.9)

Plant tissue culture is the culture and maintenance of plant cells or organs in sterile nutritionally and environmentally supportive pieces of plant tissues or the explants are known as callus. The typical explants are leaf, root, stem nodal and internodal parts, auxilliary buds, shoot tip, shoot apical meristem, flower bud anther, pollen, seeds and cotyledons. Initially, callus cells proliferate without differentiating, but eventually differentiation occurs within the tissue mass. Actively dividing cells are those uppermost and peripheral in the callus. The extent of overall differentiation usually depends on the hormone balance of the support medium and the physiological state of the tissue. The callus is formed on the original explants is called primary callus. The primary callus is dissected from pieces of tissue result in secondary callus cultures. The subculturing with new inoculums provide fresh medium for culture initiations. The period from initiation of culture to time of passage is known as passage. The plant callus has three stage of development, viz. cell division, dedifferentiation and cellular differentiation.

Step 1: Tissue sample from any region of plant is cultured

Step 2: Undefined callus culture

Step 3: Undefined callus culture grows

Step 4: Single cell culture

Step 5: Culturing results in new plant

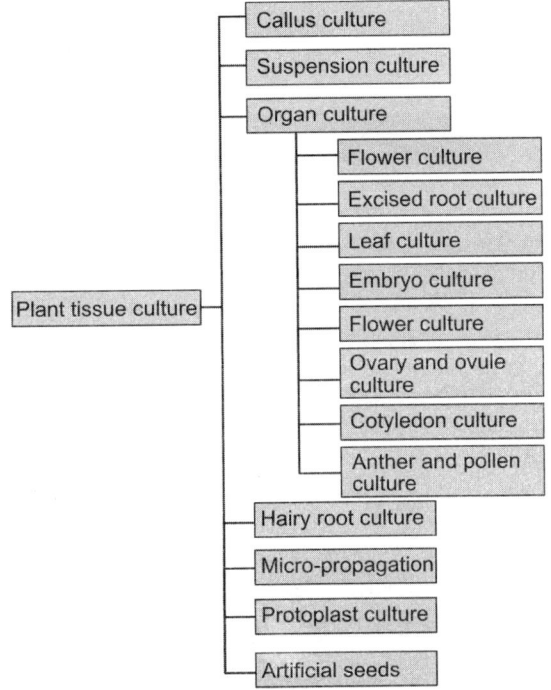

Fig. 15.9: Types of plant tissue culture

conditions (*in vitro*). Plant cell and tissue culture include the cultural techniques for regeneration of functional plants from embryonic tissues, tissue fragments, calli, isolated cells, or protoplasts.

Callus Culture (Fig. 15.10)

Callus is defined as an unorganized cell masses or tissue initiated from disorganized

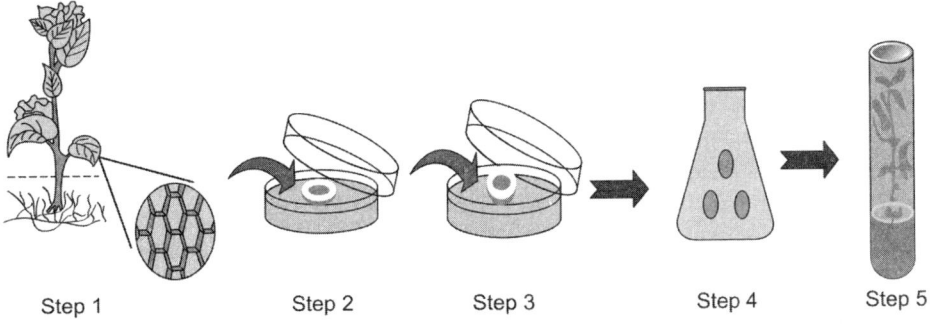

Fig. 15.10: Culture plant

Application of Callus Culture

1. Organogenesis or morphogenesis: The plant can be regenerated in large number from callus tissue through manipulation of the nutrient and hormonal constituents in the culture medium.
2. Callus tissue is good source of genetic or karyotypic variability, so it may be possible to regenerate a plant from genetically variable cells of the callus tissue.
3. Callus culture is starting material for suspension culture and vegetative propagation of the plant.
4. Cell suspension culture in moving liquid medium can be initiated from callus culture.
5. Callus culture is very useful to obtain commercially important secondary metabolites and biochemical assays can be performed from callus culture.
6. It helps in production of secondary metabolites.

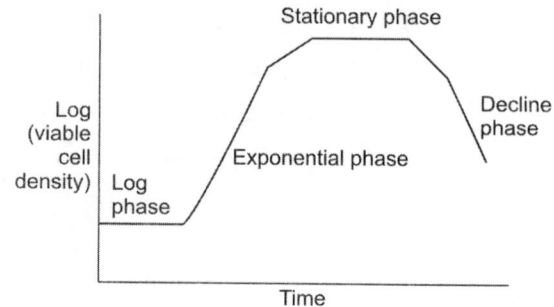

Fig. 15.11 A typical cell growth curve (cell density vs time) showing the lag, exponential, stationary, and decline phases

Suspension Culture

The suspension culture is the method of culturing isolated cell in liquid medium via two methods mechanical and enzymatic digestions. Cells of suspension culture exhibit a high rate of cell division as compared to callus culture. For the preparation of suspension culture, callus fragments are transferred to liquid medium (without agar) by continuous agitation. Agitation is achieved by rotary shaker attached to BOD incubator at rate of 50–150 rpm. Agitation is required to break up the cell aggregates, maintain uniform distribution of cells of various sizes and shapes, provide gas exchange of cells to sustain cell respiration in liquid medium.

Suspension culture is maintained under controlled condition of light temperature and aeration to follow the predictable pattern or growth curves (Figs 15.11 and 15.12).

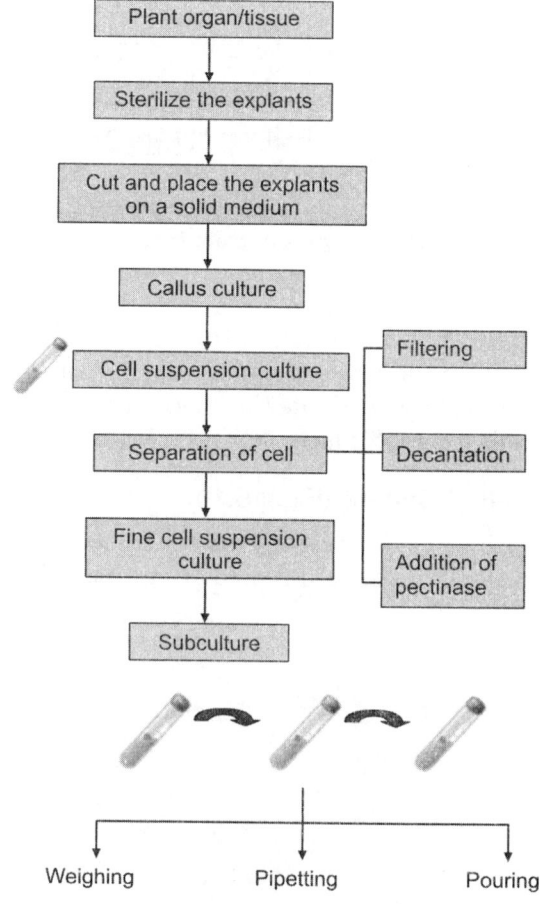

Fig. 15.12: Scheme of the procedure of initiation and maintenance of plant cell suspension cultures

1. **Lag phase:** During this stage the cells do not divide. Cells adapt to the culture conditions and the length of this phase will depend upon the growth phase of the cell line at the time of subculture and also the seeding density.
2. **Logarithmic (log) growth phase:** Cells actively proliferate and an exponential increase in cell density arises. The cell population is considered to be the most viable at this phase, therefore, it is recommended to assess cellular function at this stage. Each cell line will show different cell proliferation kinetics during the log phase and it is, therefore, the optimal phase for determining the population doubling time.
3. **Plateau (or stationary) phase:** Cellular proliferation slows down. It is at this stage the number of cells in the active cell cycle drops to 0–10% and the cells are most susceptible to injury.
4. **Decline phase:** Cell death predominates in this phase and there is a reduction in the number of viable cells. Cell death is not due to the reduction in nutrient supplements but the natural path of the cellular cycle.

Types of suspension culture are shown in Fig. 15.3 and Table 15.5.

Applications of Suspension Culture

1. To develop specific cell line or single cell clone.
2. To study effect of different chemicals.
3. For somatic embryogenesis from SC.
4. For immobilized cell cultures for secondary metabolites or for biotransformation of chemical compounds.
5. For commercial production of cell mass.

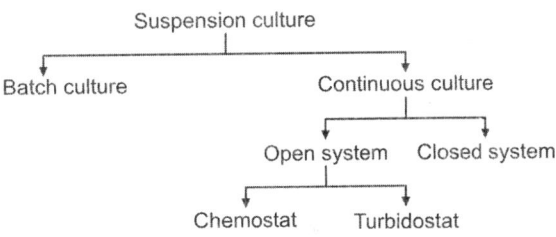

Fig. 15.13: Types of suspension culture

Table 15.5: Type of suspension culture

Batch culture: They are systems in which cells grow in a fixed volume of culture medium. **Incubation:** There is a gradual increase in cellular mass. Growth ceases due to depletion of nutrients from the medium. **Growth curve:** Sigmoid pattern of growth over a short period of time.	**Continuous culture:** Cell suspension culture can be grown in continuous culture. It involves a continuous influx of fresh medium and the withdrawal of the used medium without any cell loss. **Open continuous culture system:** The cells mass as well as the culture medium are changed periodically. Replacement is automated, i.e. addition of fresh medium occurs at a rate equaling the rate of new cell formation. **Closed continuous culture system:** This is a process in which cell mass remains unchanged. Only the composition of the medium is continuously changed.	**Chemostat:** It is the constant supply of chemical components/nutrients to get desired rate of growth. **Turbidostat:** It is the constant environment maintenance by input of medium, which is checked by measurement of turbidity of cell mass/density.

Organ Culture (Table 15.6)

Organ culture is the growth of plant organs, such as roots and shoots, beginning with the organ primordial or segments maintaining characteristic of organ in aseptic culture media. Organ culture is used principally for:
1. The maintenance of structural organization in tissues which are to be subjected to experimentally varied environments (e.g. to hormones, drugs, or radiation).
2. The study of morphogenesis, differentiation, and function in excised organs or presumptive organs; and
3. For comparison of the growth and behavior of explanted organs with the growth and behavior of similar organs *in situ*.

Hairy Root Culture (Fig. 15.14)

Hairy root cultures have been induced in many plant species leading to the *in vitro* production of numerous plant secondary metabolites and pharmacologically active compounds.

The explants exposed to ***Agrobacterium rhizogenes*** infection, hairy originate from the explants and it is termed as hairy root culture. These are fast growing, highly branched adventitious roots at the site of infection and can grow even on hormone free culture medium. Generally, hairy root cultures grow

Table 15.6: Types of organ culture with their application

Type of organ culture	Description	Applications
Meristem culture (apical tip culture/ shoot tip culture)	Meristem culture is a method in which shoot apices with a few primordial leaves are grown *in vitro*	For maintaining virus free plants, because the apical tips of shoots and roots are generally free from viruses and other microorganisms. **Examples:** Sugarcane, potatoes, banana, garlic, rhubarb, dahlias, strawberry, orchids, pineapple, and gooseberry.
Excised root culture	Root cultures can be established *in vitro* from explants of the root tip of both primary and lateral roots. Root culture requires exogenous auxins in appropriate concentration as supplements to the endogenous levels for their growth.	Cell division, cell enlargement and cellular differentiation
Leaf culture	This technique includes *in vivo* culturing of immature/ young leaves to obtain leaf discs. Dicot plants: leaf discs, fragments, leaf bases and even mesophyll protoplasts easily show regeneration of roots, shoots or somatic embryogenesis *via* callus. Monocots plants: no such potential found.	Shoot regeneration
Flower and floral meristem culture	Reproductive parts like flower are *in vitro* cultured by this method. This is generally concerned with two aspects: (a) induction of flowering in sterile culture of vegetative parts and (b) culture of floral buds and floral organs.	Flower and floral meristem culture are found in cauliflower, date palm, onion, sugar beet

(Count.)

Table 15.6: Type of organ culture with its application *(Count.)*

Type of organ culture	Description	Applications
Ovary culture	*In vitro* method to produce haploids. The nature of growth of ovaries under the influence of nutrients, vitamins and plant growth regulators	**Example:** Unpollinated ovaries of *Citrus aurantifolia* and *C. sinensis* produced embryos and plantlets in culture regenerated from the ovary wall
Embryo culture	Embryo culture can be defined as *in vitro* development of isolated mature or immature zygotic embryos from seeds in a suitable culture medium to form seedlings. Plant cells can also be induced to form embryos in plant tissue culture; these embryos are called somatic embryos. Two main steps in embryo culture: Removal or excision of the embryo. Taking care of nutritional requirement	Provides a better and direct somatic embryogenesis system. Embryo culture may help shorten the breeding cycle, the production of monoploids, testing for seed viability, study of host pathogen interaction, germination of seeds of parasitic plants as well as rare plants. *Example: Musa bulbisiona*, where seeds do not germinate in nature but can be obtained through embryo culture.
Anther and pollen culture	Generally, 2 procedures are followed to obtain haploid plants in anther and pollen culture: Direct culture of excised anthers on liquid medium or on agar. By removal of pollens from anther and its culture in a liquid medium	Used for the production of haploids, which are of immense importance for the improvement of some crop plants like coffee, fruit trees where improvements of the species is difficult due to their heterozygous nature. Important for development of mutants. Also useful material for studying somatic cell genetics, especially for cell modification by the introduction of foreign organic matter. Applied in *Datura innoxia* and Rapeseed plant.

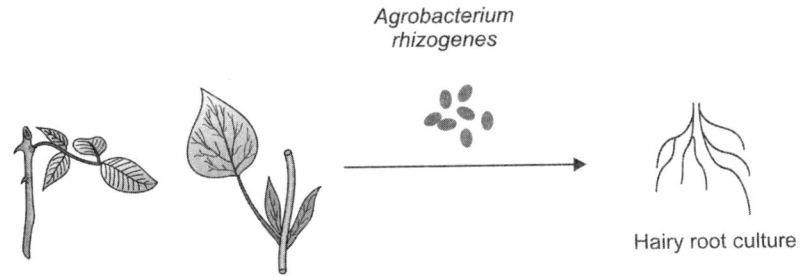

Fig. 15.14: Hairy root cultures

rapidly on media without any exogenous growth regulators and are genetically and biochemically stable, and for these reasons are promising systems for producing secondary metabolites. Growth kinetics is highly stable and of equal level in this type of culture. These cultures are usually quite stable in their biosynthetic capacity. Another benefit of hairy root cultures is that they are easily grown from small-scale shake cultures to bioreactors suitable for larger scale production of the compounds of interest.

Micropropagation

The tissue culture propagation process can be defined in four main stages as described in Table 15.7.

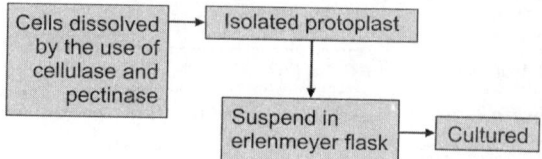

Fig. 15.15: Plasmolyticum enzymatic method

Protoplast Culture

The cell wall is thick made up of cellulose and pectin. During various process of crop improvement through various types of culture, it acts as a barrier so it is dissolved by the use of cellulase and pectinase and a naked protoplast can be freed (Fig. 15.15). Protoplast (cell without cell wall) can be developed into individual plants or they could be used to fuse

Table 15.7: Stages of microporpagation

Stages of tissue culture propagation	Description of stage
Small pieces of plant material, called explants, are carefully removed form the parent plant. Explants are obtained from the actively growing part (shoot tips, sections of leaves, stems and roots, embryos, etc.) of a desired plant.	The explants are cleaned and placed on sterile agar medium in glass bottles or test tubes.
The cells of the explants multiply in one of two ways	The sterile agar medium is a gel that contains water, sugars, nutrients, and plant hormones to support and promote plant growth.
The plantlets have developed and are ready for root formation	Tiny leaves, stems and roots make tissue culture possible.
The plantlets are removed form the glass container.	The cells may form a callus, are supplied with the correct hormones in the medium, these callus cells can develop into a normal plant. The explant may produce many new explants.
	Shoots are transplanted to another medium containing auxins, a hormone that induces the growth of roots.
	The plantlets are also given higher light intensity in preparation.
	They are divided, planted in a sterile medium, and placed in a greenhouse.
	Care must be taken during this transition to acclimatize the plant to their new environment.

with naked protoplast of other varieties or species to produce what are called somatic embryo. Crossing the protoplasts has been greatly facilitated by chemicals, such as polyethylene glycol or by other processes, such as electrofusion. Such hybridization is called somatic hybridization.

Examples: Developing somatic hybrids by crossing protoplasts of two species in crops: Brassica, Nicotiana, Petunia and Solanum.

Isolation of Protoplast

By mechanical method: Spontaneous protoplast fusion induced protoplast fusion: Treatment with calcium ions (Ca^{++}) at high pH polyethylene glycol (PEG) treatment. *Electrical fusion:* The protoplasts, which are capable of dividing, undergo first division within 2–7 days and form multicellular colonies after 2–3 weeks. After another two weeks, these colonies can be treated as standard tissue cultures.

Artificial Seeds

Synthetic can or artificial seeds are the living-seed, like structure, derived from somatic embryo or shoot buds' *in vitro* culture after encapsulation by a hydrogel. The preserved embryoids are called synthetic seeds.

Advantages

1. It could be preserved for long time at lower temperature. Rooting, hardening and conversion steps are waved off as these seeds can directly be sowed in the fields like natural seeds
2. Quality seed delivery system
3. Time and space economy
4. Global exchange of germplasm
5. Conservation and preservation of germplasm.

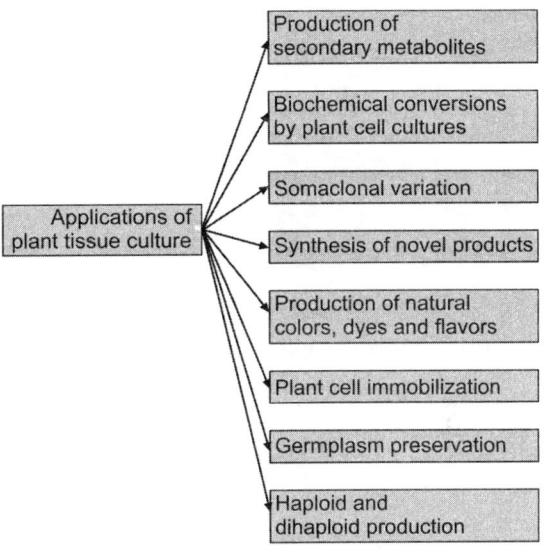

Fig. 15.16: Application of PTC

6. Analytical tool for molecular study. Uniformity in production because of identical somatic embryos.
7. Produced at any time and in any season of the year carrier for adjuvants such as micro-organisms, plant growth regulators and pesticides.

Disadvantages

1. Synthetic seeds cannot be used for soil transfer as they show very poor germination efficiency.
2. In the green houses, the efficiency is not very high, (only around 10–20%).
3. Requires encapsulation for better handling and storage.
4. High scale up for production of seeds on commercial and economic scale.
5. Requires intensive labor.

Application of PTC:

The various application of PTC is enlisted in Fig. 15.16.

16
Study of Different Families

The angiosperms or flowering plants are one of the major groups of extant seed plants and arguably the most diverse major extant plant group on the planet, with at least 260,000 living species classified in 453 families.

FLORAL FORMULA AND FLORAL DIAGRAM

The floral formula is the numerical representation of various parts of flower. This formula give information about symmetry, interrelationship of various floral parts, unisexuality as well as bisexuality in flower.

The floral diagram represents relative position and number of parts in each of the sets of organs in flower (Table 16.1). It depicts following information:

1. Sex and symmetry of flower
2. Number of floral cycles and floral parts in each cycle of flower.
3. Position of all floral parts.

FAMILIES WITH THEIR DESCRIPTION

Solanaceae

Solanaceae is commonly called as 'Brinjal family'. It includes about 90 genera and 2000 species. Members have a cosmopolitan distribution. There are around 60 species found in India.

Tables 16.2 and 16.3 describe the characteristic features and medicinal importance of Solanaceae family.

Taxonomic Classification

Class	Dicotyledonae
Subclass	Gamopetalae
Series	Bicarpellatae
Order	Polymoniales
Family	Solanaceae

Table 16.1: List of floral symbol with meanings

S.no.	Floral symbol	Meaning
1.	Br	Bracteate
2.	Ebr	Ebracteate
3.	Brl	Bracteolate
4.	0 (zero)	Absence of whorl
5.	α	Indefinite number
6.	$\oplus$	Actinomorphic
7.	$\varnothing$	Zygomorphic
8.	♂	Male flower
9.	♀	Female flower
10.	☿	Bisexual flowers
11.	K	Calyx, sepals
12.	C	Corolla, petals
13.	P	Perinath
14.	A	Androceium
15.	G	Gynoecium
16.	( )	Cohesion of floral parts of whorl
16.	C A	Epipetalous stamens
18.	P A	Epiphyllous stamens
19.	Std	Staminodes
20.	G_4	Tetracarpellary, free carpel
21.	X	Variable

Apocynaceae

Tables 16.4 and 16.5 describe the characteristic features and medicinal importance of Apocynaceae family.

Kingdom	Plantae
Subkingdom	Tracheobionta
Division	Magnoliophyta
Class	Magnoliopsida
Subclass	Asteridae
Order	Gentianales
Family	Apocynaceae

Table 16.2: Characteristic features of Solanaceae family

S.no.	Characteristic features
1.	**Habit:** Mostly annual herbs
2.	**Root:** Taproot, branched.
3.	**Inflorescence:** Solitary axillary or cymose inflorescence
4.	**Flowers:** Bracteate or ebracteate, bisexual, complete, hypogynous, pentamerous and adinomorphic
5.	**Calyx:** Sepals 5, gamosepalous, valvate aestivation and persistent. (Accrescent)
6.	**Corolla:** Petals-5, gamopetalous, aestivation valvate or imbricate with various shapes of corolla.
7.	**Androecium:** Stamens-5, polyandrous means no cohesion, epipetalous means shows adhesion, introrse, filaments basifixed and anthers dithecous
8.	**Gynoecium:** Bicarpellary, syncarpous, bilocular and axile placentation, superior.
9.	**Fruit:** Berry or capsule.
10.	**Seed:** Endospermic

Table 16.3: Medicinal importance of Solanaceae family

S.no.	Name	Part	Chemical constituents	Uses
1.	Atropa belladonna (Deadly night shade)	Roots	Atropine	Dilates the pupil of the eye
2.	Datura (Thorn apple)	Seeds	Scopolamine alkaloid	Pain reliever and sedative.
3.	Hyoscyamus niger	Leaves	Hyoscyamine alkaloid	Treatment of asthma and whooping cough
4.	Nicotiana tabacum	Leaves	Nicotine	Nerve stimulant and insecticides.
5.	Solanum xanthocarpum	Leaves		Rheumatism and cough
6.	Withania somnifera (Ashwagandha)	Root Leaves		Nerve tonic Fever
7.	Solanum nigrum	Fruit		Laxative

Table 16.4: Characteristic features of Apocynaceae family

S.no.	Characteristic features
1.	**Habit:** Flowering plants (Herbs, snobs, and woods).
2.	**Root:** Taproots and branched.
3.	**Inflorescence:** Fruit: Follicles, berry, or drupe.
4.	**Flowers:** Complete, perfect. Floral Symmetry: Radial.
5.	**Calyx:** Differentiated. Calyx
6.	**Corolla:** 5
7.	**Androecium:** Distinct, adnate to perigynous zone or to massive stigma
8.	**Gynoecium:** Syncarpous, pistil = 1, carpels/pistil=2, locules/pistil=2, ovules/locule=2-".
9.	**Leaves:** Simple. Stipules: Reduced or absent.
10.	**Fruit:** Pairs, each ovary developing into dry follicle, drupe berry.
11.	**Seed:** Flattened

Table 16.5: Medicinal importance of Apocynaceae family

S.no.	Name	Part	Chemical constituents	Uses
1.	Strophanthus kombe	Seeds	Strophanthidin	Cardiotonic
2.	Strophanthus gratus	Seeds	Ouabain	Cardiotonic
3.	Thevetia nerifolia	Seeds	Thevetin	Cardiotonic

Gramineae (Poaceae)

A monocotyledonous family containing the grasses, which number about 9000 species in about 620 genera. Grasses generally have long narrow parallel-veined leaves inserted distichously on a round hollow stem. This family contains all the cereals, like wheats (*Triticum*), maize (*Zea mays*), rice (*Oryza saliva*), barley (*Hordeum vulgare*), oats (*Avena sativa*), rye (*Secale cereale*), sugarcane (*Saccharum officinarum*), and sorghums (*Sorghum*) are all grasses.

Kingdom   – Plantae
Order   – Poales
Family   – Poaceae

Tables 16.6 and 16.7 describe the characteristic features and medicinal importance of Gramineae family.

Table 16.6: Characteristic features Gramineae family

S.no.	Characteristic features
1.	**Habit:** Annuals or perennials.
2.	**Root:** Adventitious, fibrous, branched or stilt.
3.	**Inflorescence:** Compound spike, sessile or stalked.
4.	**Flowers:** Bracteate, bracteolate, sessile, incomplete, bisexual or unisexual
5.	**Androecium:** Stamens usually three, some times six. Filaments long, anthers dithecous, versatile and linear.
6.	**Gynoecium:** Monocarpellary (presumed to be three of which two are aborted), unilocular, single ovule on basal placentation.
7.	**Leaves:** Alternate, simple, extipulate, sessile, leaf base forming tubular sheath.
8.	**Fruit:** A caryopsis with pericarp completely united with the seed coat.
9.	**Seed:** Endospermic.

Table 16.7: Medicinal Importance of Gramineae family

S.no.	Name	Part	Chemical constituents	Uses
1.	Starch	Grains and tuber	Amylose and amylopectin	Nutritive, demulcent and protective
2.	Palmarosa	Leaves and tops	Geraniol and terpenes	Rheumatism and skin diseases
3.	Corn oil	Grains	Oleic and linoleic acid	Dietary supplements
4.	Rice bran oil	Grains	Glycerides of oleic and linoleic acids	Food oil and cosmetics
5.	Wheat germ oil	Grains	Glycerides of fatty acids	Nutritive and source of Vit. E

Labiatae (Lamiaceae)

A large dicotyledonous family, commonly called the mint family, comprising some 3000 species in about 200 genera. They are often covered in aromatic hairs and many species, such as mints (*Mentha*), sage (*Salvia officinalis*), and thymes (*Thymus*), are used as pot herbs. These plants **characteristically bear essential oils** (the crushed foliage aromatic or fetid, with taxonomic predictability).

Kingdom	Plantae
Order	Lamiales
Family	Lamiaceae

Tables 16.8 and 16.9 describe the characteristic features and medicinal importance of Labiatae family.

Crucifereae

The Crucifereae family comprise roughly 3000 species of herbaceous plants within more than 300 genera.

Division	Angiospermae
Class	Dicotyledonae
Sub-class	Polypetalae
Series	Thalamiflorae
Order	Parietales

Table 16.8: Characteristic features of Labiatae family

S.no.	Characteristic features
1.	**Habit:** The herbs are annual to perennial
2.	**Inflorescence:** Flowers solitary or aggregated
3.	**Leaves:** Simple, opposite leaves, or whorled
4.	**Flowers:** Bilabiate flowers
5.	**Calyx:** 5 sepals are often with the bilabiate condition, superimposed and 1 whorled.
6.	**Corolla:** 5 more or less disguisedly sepals
7.	**Androecium:** 1 whorled, fertile stamens
8.	**Gynoecium:** 2 carpels (deeply lobed)
9.	**Fruit:** Usually non-fleshy, or fleshy (rarely); more or less a schizocarp
10.	**Seed:** Endospermic to non-endospermic, embryo well differentiated. 2 cotyledons, flat.

Table 16.9: Medicinal importance of Labiatae family

S.no.	Name	Part	Chemical constituents	Uses
1.	Rosemary	Oil	Vetivone	Stimulant, aromatic, as a flavor and stomachic
2.	Lavender	Fresh flowering tops	Linalool, pinene, geraniol	Aromatic, carminative, in perfumery
3.	Thyme	Leaves and flowering tops	Thymol, linalool	Carminative, antispasmodic and expectorant
4.	Peppermint oil	Fresh flowering tops	*l*-menthol	Carminative, stimulant and flavoring agent

Table 16.10 describes the characteristic features of Cruciferae family.

Tables 16.11 and 16.12 describe the characteristic features and medicinal importance of Papaveraceae family.

Umbelliferae (Apiaceae)

The Apiaceae (or Umbelliferae) commonly known as carrot or parsley family, mostly aromatic plants with hollow stems. The family is 16th-largest family of flowering plants, with more than 3,700 species spread across 434 genera.

Kingdom – Plantae
Order – Apiales
Family – Apiaceae

Tables 16.13 and 16.14 describe the characteristic features and medicinal importance of Umbelliferae family.

Table 16.10: Characteristic features of Crucifereae family

S.no.	Characteristic features
1.	**Habit:** The herbs are annual to perennial
2.	**Root:** Taproot
3.	**Inflorescence:** Raceme or corymbose raceme.
4.	**Leaves:** Simple, alternate, radical or cauline.
5.	**Flowers:** Ebracteate, pedicellate, mostly actinomorphic and bisexual
6.	**Calyx:** Sepals 4, polysepalous, in two whorls of two each imbricate aestivation.
7.	**Corolla:** Petals 4, arranged in single whorl alternating with sepals
8.	**Androecium:** Stamens 6, polyandrous, arranged in two whorls of 4 and 2 (tetradynamous).
9.	**Gynoecium:** Bicarpellary, syncarpous, initially unilocular and later bilocular (formation of pseudoseptum).
10.	**Fruit:** Siliqua or silicula.
11.	**Seed:** Endospermic

Table 16.11: Characteristic features of Papaveraceae family

S.no.	Characteristic features
1.	**Habit:** Annual or perennial herbs
2.	**Inflorescence:** Flowers solitary or cymes and racemes
3.	**Leaves:** Alternate to opposite or whorled, entire to lobed or dissected
4.	**Flowers:** Bisexual to bilateral
5.	**Calyx:** Sepals 2, imbricate
6.	**Corolla:** Petals 4, in 2 whorls, crumbled and deciduous
7.	**Androecium:** Stamens in whorls, anther is fixed
8.	**Gynoecium:** 2 or more carpels and ovary is superior.
9.	**Fruit:** Capsules
10.	**Seed:** Endosperm copious

Table 16.12: Medicinal importance of Papaveraceae family

S.no.	Name	Part	Chemical constituents	Uses
1.	Poppy seed oil	Poppy seeds	Glycerides of oleic and linoleic acids	Drying and iodised oil

Leguminosae (Fabaceae)

A large family of dicotyledonous plants, commonly called the pea family, and containing about 17,000 species in about 700 genera. The name of the largest subfamily Papilionoideae. The three subfamilies are: Mimosaceae, Caesalpiniaceae, and Papilionaceae.

Kingdom – Plantae
Order – Fabales
Family – Fabaceae

Tables 16.15 and 16.16 describe the characteristic features and medicinal importance of Leguminosae family.

Table 16.13: Characteristic features of Umbelliferae family

S.no.	Characteristic features
1.	**Habit:** Biennial, perennial, or annual herbs
2.	**Inflorescence:** Simple or compound umbels
3.	**Leaves:** Alternate, with oil tubes, mostly pinnately compound, sheathing base
4.	**Flowers:** Perfect or imperfect and the plants monoecious or rarely dioecious
5.	**Calyx:** 5 sepals, distinct
6.	**Corolla:** 5 petals, distinct
7.	**Androecium:** 5 stamens, distinct, alternate to petals
8.	**Gynoecium:** 2 carpels, connate; inferior;
9.	**Fruit:** Schizocarp with 2 mericarps, often strongly ribbed

Table 16.14: Medicinal importance of Umbelliferae family

S.no.	Name	Part	Chemical constituents	Uses
1.	Asafoetida	Rhizomes and roots	Resin, gum and volatile oil	Carminative, stimulant and intestinal flatulance
2.	Anise	Fruits	Anethol, methyl chavicol	Stimulant, flavoring agent, Carminative and expectorant.
3.	Cumin	Fruits	Cuminaldehyde	Stimulant, carminative and in diarrhea.
4.	Caraway	Seeds	Carvone, carvacrol	Aromatic, flavor.
5.	Coriander	Fruits	Coriandrol	Aromatic flavor, stimulant and carminative

Table 16.15: Characteristic features of Leguminosae family

S.no.	Characteristic features
1.	**Habit:** Herbs, shrubs or trees
2.	**Root:** Taproot
3.	**Inflorescence:** Racemose, rarely solitary.
4.	**Leaves:** Compound leaves
5.	**Flowers:** Five fused sepals and five petals often arranged in a shape fancifully resembling a butterfly
6.	**Calyx:** Five sepals, united
7.	**Corolla:** Five petals, usually free. Corolla is papilionaceous (butterfly-shaped)
8.	**Androecium:** Stamens (9) + 1, i.e. 9 fuse to form a round sheath around the pistil while tenth is free.
9.	**Gynoecium:** Monocarpellary, ovary unilocular, ovule numerous on marginal placenta.
10.	**Fruit:** Pod or legume

Rubiaceae

A large family of dicotyledonous plants containing about 7000 species in some 500 genera. The important products of the Rubiaceae include coffee, from *Coffea arabica* and *C. canephora*, and quinine, from species of Cinchona.

Kingdom   Plantae
Order   Gentianales
Family   Rubiaceae

Table 16.17 describes the characteristic features and medicinal importance of Rubiaceae family.

Table 16.16: Medicinal importance of Leguminosae

S.no.	Name of drug	Part	Chemical constituents	Uses
1.	Tolu balsam	Balsam	Cinnamic acid	Expectorant and antiseptic
2.	Senna leaf	Dried Leaflets	Sennosides A and B	Purgative
3.	Psoralea	Fruits	Psoralen	Treatment of leuoderma

Table 16.17: Characteristic features of Rubiaceae family

S.no.	Characteristic features
1.	**Habit:** Mostly trees, shrubs, sub-shrubs and herbs.
2.	**Inflorescence:** Cymes, head, panicle.
3.	**Leaves:** Opposite or whorled
4.	**Flowers:** Bisexual and radial
5.	**Calyx:** 4,5, Distinct or coalescent
6.	**Corolla:** Coalescent, arising from epigynous zone
7.	**Androecium:** 4,5(8–10), Distinct, adnate to epigynous zone.
8.	**Gynoecium:** Syncarpous, pistil = 1, carpels/pistil = 2(-″), locules/pistil = 2(1-″), ovules/locule = 1-″.
9.	**Fruit:** Capsule or drupe

Table 16.18: Characteristic features of Liliaceae family

S.no.	Characteristic features
1.	**Habit:** Mostly perennial herbs
2.	**Inflorescence:** Variable, mostly racemose, simple raceme or spike or umbel or panicle
3.	**Leaves:** Radical or cauline
4.	**Flowers:** Bracteate, actinomorphic, bisexual, pedicellate, homochlamydeous, trimerous, incomplete, and hypogynous.
5.	**Calyx:**
6.	**Corolla:**
7.	**Androecium:** Tamens 6, in two whorls of three each usually free or attached to tepals
8.	**Gynoecium:** Carpels 3 (tricarpellary), syncarpous, trilocular, two ovules in each
9.	**Fruit:** Berry or capsule.
10.	**Seed:** Small, endospermic.

Table 16.19: Medicinal importance of Liliaceae family

S.no.	Name	Part	Chemical constituents	Uses
1.	European squill	Leaves	Scillaren A and B	Cardiotonic
2.	Shatavari	Roots and leaves	Shatavarin I, II	Galactogogue
3.	Garlic	Bulbs	Allicin, allin	Carminative, expectorant and stimulant.
4.	Veratrum	Rhizomes	Germidine	Hypotensive, cardiac depressant.
5.	Glorisa	Rhizomes	Colchicin	Treatment of gout and cancer

Liliaceae

It is commonly called Lily family. It includes about 250 genera and 3700 species that have a cosmopolitan distribution. Around 200 species are available in India.

Division Angiospermae
Class Monocotyledonae
Series Coronarieae
Order Liliflorae
Family Liliaceae

Tables 16.18 and 16.19 describe the characteristic features and medicinal importance of Liliaceae family.

17
Quality Control and Standardization of Herbal Drugs and Formulation

PLANT IDENTIFICATION

The plants have different varieties and chemical constituents, for example, the correct botanical name should be used for identification of the plant as well as part of the plant holds the active constituent, i.e. leaf, fruit, seed, root, flower, stem, etc. or the entire plant. The method of identification of the raw material includes physical and chemical testing (Table 17.1).

Table 17.1: Parameters for plant identification

S. no.	Tests	Parameters
1.	Physical tests (organoleptic)	Color Odor and taste of the botanical loss on drying ash content, and microscopy
2.	Chemical tests	Solubility (total extractives) in water, organic solvents (ethanol, methanol, hexane); thin-layer chromatography

The proper method of extraction is important in order to maintain the innate properties of the herbal plants. Starting with the selection of proper solvent system, then method of extraction, like maceration, percolation, distillation, super-critical fluid extraction, counter-current extraction, lipidic extraction, etc.

Organized drugs: They include entire plants and consisting of flowering tops that include smaller stems, leaves, flowers and fruits, as well as others consisting of all parts of the plant growing above ground level.

Unorganized drugs: These are materials having a structure that is fairly uniform throughout and are not composed of cells built up into definite plant or animal members or organs. They are usually derived from parts of plants or animals by some process of extraction, such as incision (e.g. opium), decoction (e.g. agar), expression (e.g. olive oil), or are natural secretions (e.g. beeswax and myrrh).

Barks: Barks consist of the outermost layers of stems and roots removed by peeling them after making suitable longitudinal and transverse incisions through the outer layers. Young bark consists of following tissues:

1. *Epidermis:* A layer of closed fitted cuticularized cells with occasional stomata.
2. *Primary cortex:* A zone consisting of chlorophyll containing collenchymas and parenchyma.
3. *Endodermis:* Inner layer of cortex which frequently contains starch.
4. *Pericyclic:* It may be composed of parenchyma or fibers.
5. *Phloem:* It consists of sieve tube, companion cells and phloem parenchyma separated by radially arranged medullary rays.

Powdered bark: It possesses sieve tubes and cellulose parenchyma, cork fibers, sclerides, starch, calcium oxalates and secretory tissues. Xylem tissues are absent or only present in very small amount of chlorophyll. Aleurone grains are absent.

Leaves (Tables 17.2 to 17.5): Leaves possess neither nodes nor internodes and branches arise in their axils. The leaves are flat, thin, green appendages to the stem.

The leaves may be recognized by four well-marked characters: (1) their flattened form, (2) their thinness, (3) the presence of chlorophyll, and (4) the presence of supporting or conducting strands — the veins. Some constants are particularly useful for differentiation purposes. The blade attached to the stem by a stalk is the petiole; if there is no stalk, the leaf is termed sessile. A summary diagram of terms used for leaf description is shown in Figs 17.1.

Stomata

Stomata are structures which allow effective gas exchange and water exchange between the plant and the atmosphere. They are flanked by two guard cells which show changes in turgor in order to alter pore size, they can respond to external signals such as light, water and CO_2 and internal signals. The aperture of the stomatal pore is controlled by the two guard cells.

Table 17.2: Types of leaf margin (Fig. 17.2)

S. no.	Leaf margin	Description
1.	Entire	Smooth without teeth or lobes
2.	Undulate	Wavy
3.	Serrate	Pointed teeth that are directed upward
4.	Doubly serrate	Serrate leaf margin where the primary teeth support another set of teeth
5.	Crenate	Rounded teeth
6.	Lobed	Segmented leaf having pointed or rounded extensions separated by sinuses
7.	Sinus	Space or indentation between the lobes of a leaf blade

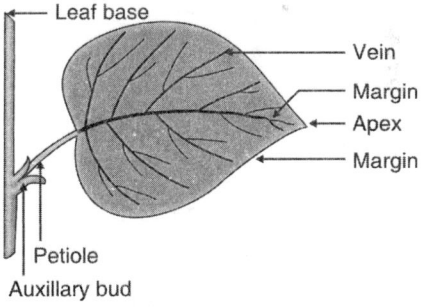

Fig.17.1: Parts of leaf

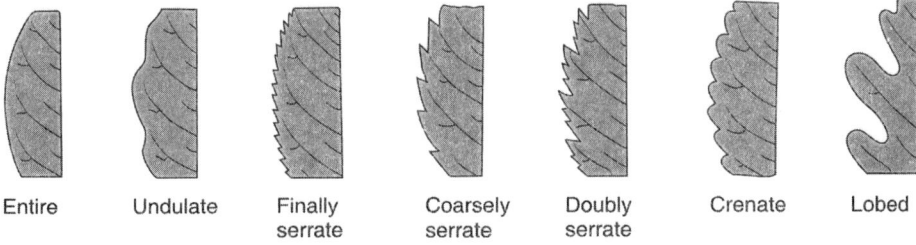

Fig.17.2: Leaf and its margins

Pharmacognosy and Phytochemistry

Table 17.3: Types of leaf tips (Fig. 17.3)

S. no.	Leaf tips	Description
1.	Acute	Slightly pointed
2.	Acuminate	Sharply pointed
3.	Bristle-tipped	Sharply pointed tip
4.	Truncate	Squared or abruptly cut off
5.	Obtuse	Rounded

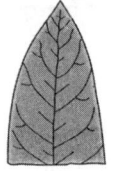 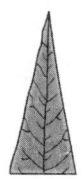 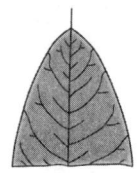

Acute　　Acuminate　　Bristle-tipped

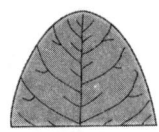

Truncate　　Obtuse

Fig.17.3: Types of leaf tips

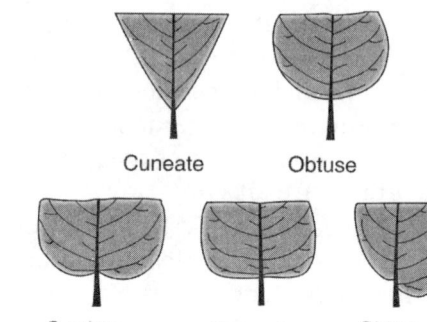

Fig.17.4: Types of leaf bases

Table 17.4: Types of leaf bases (Fig. 17.4)

S. no.	Leaf tips	Description
1.	Cuneate	Wedge-shaped
2.	Obtuse	Rounded
3.	Cordate	Heart-shaped
4.	Truncate	Squared or abruptly cut off
5.	Oblique	Asymmetrical, unequally sided

Table 17.5: Types of leaf shapes (Fig. 17.5)

S. no.	Leaf shapes	Description
1.	Asymmetrical	Completely unsymmetrical.
2.	Acuminate	Leaf that tapers into a long point
3.	Mucronate	Leaf with an extended central vein
4.	Emarginate	Notched at the end
5.	Ovoid	Egg-shaped
6.	Obovate	Resembling an upside-down egg
7.	Cordiform	Heart-shaped
8.	Oblong	Elongated shape
9.	Spatulate	Shaped like a spatula
10.	Oval	Elliptical
11.	Lanceolate	Shaped like the head of a lance
12.	Acicular	Needle-shaped

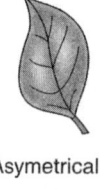 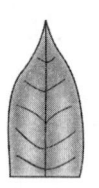 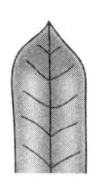 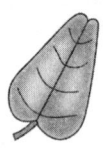 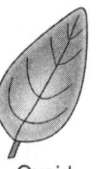 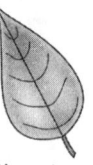

Asymetrical　Acuminate　Mucronate　Emarginate　Ovoid　Obovate

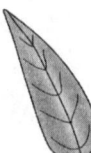 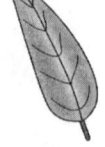 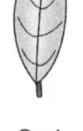 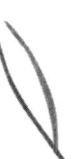

Cordiform　Oblong　Spatulate　Oval　Lanceolate　Acicular

Fig. 17.5: Types of leaf shapes

Types of stomata (Table 17.6)

In the mature leaf, four significantly different types of stoma are distinguished by their form and the arrangement of the surrounding cells, especially the subsidiary cells.

Table 17.6: Types of stomata and their description

S. no.	Types of stomata	Description
1.	Anomocytic or ranunculaceous (irregular-celled)	Stoma is surrounded by a varying number of cells, generally not different from those of the epidermis
2.	Anisocytic or cruciferous (unequal-celled)	Stoma is usually surrounded by three or four subsidiary cells, one of which is markedly smaller than the others
3.	Diacytic or caryophyllaceous (cross-celled) type	Stoma is accompanied by two subsidiary cells, the common wall of which is at right angles to the stoma
4	Paracytic or rubiaceous (parallel-celled) type	The stoma has two subsidiary cells, of which the long axes are parallel to the axis of the stoma

Trichomes

Most plants have hairs, called trichomes, on their surface that serve a number of functions ranging from protection against insect pests to heat and moisture conservation. These plant hairs, or trichomes, affect the plant in a number of ways. It has been suggested that plant hairs can change the optical properties of the leaf surface and could help to conserve heat and/or moisture. There are two main types of trichomes: Glandular and non-glandular.

Glandular trichomes contain or secrete a mixture of chemicals that have been found to have an enormous array of uses in the pesticide, pharmaceutical, and flavor/fragrance industries. Glandular trichomes which can secrete a clear viscous fluid at their tip and this exudate acts like glue and traps small-sized insects.

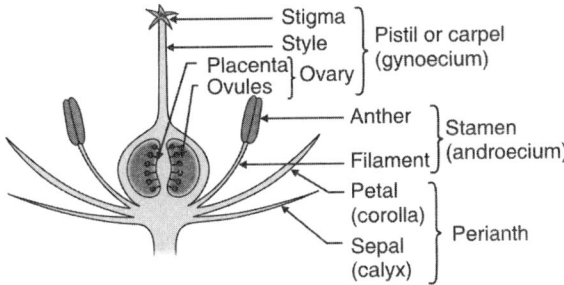

Fig.17.6: Parts of flower

Non-glandular trichome acts as a mechanical barrier to small-sized insects.

Flowers: The flowers have a short axis with undeveloped internodes, and the floral leaves are generally arranged in whorls named from below upward (Fig. 17.6), the calyx made of sepals, the corolla made of petals, the androecium made of stamens (filaments and anthers), and the gynaecium made of carpels (ovaries, styles, stigmas). Examples, saffron and corn-silk consist of styles and stigmas only; red poppy, red rose and marigold of petals only; elder flowers of petals and stamens; tilia of inflorescences and bracts.

Pistil: It is the female part of the plant, shaped like a bowling pin and located in the center of the flower. It consists of the stigma, style, and ovary.

Stigma: It is located at the top, and is connected to the ovary by the style. The ovary contains the eggs which reside in the ovules. After the egg is fertilized, the ovule develops into a seed.

Stamen: It is the male reproductive organ. It consists of a pollen sac (anther) and a long supporting filament. This filament holds the anther in position so the pollen it contains may be disbursed by wind or carried to the stigma by insects, birds or bats.

Sepals: They are small green, leaf-like structures on the base of the flower which protect the flower bud. The sepals collectively are called the calyx.

Petals: They are highly colored portions of the flower. They may contain perfume as well as nectar glands. The petals collectively are called the corolla.

Seeds

A seed is a plant member derived from a fertilized ovule; it contains an embryo and is constructed so as to facilitate its transportation. The only parts of the fruit which are genetically representative of both the male and female flowers are the seeds (mature ovules). A typical seed consists of (Fig. 17.7):

1. **Embryo:** The **embryo** is a miniature plant in an arrested state of development. The young plant within the seed consisting of:
   - Epicotyl—forms the leaf of the new plant.
   - Hypocotyl—forms the stem of the new plant.
   - Radicle—forms the root of the new plant.
2. **Endosperm:** The **endosperm** can be made up of proteins, carbohydrates or fats as well as it acts as an food reserve derived from fertilized polar nuclei.
3. **Seed coat:** A structure derived from the wall of the ovule to protect the inner parts from disease and insects.
4. **Hilum:** The funicular scar on the seed coat.
5. **Micropyle:** A hole through the seed coat.

Fruits

Fruits are mature, ripened ovaries containing seeds. Concurrently, with the development of the seed from the ovule, the ovary wall develops to form a case, called the pericarp, for the seeds, thus forming a fruit. The wall of the pericarp is usually divisible into three regions: epicarp, mesocarp, and endocarp (Table 17.7 and Fig. 17.8).

Woods

The woods consist of the tissue xylem and the maximum portion is of secondary xylem formed by the activity of the cambium. The commercial woods in larger portion consist of heartwood and dead cells. Xylem consists of conducting elements and living cells is

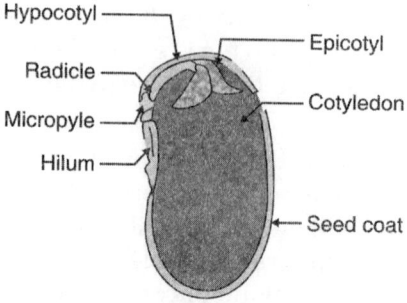

Fig.17.7: Seeds and its morphology

Table 17.7: Classification of fruits

S. no.	Types	Description and examples

1.	Simple fruits
	i. Dry fruits
	  a. Legumes
	  b. Capsules
	ii. Succulent fruits
	  c. Drupes
	  d. Berries
		Develop from a single ovary
		Senna pods, tamarind, cassia, pod, vanilla, poppy, cardamon
		
		Prune, cocculus
		capsicum, bael, orange, colocynth

2.	Aggregate fruits	Originate from a single flower which has many ovaries. Star anise, strawberry and blackberry
3.	Compound fruits	Multiple fruits are derived from a tight cluster of separate, independent flowers borne on a single structure. Hops, pineapple, fig and the beet seed

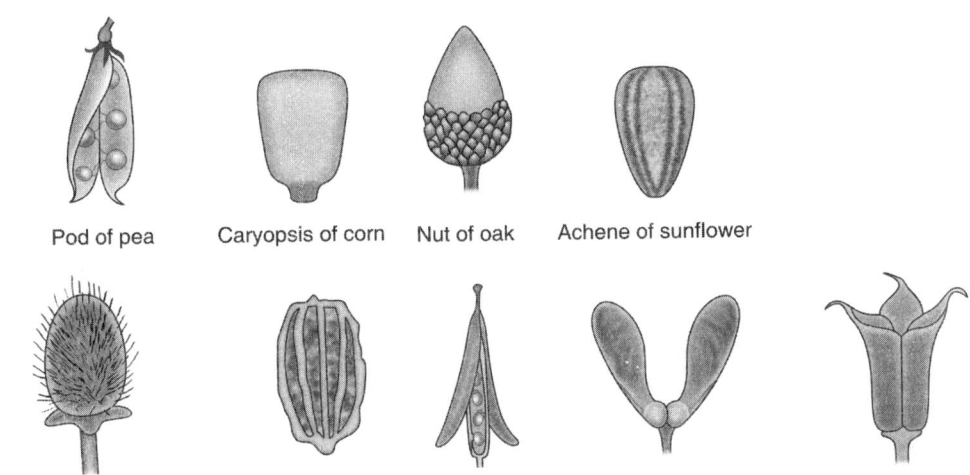

Fig. 17.8: Types of fruits

named sapwood, e.g. quassia wood. The transverse section is most useful for identification of distinguishing characters like annual rings and medullary rays.

Rhizomes and Roots

Rhizomes are stem structures growing horizontally, vertically, or in an oblique direction at the surface of the ground in which much of the lower part is embedded. The surface bears scale-leaves with occasional buds in their axils and is often marked with the encircling scars of fallen aerial leaves.

The root differs from the rhizome in that it bears only one kind of lateral appendage, namely, branches, which are similar in construction to the main root. Roots typically originate from the lower portion of a plant or cutting. They possess a root cap, have no nodes and never bear leaves or flowers directly. The principal functions of roots are to absorb nutrients and moisture, to anchor the plant in the soil, to furnish physical support for the stem, and to serve as food storage organs. Commercial rhizomes almost always contain a considerable proportion of root and, similarly, commercial roots often consist of rhizome in the upper part.

A **primary** (radical) root originates at the lower end of the embryo of a seedling plant. A taproot is formed when the primary root continues to elongate downward. This makes them difficult to transplant and necessitates planting only in deep, well-drained soil. A **lateral**, or secondary root is a side or branch root which arises from another root. A **fibrous** root system is one in which the primary root ceases to elongate, leading to the development of numerous lateral roots. These then branch repeatedly and form the feeding root system of the plant.

Stems (Fig. 17.9)

Stems are structures which support buds and leaves and serve as conducts for carrying water, minerals, and sugars. The three major internal parts of a stem are the xylem, phloem, and cambium.

The xylem and phloem are the major components of a plant's vascular system.

The vascular system transports food, water, and minerals and offers support for the plant.

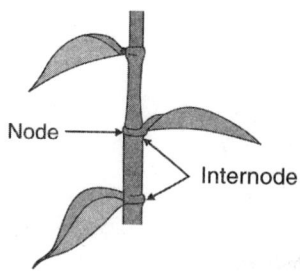

Fig. 17.9: Parts of stem

Xylem vessels conduct water and minerals, while phloem tubes conduct food.

The vascular systems of monocots and dicots differ, while both contain xylem and phloem, they are arranged differently.

MACROMORPHOLOGY

This is a valuable tool for identifying drugs and detecting many adulterants simply by an examination of calcium oxalate crystals or by the details of structure of the trichomes and other features. For the detection of adulterants in powdered drugs, knowledge of microscopical structure is essential. For microscopical measurements, stage and eyepiece micrometers, as well as camera lucida are used.

Drugs (dehydrated) should be prepared beforehand for microscopical examination by exposing them to moist atmosphere or by soaking or boiling them in water.

Alcohol should also be used for examination of mucilage or water-soluble cell contents. Structures are frequently obscured by the abundance of cell contents, the presence of coloring matters, and the shrinkage or collapse of the cell walls.

The commonly used mountants are glycerin, alcohol, carbolic acid, clove oil, and Canada balsam which have clearing effect (Table 17.8).

Table 17.8: List of clearing and bleaching agents

S. no.	Reagents	Description
1.	Chloral hydrate solution	It dissolves proteins, starch, chlorophyll, volatile oils, and resins, and expands shrunken cells. It can be used for identification of calcium oxalate crystals because does not dissolve it
2.	Potassium hydroxide solution	It is generally used as 5% aqueous solution, dissolves starch, protein, etc. and causes swelling of cell walls. It should be washed out after completion of clearing and if kept for prolonged, action is liable to cause disintegration
3.	Ether alcohol	Defatting is particularly necessary for oil seeds, such as linseed and strophanthus. The equal ratios of ether and alcohol are useful for removal of fixed and volatile oils, fats, resins, tannins, or chlorophyll
4.	Solution of chlorinated soda	It removes starch and lignin and bleaches dark-colored sections, such as those of many barks and for removing chlorophyll from leaves. Wash sections with water as soon as bleaching is complete
5.	Preparation of isolated elements	Disintegration and isolation of tissues is essential for determining the shape and size of cells and their distribution and relation in the different tissues and layers. The most important reagents used for this purpose are 5% aqueous solution of potassium hydroxide for common drugs except sclerenchymatous tissues, such as taste of capsicum and colocynth seeds or for the separation of lignified hairs, such as those of nux vomica and strophanthus; chromic/nitric is mandatory

Table 17.9: Parameters for quality control of herbal drugs

S. no	Type of standards	Examples
1.	Structural standard	**1. Macroscopic examinations:** Evaluation on the basis of morphological characteristics **i. Macromorphological evaluation** **Bark:** Curvature, transverse, in surface and fracture characteristics **Underground organs:** Shape, surface characters and transverse section **Leaves:** Surface appearance and texture (glabrous, pubescent, hispid, punctate) and lamina structure • *Shape:* Cordate, round, obovate, ovate, lanceolate, oblong, oval and linear • *Margin:* Dentate, sinuate, crenate, serrate, entire • *Incision:* Partite, fid, sect • *Composition:* Paripinnate, imparipinnate, pinnate, palmate • *Apex:* Acute, acuminate, truncate, obtuse • *Base:* Cordate, decurrent, symmetrical, asymmetrical • *Venation:* Parallel, pinnate, palmate and reticulate. **Flowers:** Receptacle, calyx, corolla and inflorescence (umbel, panicle, raceme and capitulum) **Fruits:** Shape and size (simple, aggregate and collective), type (simple dehiscent fruit, succulent fruits) **Seeds:** Size, shape, color, appearance and occurrence of any testa outgrowth. **Unorganized drug:** Solid (physical state, presence of vegetable debris, effect of heating) liquid/semisolid (colour, florescence, viscosity, density and solubility) **Cytomorphological evaluation:** Examination and arrangements of cell types parenchyma, collenchyma and sclerenchyma, epidermis and periderm, xylem and phloem **2. Microscopic examinations:** To magnify the fine structure of minute objects. **Preliminary treatment:** Dried parts of a plant may require softening in moist atmosphere, place a wad of cotton-wool moistened with water into the bottom of a test-tube and cover with a piece of filter-paper. Bark, wood and other dense and hard materials usually need to be soaked in water or equal parts of water, ethanol and glycerol for a few hours or overnight. **Preparation of specimens:** Powdered materials, surface tissues of leaves and flowers, section. **Use of clarifying agents like:** Chloral hydrate TS, lactochloral TS, lactophenol TS, sodium hypochlorite TS, solvents for fats and oils (xylene R and light petroleum R). **Histochemical detection of cell walls and contents** Iodinated zinc chloride (for detection of cellulose cell walls), phloroglucinol TS (for lignified cell wall), sudan red TS (for suberized

(Contd.)

Table 17.9: Parameters for quality control of herbal drugs *(Contd.)*

S. no	Type of standards	Examples
		or cuticular cell walls), iodine/ethanol TS (for aleurone grains), acetic acid (~60 g/l) TS or hydrochloric acid (~70 g/l) TS (for *calcium carbonate)*, chloral hydrate TS, (for calcium oxalate), potassium hydroxide (~55 g/l) TS (for *hydroxyanthraquinones)*, 1-naphthol TS and sulfuric acid (~1760 g/l) TS; (for inulin), chinese ink TS/ thionine TS (for mulicage), iodine (0.02 mol/l) VS (starch) and ferric chloride (50 g/l) TS (for tannin). **Disintegration of tissues:** *Method 1.* Nitric acid and potassium chlorate *Method 2.* Nitric acid and chromic acid *Method 3.* Caustic alkali method **Measurement of specimens:** Use a microscope with an ocular micrometer and Calibration of the ocular micrometer. **Microscopical examination:** Microchemical testing, microchemical precipitation, microsublimation.
2.	Analytical standards	**Quantitative analytical microscopy:** As per WHO, it is determining purity and botanical source of powdered drug. *Stomatal number:* It is the average number of stomata per square mm of the epidermis of the leaf. *Procedure:* Piece of leaf (middle part) is cleared by boiling with chloral hydrate solution. The upper and lower epidermes are peeled separately. The peeled epidermses are placed on slide and mounted with glycerin water. Camera lucida and drawing board are arranged for the drawings. With the help of stage micrometer, 1 sq. mm is drawn. The prepared slide is placed on the stage, epidermal cells and stomata are traced. The no. of stomata lying in the area of 1 sq. mm are counted including the cell, if at least half of its area lying within the square. Average no. of stomata per sq. mm is calculated by tracing four different fields. Stomatal number is affected by various factors like age of the plant, size of the leaf, environmental conditions, etc. Stomatal index is not much affected by these factors. It is relatively constant. Hence it is more significant in the evaluation of a leaf drug. **Determination of Stomatal Index** *Stomatal index:* It is the percentage which the numbers of stomata form to the total number of epidermal cells, each stoma being counted as one cell. Stomatal index can be calculated by using following equation. $$\text{Stomatal index} = S \times 100/E + S$$ where S = the number of stomata in a given area of leaf; and E = the number of epidermal cells (including trichomes) in the same area of leaf. *Procedure:* The first seven steps are similar as mentioned in the determination of stomatal number. The no. of stomata and the no. of epidermal cells in each field are counted. Stomatal index is calculated

(Contd.)

Table 17.9: Parameters for quality control of herbal drugs *(Contd.)*

S. no	Type of standards	Examples

using the above formula. Values for upper and lower surfaces (epidermises) are determined separately.

Vein-islet number: A vein islet is the small area of green tissue surrounded by the vein-lets. The vein-islet number is the average number of vein-islets per square mm of a leaf surface. It is determined by counting the number of vein-islets in an area of 4 sq. mm of the central part of the leaf between the midrib and the margin.

Procedure: A piece of leaf is cleared by boiling in chloral hydrate solution. Camera lucida and drawing board are arranged for the drawings. With the help of stage micrometer, 1 sq. mm is drawn. The cleared leaf is mounted on the slide and a drop of glycerin water was added then covered with cover slip. The above prepared slide is placed on the stage of the microscope. Veins are traced which are included within the square. The outlines of those islets which overlap two adjacent sides of the square are also traced. The no. of vein-islets in the sq. mm is counted. The islets which are intersected by the sides of square are included on two adjacent sides and excluded on other two sides.

The average no. of vein islets from four squares are found, and average no. of vein islets are calculated.

Vein termination: It is defined as the no. of vein let termination per sq. mm of the leaf surface, midway between midrib of the leaf and its margin. A vein termination is the ultimate free termination of vein-let.

Procedure: The average no. of vein terminations present within the square is counted from four different squares to get the value for one sq. mm.

Palisade ratio: Palisade ratio is the average number of palisade cells beneath one epidermal cell of a leaf. It is determined by counting the palisade cells beneath four continuous epidermal cells.

Procedure: A piece of leaf is cleared by boiling in chloral hydrate solution. Camera lucida and drawing board are arranged for the drawings. The four cells of the epidermis are traced off. By focusing down to palisade layer, sufficient cells are traced off to cover the epidermal cells. The no. of palisade cells under the four epidermal cells is counted.

Average no. of cells beneath a single epidermal cell is calculated which gives the palisade ratio. By focusing different part of the leaf, the same is traced and the average is calculated to get the palisade c ratio of the leaf.

Lycopodium spore method

Standardization parameters

Ash value: Ignition of medicinal plant material yields total ash constituting both physiological (from the plant tissue) and non-physiological (extraneous matter adhering to the plant) ash.

Determination of ash: Ignition of medicinal plant materials

Total ash: Measure the total amount of material remaining after ignition.

(Contd.)

Table 17.9: Parameters for quality control of herbal drugs *(Contd.)*

S. no	Type of standards	Examples
		This includes both "physiological ash", which is derived from the plant tissue itself, and "non-physiological" ash, which is the residue of the extraneous matter (e.g. sand and soil) adhering to the plant surface. **Acid-insoluble ash:** Residue obtained after boiling the total ash with dilute hydrochloric acid, and igniting the remaining insoluble matter. This measures the amount of silica present, especially as sand and siliceous earth. **Water-soluble ash** is the difference in weight between the total ash and the residue after treatment of the total ash with water. **Determination of extractable matter:** This method determines the mount of active constituents extracted with solvents from a given amount of medicinal plant material. It is the amount of soluble constituents (active or otherwise) extracted with solvents like alcohol and water from a given amount of medicinal plant material. **Hot Extraction and Cold Maceration** **Hot extraction:** Place about 4.0 g of coarsely powdered air-dried material, accurately weighed, in a glass-stoppered conical flask. Add 100 ml of water and weigh to obtain the total weight including the flask. Shake well and allow to stand for 1 hour. Attach a reflux condenser to the flask and boil gently for 1 hour; cool and weigh. Readjust to the original total weight with the solvent specified in the test procedure for the plant material concerned. Shake well and filter rapidly through a dry filter. Transfer 25 ml of the filtrate to a tared flat-bottomed dish and evaporate to dryness on a water-bath. Dry at 105°C for 6 hours, cool in a desiccator for 30 minutes, then weigh without delay. Calculate the content of extractable matter in mg per g of air-dried material. **Cold maceration:** Place about 4.0 g of coarsely powdered air-dried material, accurately weighed, in a glass-stoppered conical flask. Macerate with 100 ml of the solvent specified for the plant material concerned for 6 hours, shaking frequently, then allow to stand for 18 hours. Filter rapidly taking care not to lose any solvent, transfer 25 ml of the filtrate to a tared flat-bottomed dish and evaporate to dryness on a water bath. Dry at 105°C for 6 hours, cool in a desiccator for 30 minutes and weigh without delay. Calculate the content of extractable matter in mg per g of air-dried material. For ethanol-soluble extractable matter, use the concentration of solvent specified in the test procedure for the plant material concerned; for water-soluble extractable matter, use water as the solvent. Use other solvents as specified in the test procedure. **Determination of Water and Volatile Matter** Limits for water content should, therefore, be set for every given plant material. This is especially important for materials that absorb moisture easily or deteriorate quickly in the presence of water. **Preparation of material** (cutting, granulating or shredding) **Azeotropic method** (toluene distillation) **Loss on drying** (gravimetric determination)

(Contd.)

Table 17.9: Parameters for quality control of herbal drugs *(Contd.)*

S. no	Type of standards	Examples
		Determination of volatile oils: By steam distillation, with Clevenger apparatus, volatile oils are characterized by their odor, oil-like appearance and ability to volatilize at room temperature. Chemically, they are usually composed of mixtures of, for example, monoterpenes, sesquiterpenes and their oxygenated derivatives. In order to determine the volume of oil, the plant material is distilled with water and the distillate is collected in a graduated tube. The aqueous portion separates automatically and is returned to the distillation flask. If the volatile oils possess a mass density higher than or near to that of water, or are difficult to separate from the aqueous phase owing to the formation of emulsions, a solvent with a low mass density and a suitable boiling-point may be added to the measuring tube. The dissolved volatile oils will then float on top of the aqueous phase.
		Determination of bitterness value: Bitter drugs are used therapeutically, mostly as appetizing agents. Their bitterness stimulates secretions in the gastrointestinal tract, especially of gastric juice, compared by that of a dilute solution of quinine hydrochloride.
		Determination of hemolytic activity: Medicinal plant with Caryophyllaceae, Araliaceae, Sapindaceae, Primulaceae, and Dioscoreaceae contain saponins. When added to a suspension of blood, saponins produce changes in erythrocyte membranes, causing hemoglobin to diffuse into the surrounding medium. The hemolytic activity of plant materials, or a preparation containing saponins, is determined by comparison with that of a reference material, saponin R, which has a hemolytic activity of 1000 units per g. A suspension of erythrocytes is mixed with equal volumes of a serial dilution of the plant material extract. The lowest concentration to effect complete hemolysis is determined after allowing the mixtures to stand for a given period of time. A similar test is carried out simultaneously with saponin R.
		Determination of tannins: By hide powder method.
		Determination of swelling index: The swelling index is the volume in ml taken up by the swelling of 1 g of plant material under specified conditions. Its determination is based on the addition of water or a swelling agent as specified in the test procedure for each individual plant material (either whole, cut or pulverized). Using a glass-stoppered measuring cylinder, the material is shaken repeatedly for 1 hour and then allowed to stand for a required period of time.
		Determination of foaming index: The foaming ability of an aqueous decoction of plant materials and their extracts is measured in terms of a foaming index. Reduce about 1 g of the plant material to a coarse powder (sieve size no. 1250), weigh accurately and transfer to a 500 ml conical flask containing 100 ml of boiling water. Maintain at moderate boiling for 30 minutes. Cool and filter into a 100-ml volumetric flask and add sufficient water through the filter to dilute to volume.

(Contd.)

Table 17.9: Parameters for quality control of herbal drugs *(Contd.)*

S. no	Type of standards	Examples
		Determination of pesticide residues: Limits for pesticide residues should be established following the recommendations of the Food and Agriculture Organization of the United Nations (FAO) and the World Health Organization (WHO) which have already been established for food and animal feed. These recommendations include the analytical methodology for the assessment of specific pesticide residues.
		Determination of arsenic and heavy metals—limit test for arsenic: The amount of arsenic in the medicinal plant material is estimated by matching the depth of color with that of a standard stain. The contents of lead and cadmium may be determined by inverse voltametry or by atomic absorption spectrophotometry.
		Determination of microorganisms—radioactive contamination: The amount of exposure to radiation depends on the intake of radio-nuclides and other variables, such as age, metabolic kinetics, and weight of the individual (also known as the dose conversion factor).
		Culture media and strains of micro-organisms—culture media: Baird-Parker agar, brilliant green agar, buffered sodium chloride-peptone solution pH 7.0, casein-soybean digest agar, cetrimide agar, deoxycholate citrate agar, Enterobacteriaceae enrichment broth-mossel, lactose broth, MacConkey agar, MacConkey broth, Sabouraud glucose agar with antibiotics, soybean-casein digest medium, Tetrathionate bile brilliant green broth, triple sugar iron agar, violet-red bile agar with glucose and lactose, xylose, lysine, deoxycholate agar.
3.	Standard relating to physical constants	**Determination of density:** Pycnometer and Oscillating U-tube. **Determination of refractive index:** Refractometer. **Determination of viscosity:** Viscometer. **Determination of optical rotation:** Polarimeter.

Quality can be defined as the status of a drug that is determined by identity, purity, content, and other chemical, physical, or biological properties, or by the manufacturing processes. *Quality control* is a set of activities intended to ensure efficacy and safety of herbal products (Table 17.9). It refers to processes involved in maintaining the quality and validity of a manufactured product.

In general, quality control is based on three important pharmacopoeial definitions:

1. *Identity:* Is the herb the one it should be?
2. *Purity:* Is their contaminants, e.g. in the form of other herbs which should not be there?
3. *Content or assay:* Is the content of active constituents within the defined limits?

To prove identity and purity, criteria such as type of preparation, physical constants, adulteration, contaminants, moisture, ash content and solvent residues have to be checked.

CHROMATOGRAPHIC METHODS

The chromatographic techniques used in the isolation of various types of natural products can be broadly classified into two categories: classical or older, and modern.

Classical or older chromatographic techniques include:
1. Thin-layer chromatography (TLC).
2. Preparative thin-layer chromatography (PTLC).
3. Open-column chromatography (CC).
4. Flash chromatography (FC).

Modern chromatographic techniques are:
1. High-performance thin-layer chromatography (HPTLC).
2. Multiflash chromatography.
3. Vacuum liquid chromatography (VLC).
4. Chromatotron.
5. Solid-phase extraction
6. Droplet countercurrent chromatography (DCCC).
7. High-performance liquid chromatography (HPLC).
8. Hyphenated techniques (e.g. HPLC-PDA, LC-MS, LC-NMR and LC-MS-NMR).

Traditional herbal medicines make excellent leads for new drug development. New plant-derived medicines can come from three sources: single active principles, active fractions, and validated prescriptions. Conventionally, for single active compounds, lead discovery and drug development involve highly efficient bioactivity-directed fractionation and isolation (BDFI) coupled with structural characterization, analog synthesis, and mechanism of action studies. Today, new scientific technologies, including biological screening methods, continue to improve this process. For multi-component herbal prescriptions standardization and quality control, including GAP (good agricultural practice), GMP (good manufacturing practice) and GCP (good clinical Practice), must be performed to guarantee high quality and consistency. To validate herbal efficacy and safety reliable chemical, pharmacological, as well as drug administration, distribution, metabolism, excretion, and toxicological (ADMET) studies are needed.

18
Morphological, Microscopic and Analytical Profile of Important Herbs

Asokha (Table 18.1)

Synonyms: Sanskrit: Kankeli; **English:** Asok Tree; **Gujrati:** Ashoka; **Hindi:** Ashoka

Biological source: Ashoka consists of dried stem bark of the plant *Saraca asoca* (Rose.) De. Willd, Syn. *Saraca indica* Linn (Family Leguminosae).

Classification

- Kingdom   Plantae
- Division   Magnoliophyta
- Class   Mgnoliopsida
- Order   Fabales
- Family   Caesalpinaceae
- Genus   *Saraca*
- Species   *asoca*

Habitat: It is found throughout India. Specially in Himalaya, Kerala, Bengal and whole south region.

Description

a. **Macroscopic characters of stem bark:**
Color: Externally, dark green to greenish grey. Internally reddish-brown.
Odor: Characteristic
Taste: Astringent and bitter
Fracture: Splintery exposing striated surface
Extra features: Stem barks are rough and uneven due to the presence of rounded or projecting lenticles.

b. **Microscopic section:**
Bark: Transverse section of stem bark shows periderm consisting of a wide layer of cork, radially flattened narrow cork cambium, secondary cortex wide with one or two continuous layers of stone cells with many patches of sclereids, parenchymatous tissue contains yellow masses and prismatic crystals: secondary phloem consists of phloem parenchyma, sieve tubes with companion cells and phloem fibers occurring in groups, crystal fibers present.

Stem: Transverse section of stem is circular. Small rounded to oval projecting lenticles are present on the surface. Epidermis is single-layered with thin cuticle. Below the epidermis, 5–6 layers of cork are seen. Cortex is 12–16- layered. In the middle region of cortex, 3–5 layers of stone cells are clearly visible. Just above, the phloem region is very distinct and contains tannin cells. Cambium is very clear and is 2–3-layered. Xylem region is composed mostly of tracheids and a few vessels. Primary xylem is prominent. There is prominent pith, composed of thin-walled parenchyma and many of the pith cells contain polygonal calcium oxalate crystals.

Powder characters: Ashoka bark powder brown in color, under microscope it contains some tracheids, large quantity of fibers, stone cells, parenchyma cells, sieve tube fragments and many unidentified cells.

Table 18.1: Identity, purity and strength of ashoka

Solubility	In water NLT 60% w/w In alcohol NLT 40% w/w
Foreign matter	NMT 2%
Total ash	NMT 11%
Acid-insoluble ash	NMT 1%
Alcohol-soluble extractive (90%)	NLT 15%
Water-soluble extractive	NLT 11%
pH (1% w/v solution)	5 to 7
Loss on drying	NMT 5%
Moisture content	NMT 5%
Microbiological analysis	
A. Pathogens (*E. coli, S. aureus*)	Absent
B. Total bacterial count (CFU/gm)	NMT 800 CFU/gm
C. Total fungal count (CFU/gm)	NMT 500 CFU/gm
Heavy metal	
A. Arsenic	NMT 1 ppm
B. Lead	NMT 5 ppm

TLC profile: Assay of active principle by HPTLC/HPLC: Tannins NLT 30% w/w.

Constituents: The phytochemical study shows presence of (–) epicatechin, tannins, crystalline glycoside, flavonoids and saponins in the bark of plant.

Therapeutic uses: *Saraca asoca* is highly regarded as an universal panacea in the ayurvedic medicine. It is used as spasmogenic, oxytocic, uterotonic, antibacterial, anti-implantation, antitumor, anti-progestational, antiestrogenic activity against menorrhagia and anticancer. It has many uses, like to treat skin infections, CNS function, genitourinary functions. Dried root is used in paralysis, hemiplegia and visceral numbness. It acts as a vulnerary and hastens healing time of skin trauma and broken bones.

Adulterants: The drug is widely adulterated with the bark of *Polyalthia longifolia* (Devdaru).

Ashwagandha (Table 18.2)

Synonyms: Sanskrit: Hayagandha; **Gujrati:** Asgandha; **Hindi:** Asgandh.

Biological source: Asvagandha consists of dried mature roots of *Withania somnifera* Dunal (Family Solanaceae).

Habitat: Cultivated in field and open grounds throughout India, widely cultivated in certain areas of Madhya Pradesh and Rajasthan.

Classification

- Kingdom   Plantae
- Division   Angiosperma
- Class   Dicotyledoneae
- Order   Tubiflorae
- Family   Solanaceae
- Genus   *Withania*
- Species   *somnifera* Dunal

Description

a. Macroscopy characters of root:

Color: Outer surface buff to grey-yellow color with longitudinal wrinkles

Odor: Characteristic

Taste: Bitter and acrid.

Fracture: Smooth and powdery

Extra features: Roots straight conical, unbranched and some of them bear a crown, thickness varying with age.

b. Microscopic characters of root:

Transverse section of root shows exfoliated cork or crushed, when present isodiametric and non-lignified, cork cambium 2–4 layers of phellogen and about 15–20 rows of phelloderm. It prominently shows parts of vascular tissue like cambium, consisting of 3–5 layers of tangentially elongated cells. Secondary cortex about 20 layers of compact parenchymatous cells. Secondary xylem is hard which forms continuous vascular ring interrupted by medullary rays. Phloem consists of sieve tubes, companion cells, phloem parenchyma, cambium 4–5 rows of tangentially elongated cells.

Table 18.2: Identity, purity and strength of ashwagandha

Foreign matter	NMT 2%
Total ash	NMT 7%
Acid-insoluble ash	NMT 1%
Alcohol-soluble extractive (25%)	NLT 15%
Water-soluble extractive	Nil
Moisture content	<8.0%w/w
Phytochemical analysis	
Total saponins	>4.0%w/w
Total alkaloids	>0.15%w/w
Free withanolides	0.5–1.2%w/w
Conjugated withanolides	0.3–1.0%w/w

TLC: Adsorbent: Silicagel G

Mobile phase: Benzene: Ethyl acetate 2: 1

Sample preparation: The conjugated and free withanolide fractions isolated from *Withania somnifera* extract was dissolved in chloroform and applied on TLC plate.

Detection: Vanillin boric acid and sulphuric acid reagent

Rf: 0.05, 0.15, 0.2, 0.6, 0.9 Withanolides (dark pink color spots).

Constituents: The principle constituents are alkaloids and withanolides. Ashwagandha root contains 13 types of alkaloids including cusehygrine, anahgrine, tropin, anaferin, withasomine, visamine, withanone and withaferin.

Therapeutic uses: *Withania somnifera* Dunal (ashwagandha, WS) is widely used in Ayurvedic medicine, the traditional medical system of India. It is an ingredient in many formulations prescribed for a variety of musculoskeletal conditions (e.g. arthritis, rheumatism), and as a general tonic to increase energy, improve overall health and longevity, and prevent disease in athletes, the elderly, and during pregnancy.

Bael Fruit (Table 18.3)

Synonyms: Sanskrit: Sriphala; **English:** Bengal quince, bael fruit; **Hindi:** Bel

Biological source: Bilva consists of pulp of entire, unripe or half-ripe fruits of *Aegle marmelos* Carr. (Family Rutaceae).

Habitat: It is cultivated throughout the country, rind of fruit is removed and pulp is bruised and dried.

Description

a. Macroscopic characters of fruit

Color: Externally greenish when young yellowish-brown when ripe

Odor: Faintly aromatic

Taste: Mucilaginous and slightly bitter and astringent.

Size: 5–18 cm in diameter

Shape: Sub-globose

b. Macroscopic characters of seed

Color: Brown

Size: Oblong

Extra features: Dried pulp hard and pale to dark red in color, frequently breaks away from the rind during drying, leaving a thin layer attached to it.

Table 18.3: Identity, purity and strength of bael fruit

Total ash	NMT 4%
Acid-insoluble ash	NMT 1%
Alcohol-soluble extractive	NLT 6%
Water-soluble extractive	NLT 50%

TLC of Alcoholic Extract of Bael

Adsorbant: Silica gel 'G'

Solvent system: Toluene: Ethyl acetate (95:5)

Detection: UV and iodine vapor

Spraying agent: Dragendorff reagent

Relative front: 0.07 (greenish blue), 0.14 (greenish blue), 0.25, 0.39 and 0.67 (all blue) under UV On exposure to iodine vapor, three spots appear at Rf. 0.14, 0.25 and 0.97 (all yellow). On spraying with dragendorff reagent, one spot appears at Rf. 0.25 (orange).

Constituents: The medicinal value of bael fruit is enhanced due to presence of tannins, the evaporating substance in its rind. The rind contains 20% and the pulp has only 9% of tannin. Additionally, it also contains marmalosin, mucilage, fatty oil and sugar. A major constituent of the fruit is the mucilage and marmelosin (0.5%) a coumarin, in addition to the minor constituents, like reducing sugar, essential oils, ascorbic acid and various minerals. Bitter, light-yellow oil contains 15.6% palmitic acid, 8.3% stearic acid, 28.7% linoleic and 7.6% linolenic acid. The seed residue contains 70% protein.

Therapeutic uses: The ripe fruit has cooling effect and is constipative. Raw bael fruit is consumed for treatment of ailments, such as arthritis and gout. Ripe fruit is taken during summer to keep the body and mind cool. Bael also helps to sharpen intellect and concentration of mind.

Citraka (Table 18.4)

Synonyms: Sanskrit: Agni, Vahni; **English:** Lead war; **Hindi:** Chira, Chitra; **Gujrati:** Chitrakmula.

Biological source: Citraka consists of dried mature root of *Plumbago zeylanica* Linn, belonging to family Plumbaginaceae.

Habitat: A large perennial sub-scandent shrub, found throughout India in wile state in Peninsular India and occasionally cultivated in gardens throughout India.

Description

a. Macroscopic characters of root:

Color: Reddish to deep brown

Odor: Disagreeable

Taste: Acrid

Size: 30 cm or more in length, 6 mm or more in diameter

Extra features: Bark is thin and brown, internal structure striated.

b. Microscopic characters of root: It shows outer most tissue of cork consisting of 5–7 row, of cubical to rectangular dark brown cells, secondary cortex consists of 2–3 rows of thin-walled rectangular, light brown cells, most of the cortex cells contain starch grains, secondary cortex followed by a wide zone of cortex, composed of large polygonal to tangentially elongated parenchymatous cells varying in size and shape, containing starch grains and some cells with yellow contents, fibers scattered singly or in groups of 2–6, phloem a narrow zone of polygonal, thin-walled cells, consisting of usual elements and phloem fibers, similar to cortical zone, phloem fibers usually in groups of 2–5 or more but occasionally occurring singly, lignified with pointed ends and narrow lumen, similar in shape and size to those of secondary cortex, cambium indistinct, xylem light yellow to 39

Table 18.4: Identity, purity and strength of chitraka

Foreign matter	NMT 3%
Total ash	NMT 3%
Acid-insoluble ash	NMT 1%
Alcohol-soluble extractive	NLT 12%
Water-soluble extractive	NLT 12%

whitish, vessels radially arranged with pitted thickenings, medullary rays straight, 1–6 seriate cells, radially elongated starch filled with starch grains, stone cells absent.

Constituents: The root yielded naphthoquinone derivatives, plumbagin being the most important active principle.

Therapeutic uses: Roots are used as intestinal flora normalizer, stimulates digestive processes; used for dyspepsia. Root paste is applied in order to open abscesses; it is used externally in leprosy and other obstinate skin diseases. A cold infusion is used for influenza and black-water fever.

Coriander (Table 18.5)

Synonyms: Sanskrit: Dhanika, Kustumburu; **English:** Coriander fruit; **Hindi:** Dhaniya; **Gujrati:** Dhana

Biological source: Coriander consists of dried ripe fruits of *Coriandrum sativum* Linn, belonging to family Umbelliferae.

Habitat: A slender, glabrous, branched, annual herb, cultivated all over India. Cultivated chiefly in Madhya Pradesh, Karnataka, Rajasthan, Maharashtra, Tamil Nadu and Bihar.

Description

a. Macroscopic characters of fruit:
Color: Brownish-yellow or brown
Odor: Aromatic
Taste: Spicy and characteristic
Shape: Globular
Size: Cremocarp about 2–4 mm in diameter
Extra features: Fruit is crowned by sepals and styles. It consists of primary ridges (10) and secondary ridges (8).

b. Microscopic characters of fruit:
Epicarp: It is composed of a layer of polygonal, colorless, thin-walled cells, with a smooth cuticle. Most of the cells contain small prisms of calcium oxalate.

Mesocarp: The sclerenchyma of the mesocarp consists of two types of cells masses of very thick-walled, sinuous, fusiform cells with a narrow lumen and two or three layers of large, rectangular or polygonal cells with only slightly thickened walls.

Endocarp: The endocarp composed of a layer of thin-walled, lignified cells, elongated. It is usually found adherent to the rectangular sclereids of the mesocarp.

Vittae: The brown fragments of the vittae composed of thin-walled cells, polygonal.

Testa: It is a single layer of brown, very thin-walled polygonal cells.

Endosperm: The endosperm is composed of thick-walled cells containing microrosette crystals of calcium oxalate and aleurone grains.

Powder: Fawn to brown, epidermal cells of pericarp when present, slightly thick-walled and may containing small prism of calcium oxalate, parenchymatous cells of mesocarp without reticulate thickening, masses of sclerenchymatous cells of mesocarp in sinuous rows, often crossing at right angles, large tubular hexagonal rather thin-walled sclerenchymatous cells of endocarp, cells of inner epidermis with slightly sinnous anticlinal walls, thick-walled polygonal parenchymatous cells of endosperm, containing fixed oil and numerous small aleurone grains, microrosettes of calcium oxalate.

Table 18.5: Identity, purity and strength of coriander	
Foreign matter	NMT 2%
Total ash	NMT 6%
Acid-insoluble ash	NMT 1.5%
Alcohol-soluble extractive	NLT 10%
Water-soluble extractive	NLT 19%
Volatile oil	NLT 0.3%

Constituents: Coriander contains 0.5 to 1% volatile oil, consisting mainly of delta-linalool (55–74%), alpha-pinene and terpinine. It also contains flavonoids, coumarins, phthalides and phenolic acids.

Therapeutic uses: It is used as a sedative, spasmolytic, hypotensive, nervine, antiseptic. Used in cutaneous and scrofulous affections, chronic fever and liver complaints.

Vasaka (Table 18.6)

Synonyms: Sanskrit: Vrsa, Vasaka; **English:** Vasaka; **Hindi:** Aduss, Arusa

Biological source: Vasaka consists of fresh, dried, mature leaves of *Adhatoda vasica* Nees, belonging to family Acanthaceae.

Habitat: A sub-herbaceous bush, found throughout the year in plains and sub-Himalayan tracts in India.

Classification

- Kingdom   Plantae
- Order   Lamiales
- Family   Acanthaceae
- Genus   *Justicia*
- Species   *adhatoda*

Description

a. Macroscopic characters of leaves:

Color: Dried leaves dull brown above, light greyish brown below

Odor: Characteristic

Taste: Bitter

Size: 10–30 cm long and 3–10 cm broad

Shape: Lanceolate to ovate-lanceolate

b. Microscopic characters of leaf: Transverse section of leaf shows, dorsiventral surface with 2 layers of palisade cells, in surface view, epidermal cells sinuous with anomocytic stomata on both surfaces, more numerous on the lower, clothing trichomes few, 1–3, rarely up to 5-celled, thin-walled, uniseriate, up to 500 µ and glandular trichomes with unicellular stalk and 4 celled head measuring, 25–36 µ in diameter in surface view, cystoliths in mesophyll layers, elongated and cigar-shaped, acicular and prismatic forms of calcium oxalate crystals present in mesophyll, palisade ratio, 5–6, 5–8.5, stomatal index, 10.8–14.2–18.1 for lower surface.

Table 18.6: Identity, purity and strength of vasaka

Foreign matter	NMT 2%
Total ash	NMT 21%
Acid-insoluble ash	NMT 1%
Alcohol-soluble extractive	NLT 3%
Water-soluble extractive	NLT 22%

TLC of Methanolic Extract

Adsorbent: Silica gel G

Solvent system: 1, 4 Dioxane: Ammonia solution (9:1)

Detection: Drangendroff reagent

Densitometric scan: 254 nm

Rf: 0.58 (Vasicine)

Constituents: The chief quinazoline alkaloid vasicine and essential oil. The leaves contain two major alkaloids called vasicine and vasicinone.

Therapeutic uses: It is a bitter bronchodilator, respiratory stimulant, hypotensive, cardiac depressant, uterotonic and abortifacient.

Brahmi (Whole Plant) (Table 18.7)

Synonyms: Sanskrit: Sarasvati, Kapotavanka; **English:** Thyme leaved gratiola; **Hindi:** Manduka Parni.

Biological source: Brahmi consists of dried whole plant of *Bacopa monnieri* (Linn.) Wettst., Syn. *Herpestis monnieria* (LiM.) H.B. and K. (Family Scrophulariaceae).

Habitat: A glabrous, succulent, small, prostrate or creeping annual herb, found throughout India in wet and damp places.

Classification

- Kingdom   Plantae
- Order   Lamiales
- Family   Scrophulariaceae
- Genus   *Bacopa*
- Species   *monnieri*

Description

a. Macroscopic characters of parts of Brahmi:

Root: Thin, wiry, small, branched creamish-yellow.

Stem: Thin, green or purplish green, about 1–2 mm thick, soft, nodes and internodes prominent, glabrous; taste—slightly bitter.

Leaf: Simple, opposite, decussate, green, sessile, 1–2 cm long, obovate-oblong; taste—slightly bitter.

Flower: Small, axillary and solitary, pedicels 6–30 mm long, bracteoles shorter than pedicels.

Fruit: Capsules up to 5 mm long, ovoid and glabrous.

b. Microscopic characters of Brahmi:

Root: Shows a single layer of epidermis, cortex having large air cavities; endodermis single-layered; pericycle not distinct; stele consists of a thin layer of phloem with a few sieve elements and isolated material from xylem shows vessels with reticulate thickenings.

Stem: Shows single layer of epidermis followed by a wide cortex of thin-walled cells with very large intercellular spaces; endodermis single-layered; pericycle 3 consisting of 1–2 layers; vascular ring continuous, composed of a narrow zone of phloem towards periphery and a wide ring of xylem towards center; center occupied by a small pith with distinct intercellular spaces; starch grains simple, round to oval, present in a few cells of cortex and endodermis, measuring 4–14 µ in diameter, and 8.0–14.0 × 2.5–9.0 µ in diameter, respectively.

Leaf: Shows a single layer of upper and lower epidermis covered with thin cuticle; glandular hairs sessile, subsidiary cells present on both surfaces; a few prismatic crystals of calcium oxalate occasionally found distributed in mesophyll cells; mesophyll traversed by small veins surrounded by bundle sheath; no distinct midrib present.

Powder: Yellowish-brown; shows xylem vessels with reticulate thickening, glandular hairs, simple, round and oval starch grains, measuring 4–14 µ in diameter.

Table 18.7: Identity, purity and strength of Brahmi

Foreign matter	NMT 2%
Total ash	NMT 18%
Acid-insoluble ash	NMT 6%
Alcohol-soluble extractive	NLT 6%
Water-soluble extractive	NLT 15%

TLC

Adsorbent: Silica gel G

Solvent system: Chloroform: methanol (9:1)

Ethyl acetate: Methanol: water (7:2:1)

Sample: The powdered drug is successively treated with petroleum ether, chloroform and methanol. Three solutions are concentrated separately.

Detection: Anisaldehyde sulfuric acid reagent

Rf: 0.52 (Bacoside)

Constituents: The herb contains the alkaloids brahmine, herpestine, and a mixture of three bases. The herb also contains the saponins, monnierin, hersaponin, bacosides A and B.

HPTLC: It can be performed on 20 cm × 10 cm aluminium-backed HPTLC plates coated with 200 μm layers of RP-18F254 silica gel. Before use, the plates should be prewashed with methanol and activated at 60°C for 5 min. A constant application rate of 0.1 μL s^{-1} was used. Plates were developed to a distance of 8 cm, in the dark, with toluene–methanol–ethyl acetate, 7.5:2.5:2.0 (v/v), as mobile phase. Before development, the chamber was saturated with mobile phase for 30 min at room temperature (25 ± 2°C). These conditions resulted in good resolution. Densitometric scanning absorbance mode at 344 nm, the slit dimensions were 5 mm × 0.45 mm and the scanning speed was 10 mm s^{-1}.

Therapeutic uses: Adaptogenic, astringent, diuretic, sedative, potent nervine tonic, antianxiety agent (improves mental functions, used in insanity, epilepsy), antispasmodic used in bronchitis, asthma and diarrhea).

Methi (Seed) (Table 18.8)

Synonyms: Sanskrit: Methini; **English:** Fenugreek; **Gujrati:** Methi; **Hindi:** Methi

Biological source: Methi consists of seeds of *Trigonella foenum-graecum* Linn, belonging to family Fabaceae.

Habitat: An aromatic, 30–60 cm tall, annual herb, widely cultivated in many parts of India.

Classification

- Kingdom — Plantae
- Division — Magnoliophyta
- Class — Magnoliopsida
- Order — Fabales
- Family — Fabaceae
- Subfamily — Faboideae
- Tribe — Trifolieae
- Genus — *Trigonella*

Description

a. Macroscopic characters of seed:

Color: Dull yellow
Odor: Pleasant
Taste: Bitter
Shape: Oblong, rhomboidal with deep furrow running obliquely dividing seed into a larger and smaller part.
Size: 30.2–0.5 cm long, 0.15–0.35 cm broad
Extra features: Seed is smooth and hard, becomes mucilaginous when soaked in water.

b. Microscopic characters of seed: Seed shows a layer of thick-walled, columnar palisade, covered externally with thick cuticle; cells flat at base, mostly pointed but a few flattened at apex, supported internally by a tangentially wide bearer cells having radial rib-like thickenings; followed by 4–5 layers of tangentially elongated, thin-walled, parenchymatous cells; endosperm consists of a layer of thick-walled cells containing aleurone grains, several layers of thin-walled, mucilaginous cells, varying in size, long axis radially elongated in outer region and tangentially elongated in inner region; cotyledons consists of 3–4 layers of palisade cells varying in size with long axis and a few layers of rudimentary spongy tissue; rudimentary vascular tissue situated in spongy mesophyll; cells of cotyledon contain aleurone grains and oil globules.

Powder: Yellow; shows groups of palisade parenchymatous cells, aleurone grains, oil globules, endosperm and epidermal cells of testa.

Table 18.8: Identity, purity and strength of fenugreek	
Foreign matter	NMT 2%
Total ash	NMT 4%
Acid-insoluble ash	NMT 0.5%
Alcohol-soluble extractive	NLT 5%

Constituents: The fenugreek contains 45–60% carbohydrates, mainly mucilaginous fiber (galactomannans); 20–30% proteins high in lysine and tryptophan; 5–10% fixed oils (lipids). The alkaloids, like pyridine-type alkaloids mostly trigonelline, choline, gentianine, and carpaine. Flavonoids, like apigenin, luteolin, orientin, quercetin, vitexin, and isovitexin. Free amino acids like 4-hydroxyisoleucine, arginine, histidine, and lysine. The other constituents are calcium, iron, saponins, glycosides yielding steroidal sapogenins on hydrolysis (diosgenin, yamogenin, tigogenin, neotigogenin); cholesterol and sitosterol, vitamins A, B1, C, and nicotinic acid; and volatile oils (n-alkanes and sesquiterpenes).

TLC

Adsorbent: Silica gel

Solvent system: Butanol: acetone: water (45:5:50)

Rf: 0.06

Therapeutic uses: The several health beneficial physiological attributes of fenugreek seeds have been seen in animal studies as well as human trials. These include antidiabetic effect, hypocholesterolemic influence, antioxidant potency, digestive stimulant action, and hepatoprotective effect. Fenugreek seeds have been used to increase lactation, and to treat pellagra, appetite loss, indigestion, dyspepsia, bronchitis, fever, hernia, impotence, vomiting, and stomach ulcers.

Neem (Leaf) (Table 18.9)

Synonyms: Sanskrit: Aristha, Picumarda; **English:** Margosa tree; **Gujrati:** Limba, Limbado; **Hindi:** Nim, Nimba.

Biological source: Nimba (leaf) consists of dried leaf of *Azadirachta indica* A. Juss Syn. *Melia azadirachta* Linn, belonging to family Meliaceae.

Habitat: A moderate sized to fairly large evergreen tree, attaining a height of 12–15 m with stout trunk and spreading branches, native to Burma; found all over India at elevation of 900 m.

Classification

- Kingdom   Plantae
- Division   Magnoliophyta
- Class   Magnoliopsida
- Order   Sapindales
- Family   Meliaceae
- Genus   *Azadirachta*
- Species   *indica*

Description

a. Macroscopic characters of leaves:

Color: Slightly yellowish-green

Odor: Indistinct

Taste: Bitter

Size: 15–25 cm long, 0.1 cm thick

Shape: Lanceolate

Extra features: Compound, alternate and leaflets with oblique base.

b. Microscopic characters of leaf:

Midrib: Leaflet through midrib shows a biconvex outline; epidermis on either side covered externally with thick cuticle; below epidermis, 4–5-layered collenchyma present; stele composed of one crescent-shaped vascular bundles towards lower and two to three smaller bundles towards upper surface; rest of tissues composed of thin-walled, parenchymatous cells having secretory cells and rosette crystals of calcium oxalate; phloem surrounded by non-lignified fiber strand; crystals also present in phloem region.

Lamina: Shows dorsiventral structure; epidermis on either surface, composed of thin-walled, tangentially elongated cells, covered externally with thick cuticle; anomocytic stomata present on lower surface only; palisade single-layered; spongy parenchyma composed of 5–6-layered, thin-walled cells, traversed by a number of veins; rosette crystals of calcium oxalate present in a few cells; palisade ratio 3.0–4.5; stomatal index 13.0–14.5 on lower surface and 8.0–11.5 on upper surface.

Powder: Green; shows vessels, fibers, rosette crystals of calcium oxalate, fragments of spongy and palisade parenchyma.

Table 18.9: Identity, purity and strength of neem	
Foreign matter	NMT 2%
Total ash	NMT 10%
Acid-insoluble ash	NMT 1%
Alcohol-soluble extractive	NLT 13%
Water-soluble extractive	NLT 19%

TLC: TLC on silica gel with petroleum ether-acetone 25:2; detection by spraying with 50% ethanolic sulfuric acid and heating at 200°C. Quantitative TLC by densitometry at 450 nm.

Constituents: Neem mainly contains triterpenoids and sterols.

Therapeutic uses: Leaf, bark is used as antimicrobial, antifungal, anthelmintic, insecticidal, antiviral, antipyretic, antimalarial, antiperiodic, mosquito larvicidal, anti-inflammatory, antifertility, spermicidal, hypoglycemic; used in inflammation of gums, gingivitis, periodontitis, sores, boils, enlargement of spleen, malarial fever, fever during childbirth, measles, smallpox, head scald and cutaneous affections.

Tulsi (Whole Plant) (Table 18.10)

Synonyms: Sanskrit: Surasa; **English:** Holy basil; **Gujrati:** Tulasi, Tulsi; **Hindi:** Tulasi

Biological source: Tulsi consists of dried whole plant of *Ocimum sanctum* Linn., belonging to family Lamiaceae.

Habitat: An erect, 30–60 cm high, much branched, annual herb, found throughout India; grown in houses, gardens and temples.

Description

a. Macroscopic features of whole plant:

Root

Color: Blackish-brown externally and pale violet internally

Extra features: Thin, wiry, branched, hairy and soft

Stem

Color: Externally, purplish-brown to black; internally, cream-coloured.

Odor: Faintly aromatic

Fracture: Fibrous

Extra features: Erect, herbaceous, woody, branched and sub quadrangular,

Leaf

Color: Greenish

Odor: Aromatic

Taste: Characteristic.

Size: 2.5–5 cm long 1.6–3.2 cm wide

Shape: Elliptic oblong and entire or serrate

Flower

Color: Purplish or crimson

Odor: Aromatic

Taste: Pungent

Pedicels: Longer than calyx

Calyx: Ovoid

Corolla: About 4 mm long and pubescent.

Fruit

Color: Pale brown or reddish

Odor: Aromatic

Taste: Pungent.e:

Shape: Sub-globose, smooth and slightly compressed

Seed

Shape: Rounded to oval

Color: Brown

Odor: None

Taste: Pungent

Extra features: Mucilaginous when soaked in water.

b. Microscopic features:

Root: Shows a single layered epidermis followed by cortex, consisting of seven or more layers of rectangular, round to oval polygonal, thin-walled, parenchymatous cells, filled with brown content, inner layers of cortex devoid of contents; phloem consisting of sieve elements, thin-walled, rectangular parenchyma cells and scattered groups of fibers, found scattered in phloem; xylem consists of vessels, tracheids, fibers and parenchyma; vessels pitted; fiber tracheides, long, pitted with pointed ends; fibers thick-walled and with pointed ends.

Stem: Shows a single-layered epidermis with uniseriate, multicellular covering trichomes having 5–6 cells, occasionally a few cells collapsed; cortex consists of 10 or more layers of thin-walled, rectangular, parenchymatous cells; phloem consists of sieve elements, thin-walled, rectangular parenchyma cells and fibers; fibers found scattered mostly throughout phloem, in groups and rarely in singles; xylem occupies major portion of stem consisting of vessels, tracheids, fibers and parenchyma; vessels pitted; fibers with pointed ends; center occupied by pith consisting of round to oval, thin-walled, parenchymatous cells.

Leaf

Petiole: Shows somewhat cordate outline consisting of single-layered epidermis composed of thin-walled, oval cells having a number of covering and glandular trichomes covering trichomes multicellular 1–8-celled long, rarely slightly reflexed at tip; glandular trichomes short, sessile with 1–2-celled stalk and 2–8 celled balloon-shaped head measuring 22–27 in diameter; epidermis followed by 1 or 2 layers and 2 or 3 layers of thin-walled, elongated, parenchyma cells towards upper and lower surfaces respectively; three vascular bundles situated centrally, middle one larger than other two, xylem surrounded by phloem.

Midrib: Epidermis, trichomes and vascular bundles similar to those of petiole except cortical layers reduced towards apical region.

Lamina: Epidermis and trichomes similar to those of petiole; both anomocytic and diacytic type of stomata present on both surfaces, slightly raised above the level of epidermis; palisade single-layered followed by 4–6 layers of closely packed spongy parenchyma with chloroplast and oleoresin; stomatal index 10–12–15 on upper surface and 14–15–16 on lower surface; palisade ratio 3.8; vein islet number 31–35.

Powder: Greenish, shows thin-walled, parenchymatous cells, a few containing reddish-brown contents, unicellular and multicellular-trichomes either entire or in pieces; thin-walled fibers, xylem vessels with pitted thickenings, fragments of epidermal cells in surface view having irregular shape, oil globules, rounded to oval, simple as well as compound starch grains having 2–5 components, measuring 3–17 μ in diameter.

Table 18.10: Identity, purity and strength of Tulsi

Foreign matter	NMT 2%
Total ash	NMT 10%
Acid-insoluble ash	NMT 1.5%
Alcohol-soluble extractive	NLT 4%
Water-soluble extractive	NLT 8%

TLC of tulsi oil diluted in chloroform-toluene (1:10) (obtained by steam distillation):

Adsorbent: Silica gel 'G'

Solvent system: Toluene: ethyl acetate (93:7)

Standard: Eugenol to be applied as standard also diluted in 130 ratio and 10 μl of each to be applied in band form.

Spraying agent: Vanillin-sulfuric acid reagent and heat the plate at 110°C for 5 minutes.

Standard Rf: Eugenol (orange-brown) approx. Rf. value 0.7.

Constituents: The major components of Tulsi is the essential oil like eugenol, carvacrol, nerol and eugenolmethylether. Leaves contain ursolic acid, apigenin, luteolin, apigenin-7-O-glucuronide, luteolin-7-O-glucuronide, orientin and molludistin.

Therapeutic Uses

Leaf: Carminative, stomachic, antispasmodic, antiasthmatic, antirheumatic, expectorant, stimulant, hepatoprotective, antiperiodic, antipyretic and diaphoretic.

Seed: Used in genitourinary diseases.

Root: Antimalarial.

Plant: Adaptogenic and antistress.

Essential oil: Antibacterial and antifungal.

Apamarga (Root) (Table 18.11)

Synonyms: Sanskrit: Adhahsalya, Sikhari; **English:** Prickly chaff flower; **Hindi:** Chirchira, Latjira

Biological source: Apamarga consists of dried root of *Achyranthes aspera* Linn., belonging to family Amaranthaceae.

Habitat: A stiff erect herb found commonly throughout the tropical and subtropical regions as a weed up to 900 m, up to an altitude of 2,100 m in the southern Andaman Islands.

Description

a. Macroscopic characters of root:

Color: Yellowish-brown

Odor: Not distinct

Taste: Not characteristic

Shape: Cylindrical slightly ribbed

Extra features: Rough due to presence of some root scars, secondary and tertiary roots are also present.

b. Microscopic characters of root: Mature root shows 6–10-layered, rectangular, tangentially elongated, thin-walled cork cells; secondary cortex consisting of 6–9 layers, oval to rectangular, thin-walled parenchymatous cells having scattered, thick-walled, irregular lignified stone cells, followed by 5–6 discontinuous rings of anomalous secondary thickening, composed of vascular tissues; small patches of sieve tubes are distinct in the phloem parenchyma demarcating the xylem rings; secondary xylem composed of tracheids, fibers and parenchyma; vessels with both simple and bordered pits and with scalariform thickening, measuring 135–348 μ in length and 32–64 μ in width; fibers pointed at both ends with walls moderately thickened, measuring 260–740 μ in length and 12–24 μ in width; tracheids have tapering ends, measuring 165–535 µ in length and 17–34 µ in width. In *A. bidentata* BL., vessels show bordered pits and reticulate thickening; medullary rays not distinct; stone cells and prismatic crystals absent in cortex.

Powder: Yellowish-brown; shows fragments of rectangular cork cells, stone cells, vessels showing bordered pits and scalariform thickening, fibers and a few prismatic crystals of calcium oxalate.

Table 18.11: Identity, purity and strength of apamarga

Foreign matter	NMT 1%
Total ash	NMT 9%
Acid-insoluble ash	NMT 1%
Alcohol-soluble extractive	NLT 2%
Water-soluble extractive	NLT 10%

TLC of alcoholic extract of apamarga

Adsorbent: Silica gel 'G'

Solvent system: Chloroform: methanol (95:5)

Detecting agent: UV (366 nm) and iodine chamber

Rf: Five fluorescent zones at Rf. 0.05, 0.19, 0.43, 0.50 and 0.97 (all light blue under UV), six spots appear at Rf. 0.05, 0.12, 0.43, 0.50, 0.92 and 0.97 (all yellow in iodine chamber).

Spraying agent: Dragendorff reagent followed by 5% methanolic-sulfuric acid reagent, two spots appear at Rf 0.12 and 0.97 (both light orange).

Constituents: The whole plant contains the alkaloids achyranthine and betaine, ecdysterone and oleanolic acid, tannins and glycosides. The ashes of the plant yield large quantities of potash. The roots contain free oleanolic acid (0.096%) and its saponins (1.93%).

Therapeutic uses: Astringent, pectoral (ashes of the plant used in asthma and cough), diuretic, hepatoprotective, emmenagogue, abortifacient activity, emetic and antifungal.

Dhatura (Seed) (Table 18.12)

Synonyms: Sanskrit: Kanaka, Ummatta; **English:** White thorn apple; **Hindi:** Dhatura

Biological source: Dhatura consists of dried seeds of *Datura metel* Linn.; Syn. *D. fastuosa* L., *D. alba* Ramph; *D. cornucopaea* Hort, belonging to family Solanaceae.

Habitat: It occurs wild throughout India, particularly in waste place.

Description

a. Macroscopic characters of seed:

Color: Yellowish-brown

Odor: Odorless

Taste: Bitter

Size: 0.6 cm long, 0.4 cm wide

Extra features: Surface finely pitted, reniform, compressed and flattened.

b. Microscopic characters of seed: Shows in outline more or less elongated, irregular or wavy structure having bulgings at either side; testa single-layered consists of thick-walled, lignified, sclerenchymatous cells forming club-shaped structure, followed by 3–5-layered more or less tangentially elongated, thin-walled, parenchymatous cells; endosperm encloses more or less curved embryo composed of polygonal, thin-walled, parenchymatous cells, filled with aleurone grains and abundant oil globules.

Powder: Brown and oily; shows fragments of testa of groups of thick-walled, light brown sclerenchymatous cells; polygonal, thin-walled parenchymatous cells containing oil globules and aleurone grains.

Table 8.12: Identity, purity and strength of datura	
Foreign matter	NMT 2%
Total ash	NMT 6%
Acid-insoluble ash	NMT 1%
Alcohol-soluble extractive	NLT 5%
Water-soluble extractive	NLT 7%

TLC of Alcoholic Extract

Adsorbent: Silica gel 'G' plate.

Solvent system: Toluene: Ethylacetate: diethylamine (7:2:1).

Detecting agent: U.V. (366 nm) and iodine chamber.

Spraying agent: Dragendorff reagent.

Rf: Three fluorescent zones at Rf 0.18, 0.33 (both light blue) and 0.93 (blue) in UV, three spots appear at Rf 0.33, 0.47 and 0.93 (all yellow) in iodine vapor, two spots appear at Rf 0.33 and 0.47 (both orange) with spraying agent.

Constituents: It mainly contains tropane alkaloids like hyoscyamine and fixed oil.

Therapeutic uses: It is used in headache, hemiplegia, epilepsy, delirium, convulsions, cramps, rigid thigh muscles and rheumatism.

Garlic (Bulb) (Table 18.13)

Synonyms: Sanskrit: Rasona; **English:** Garlic; **Gujrati:** Lasan; **Hindi:** Lahasun

Biological source: Garlic consists of bulb of *Allium sativum* Linn., belonging to family Liliaceae.

Habitat: A perennial bulbous plant, cultivated as an important condiment crop native to central Asia, cultivated all over India.

Description

a. Macroscopic characters of bulb:
- *Color:* Thin papery whitish and brittle scales having 2–3 yellowish green folded leaves.
- *Shape:* Sub-globular
- *Size:* 4–6 cm in diameter, consisting of 8–20 cloves, 2–3 cm long and 0.5–0.8 cm wide.
- *Odor:* Peculiarly pungent and disagreeable
- *Taste:* Acrid gives warmth to the tongue.

b. Microscopic characters of bulb:

A clove of bulb shows tri to tetrangular appearance in outline; outer scale consists of an outer epidermis, followed by hypodermal crystal layer, mesophyll made of parenchyma cells and an inner epidermis; both outer and inner epidermises consist of subrectangular cells; hypodermis consists of compressed, irregular, tangentially elongated cells, each cell having large prismatic crystals of calcium oxalate, while many cells contain small prismatic crystals also, mesophyll several layers of parenchymatous cells having a few vascular tissues with spiral vessels; inner epidermis similar to outer one; inner scale similar to outer scale but outer epidermis composed of sclerenchymatous cells; prismatic crystals in hypodermis slightly smaller. In surface view, cells of outer epidermis elongated, narrow with thin porous wall while those of inner epidermis similar to outer one but non-porous; cells of hypodermal crystals layer ellipsoidal with thick porous walls, each cell having large prismatic crystals of calcium oxalate, many cells also contain small prismatic crystals in addition to bigger ones; inner scale shows markedly sclerenchymatous cells with greatly thickened walls and very narrow lumen; cells of

Table 18.13: Identity, purity and strength of garlic	
Foreign matter	NMT 2%
Total ash	NMT 4%
Acid-insoluble ash	NMT 1%
Alcohol-soluble extractive	NLT 2.5%
Loss on drying	NLT 60%
Volatile oil	NLT 0.1%

hypodermal crystal layer somewhat smaller with walls more frequently pitted, size of crystals also smaller.

TLC of the Alcoholic Extract

Adsorbent: Silica gel 'G' plate

Solvent system: n-Butanol: isopropanol: acetic acid: water (3 : 1 : 1 : 1)

Detecting agent: Under UV (366 nm) and iodine chamber.

Spraying agent: Ninhydrin and vanillin-sulfuric acid reagent, heating the plate for 10 minutes at 110°C.

Rf: Two fluorescent zones at Rf. 0.58 and 0.72 (both light blue under UV), nine spots appear at Rf. 0.18, 0.26, 0.34, 0.38, 0.46, 0.58, 0.72, 0.77 and 0.93 (all yellow in iodine chamber), seven spots appear at Rf. 0.26, 0.38, 0.46, 0.58, 0.67, 0.72 and 0.93 (all pink with ninhydrin). Seven spots appear at Rf. 0.26, 0.38, 0.46, 0,58, 0.67, 0.72 and 0.93 (all gery with vanillin-sulfuric acid reagent).

Constituents: Volatile oil containing allyl disulphide and diallyl disulphide. It also contains allin, allicin, mucilage and albumin.

Therapeutic uses: It is used as antibiotic, bacteriostatic, fungicide, anthelmintic, antithrombic, hypotensive, hypoglycemic, hypocholesterolemic. Also used for upper respiratory tract infections and catarrhal conditions.

Black Pepper (Table 18.14)

Synonyms: Sanskrit: Vellaja; **English:** Black pepper; **Hindi:** Kalimirch

Biological source: It consists of fully mature dried fruit of *Piper nigrum* Linn., belonging to family Piperaceae.

Habitat: A climber, cultivated from Konkan Southwards, especially in North Konkan Kerala, and also in Assam, Karnataka, Maharashtra, and Kerala.

Description

a. Macroscopic characters of fruit:
Color: Greyish-black to black
Odor: Aromatic
Taste: Pungent.
Size: 0.4–0.5 cm in diameter.
Extra features: Fruit is hard and wrinkled.

b. Microscopic characters of fruit: Fruit consists of a thick pericarp for about one-third of fruit and an inner mass of perisperm, enclosing a small embryo; pericarp consists of epicarp, mesocarp and endocarp. Epicarp composed of single layered, slightly sinuous, tabular cells forming epidermis, below which, are present 1 or 2 layers of radially elongated, lignified stone cells adjacent to group of cells of parenchyma. Mesocarp wide, composed of band of tangentially elongated parenchymatous cells having a few isolated, tangentially elongated oil cells present in outer region and a few fibrovascular bundles, a single row of oil cells in the inner region of mesocarp. Endocarp composed of a row of beaker-shaped stone cells; testa single-layered, yellow-colored, thick-walled sclerenchymatous cells; perisperm contains parenchymatous cells having a few oil globules and packed with abundant, oval to round, simple and compound starch grains measuring 5.5–11.0 μ in diameter; having 2–3 components and a few minute aleurone grains.

Powder: Blackish-grey; shows debris with a characteristic, in groups, more or less isodiametric or slightly elongated stone cells, interspersed with thin-walled, polygonal hypodermal cells; beaker-shaped stone cells from endocarp and abundant polyhedral, elongated cells from perisperm, packed tightly with masses of minute compound and single, oval to round, starch grains measuring 5.5–11.0 μ in diameter; having 2–3 components and a few aleurone grains and oil globules.

Table 18.14: Identity, purity and strength of black pepper

Foreign matter	NMT 2%
Total ash	NMT 5%
Acid-insoluble ash	NMT 0.5%
Alcohol-soluble extractive	NLT 6%
Water-soluble extractive	NLT 6%

TLC of the Alcoholic Extract

Adsorbent: Silica gel 'G' plate

Solvent system: Toluene: ethylacetate (7 : 3)

Detecting agent: UV (366 nm), iodine chamber

Spraying agent: Dragendorff reagent followed by 5% methanolic-sulfuric acid and vanillin-sulfuric acid reagent and heating the plate for 10 minutes at 110°C.

Rf: Visible light four spots at Rf. 0.05, 0.08 (both light green), 0.27 (light yellow) and 0.52 (yellow). Under UV (366 nm) 10 fluorescent zones are visible at Rf. 0.05, 0.08 (both light brown), 0.20 (light blue), 0.46 (blue), 0.52 (greenish-yellow), 0.57 (bluish-yellow), 0.66 (light-blue), 0.74 (light pink), 0.82 and 0.97 (both blue). On exposure to iodine vapor, eleven spots appear at Rf. 0.05, 0.08, 0.14, 0.20, 0.27, 0.34, 0.46, 0.57, 0.66, 0.74 and 0.97 (all yellow). On spraying with Dragendorff reagent followed by 5% methanolic-sulfuric acid reagent, nine spots appear at Rf. 0.05 (light-orange), 0.14, 0.20, 0.27 (all orange), 0.46, 0.57 (both yellowish-orange), 0.66, 0.74 (both orange) and 0.97 (light-orange). On spraying with vanillin-sulfuric acid reagent and heating the plate for 10 minutes at 110°C, 12 spots appear at Rf. 0.05, 0.08, 0.20, 0.27, 0.46, 0.52, 0.57, 0.66, 0.74, 0.82, 0.90.and 0.97 (all violet).

TLC of Piperine

Preparation of the extract: Extract 1 g of pepper powder by heating under reflux for 15 minutes with 10 ml methanol. Filter, evaporate the filtrate so as to reduce it to 2 ml and use for TLC application.

Standard Piperine

Dilute 5 gm in 5 ml methanol.

Adsorbent: Silica gel plate

Solvent system: Toluene: ethylacetate (7:3) (saturate the chamber for at least 30 minutes)

Application: Pepper extract: 20 µ

Piperine: 10 µ

Running distance: 10 to 12 cm

Drying: Air drying for 15 to 20 min and then in an oven for 5 min.

Detection: Cool and spray the plate thoroughly with vanillin-sulfuric acid reagent and heat at 110°C for 5–10 min under observation. When piperine spots appear lemon yellow, the plate is to be taken out. Over-heating turns yellow spots to violet.

Rf. of piperine: Approximately 0.5 in case of hand made plates.

Constituents: The fruit yielded alkaloids like piperine, piperatine and piperidine; amides, piperyline, piperoleins A and B, N-isobutyl- cicosa-*trans*-2-*trans*-4-dienamide and essential oil.

Therapeutic uses: It is used as stimulant, carminative, diuretic, anticholerin, sialogogue and antiasthmatic. It is also used in fevers, dyspepsia, flatulence, indigestion, and as mucous membrane and gastrointestinal stimulant. Externally, as an rubefacient and stimulant to the skin.

19

Chromatography

The term chromatography refers to several related techniques for analyzing, identifying, or separating mixtures of compounds. Separation of two sample components in chromatography is based on their different distribution between two non-miscible phases. In each technique, a sample mixture is placed into a liquid or gas, called a mobile phase, a fluid, is streaming through the chromatographic system. The mobile phase carries the sample through a solid support, called the stationary phase, which contains an adsorbent or another liquid. The different compounds in the sample mixture move through the stationary phase at different rates, due to different attractions for the mobile and stationary phases. In gas chromatography, the mobile phase is a gas, in liquid chromatography, it is a liquid.

Theory of Chromatography

Typical response obtained by chromatography (i.e. a chromatogram):

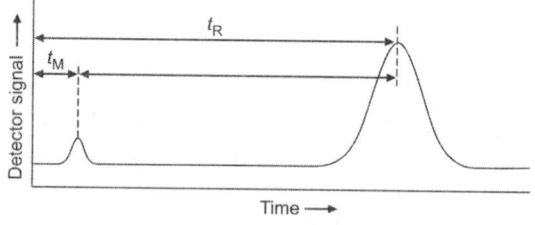

Where:
t_R = retention time (analyte peak)
t_M = void time (unretained peak)
t'_R = Corrected retention time

The separation of solutes in chromatography depends on two factors:

1. A difference in the retention of solutes (i.e. a difference in their time or volume of elution).
2. A sufficiently narrow width of the solute peaks (i.e. good efficiency for the separation system).

Solute Retention

A solute's retention time or retention volume in chromatography is directly related to the strength of the solute's interaction with the mobile and stationary phases.

Retention on a given column pertains to the particulars of that system:
1. Size of the column
2. Flow rate of the mobile phase

Capacity factor (k'): It is to measure of retention, determined from t_R or V_R.

$$k' = (t_R - t_M)/t_M$$

or

$$k' = (V_R - V_M)/V_M$$

Capacity factor is useful for comparing results obtained on different systems since it is independent on column length and flow-rate.

Efficiency

Efficiency is related theoretically to the various kinetic processes that are involved in solute retention and transport in the column. It is needed to determine the width or standard deviation (s) of peaks.

Chromatographic separations are a result of the interactions between the analyte and the two phases. In general, there are five types of interactions (Table 19.1).

1. Adsorption chromatography (Fig. 19.1)
2. Partition chromatography (Fig. 19.2)
3. Ion-exchange chromatography (Fig. 19.3)
4. Affinity chromatography (Fig. 19.4)
5. Size-exclusion chromatography (Fig. 19.5)

Table 19.1: Types of chromatography with their description

S. no.	Type of chromatography	Details	Examples
1.	**Adsorption chromatography** (also known as displacement, liquid/solid chromatography)	Adsorption chromatography is another technique that uses a solid stationary phase, the adsorbent, packed in a glass column, and a solvent, the mobile phase, that moves slowly through the packed column. A solvent used as a mobile phase is called an eluent. It is based on interactions between the solute and fixed active sites on the stationary phase. The active sites of the stationary phase interact with the functional groups of the compounds to be separated by non-covalent bonds, non-polar interactions, Van der Waals forces, and hydrophobic interactions. **Stationary phase:** A solid adsorbent packed in a column, spread on a plate, or on a porous paper. **Mobile phase:** Usually a liquid solvent.	Separation of alcohols from hydrocarbons using silica gel, Silanol groups on the gel interacts with the polar functional groups on the alcohols.
2.	**Partition chromatography**	It is a very useful technique because it can resolve minute differences in the solubility of the solutes. It is well suited for separating homologues and isomers. The solute molecules interact between	Separation of polar compounds, such as amino acids, carbohydrates, and water-soluble plant pigments.

(Contd.)

Table 19.1: Types of Chromatography with their description (*Contd.*)

S. no.	Type of chromatography	Details	Examples
		two non-miscible liquid phases according to their relative solubility. This process is also referred to as liquid/liquid chromatography. **Stationary phase:** A film of liquid that is strongly adsorbed to an inert support **Mobile phase:** A different liquid with a different polarity	
3.	Ion-exchange chromatography	The ion-exchange chromatography process allows the separation of ions and polar molecules based on the electrical properties of the molecules. **Stationary phase:** A resin or gel matrix contains covalently bound positive or negative functional groups. Cation exchange column carries negatively charged groups. Anion exchange column carries positively charged groups **Mobile phase:** A buffered aqueous solution carries a counter-ion whose charge is opposite and in equilibrium with the total charge of the resin.	—
4.	Affinity chromatography	In affinity chromatography, separations are based on specific interactions between interacting pairs of substance. such as a macromolecule and its substrate, cofactor, allosteric effector, or inhibitor. **Stationary phase:** A gel matrix to which a specific ligand is attached **Mobile phase:** A buffered solution	—

(*Contd.*)

Table 19.1: Types of Chromatography with their description (Contd.)

S. no.	Type of chromatography	Details	Examples
5.	**Size-exclusion chromatography:** (Known as gel filtration, gel permeation chromatography, and molecular sieve chromatography)	In size-exclusion chromatography, no chemical attraction or interaction occurs between the solutes and the stationery phase. The molecules are separated according to their size. High molecular weight molecules ranging between 2000 and 25,000,000 daltons can be separated. **Stationary phase:** A chemically inert material, such as a gel or a porous inorganic solid. Common examples are polyacrylamide polymers, porous glass or porous silica beads. **Mobile phase:** Water or an aqueous solution that solely serves as a carrier for the analyte.	—

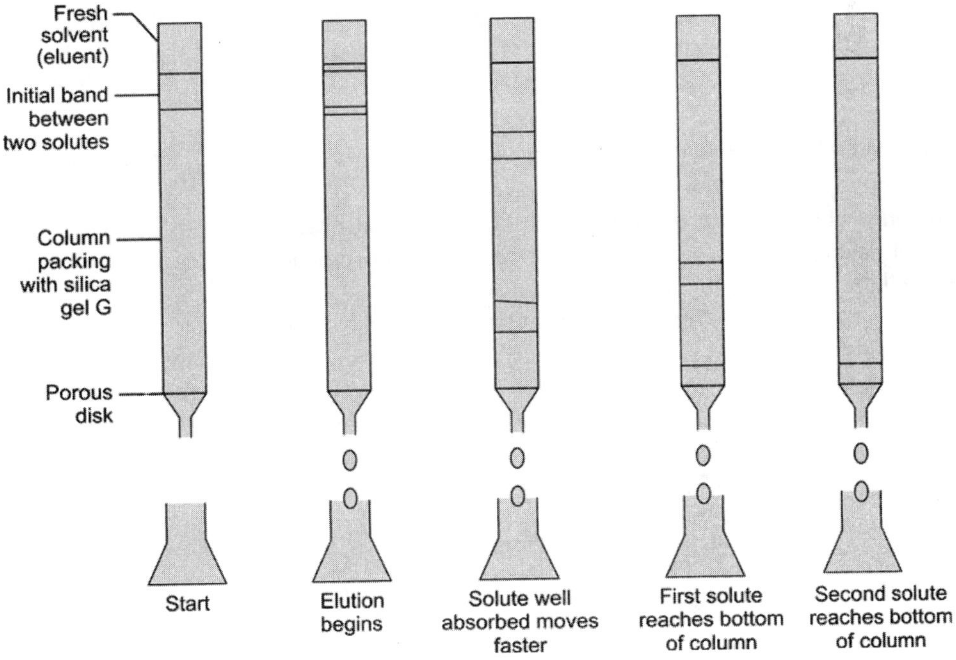

Fig. 19.1: Adsorption chromatography

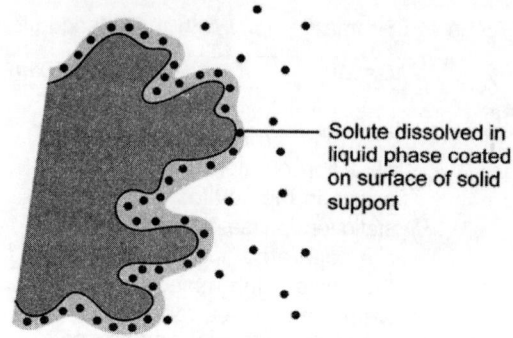

Fig. 19.2: Partition chromatography

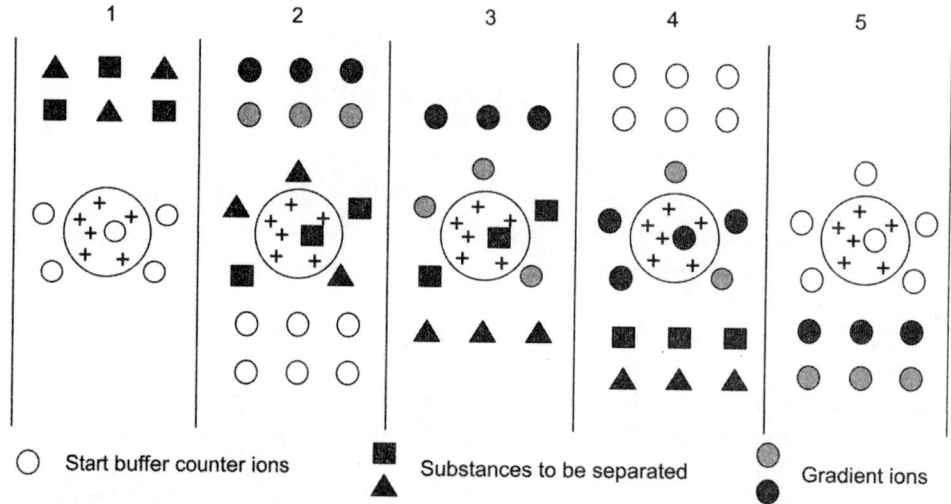

1. Ion exchange chromatography begins
2. Adsorption phase
3. Starting of desorption
4. End of desorption
5. Regeneration

Fig. 19.3: Ion-exchange chromatography

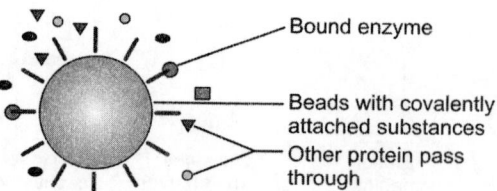

Fig. 19.4: Affinity chromatography

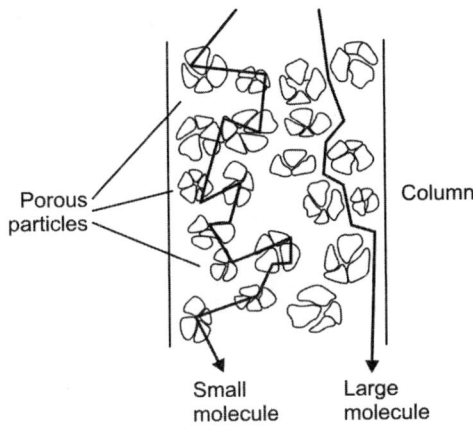

Fig. 19.5: Size-exclusion chromatography

Paper Chromatography (Fig. 19.6)

Principle

The principle of separation in paper chromatography is partition chromatography. Analytes are separated based on the interactions between two non-miscible liquid phases according to their relative solubility. The main difference of paper chromatography is that sheet of paper is used for the inert phase.

The paper usually contains pure cellulose and no lignin, copper, or other impurities and is available in strips or in sheets. Low-porosity paper will produce a slow rate of movement of the solvent and thick papers have increased sample capacity.

Stationary phase: Water that is tightly bound to the cellulose structure and fill interspaces of the paper fibers.

Mobile phase: Any solvent (also known as a developing solvent) that is partially miscible in water. Choice of the solvent will depend on the nature of the substances to be separated. Often, a mixture of two or three solvents is required.

1. **Capillary action:** The movement of liquid within the spaces of a porous material due to the forces of adhesion, cohesion, and surface tension. The liquid is able to move up the filter paper because its attraction to itself is stronger than the force of gravity.

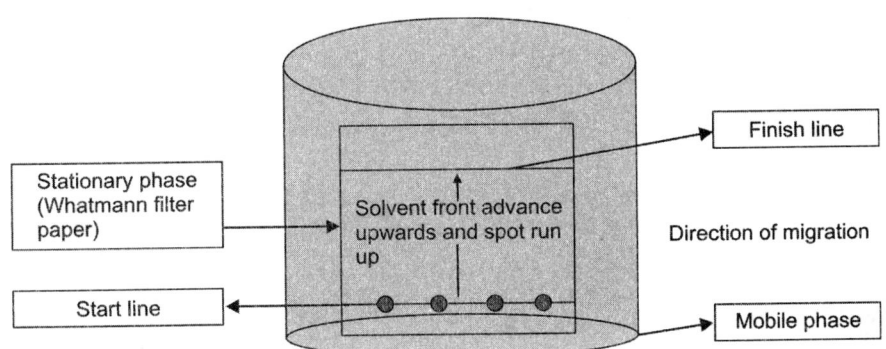

Fig. 19.6: Paper chromatography

2. **Solubility:** The degree to which a material (solute) dissolves into a solvent. Solutes dissolve into solvents that have similar properties. This allows different solutes to be separated by different combinations of solvents. Separation of components depends on both their solubility in the mobile phase and their differential affinity to the mobile phase and the stationary phase.

Techniques Used in Paper Chromatography

Ascending technique: In a chromatographic chamber, the solvent rises up the paper by capillary action and allows a separation of the components as it ascends.

Descending technique: In a chromatographic chamber, a paper strip is hanged vertically with the spotted end be up. The solvent rises up the wick and descends across the spot and down the paper. This technique permits a separation over a longer distance and allows an increase in resolution.

Applications

1. It is used for diagnosis of presence of amino acids in urine.
2. In food industry, paper chromatography is usually used for highly polar compounds, such as sugars, amino acids, and natural pigments.

The analytes that are highly water-soluble or have the greater hydrogen-bonding capacity can move slower along the paper, while less polar compounds will travel faster with the solvent.

The degree of retention of a component is called the retardation factor (R_f).

$$(R_f) = \frac{\text{Distance migrated by an analyte } (Da)}{\text{Distance migrated by the solvent } (Ds)}$$

Thin Layer Chromatography (Fig. 19.7)

The stationary phase is a thin layer of a solid, such as alumina or silica supported on an inert base such as glass, aluminum foil or insoluble plastic. The mixture is 'spotted' at the bottom of the TLC plate and allowed to dry. The plate is placed in a closed vessel containing solvent (the mobile phase) so that the liquid level is below the spot.

The solvent ascends the plate by capillary action, the liquid filling the spaces between the solid particles. This technique is usually done in a closed vessel to ensure that the atmosphere is saturated with solvent vapor and that evaporation from the plate is minimized before the run is complete. The plate is removed when the solvent front approaches the top of the plate and the position of the solvent front recorded before it is dried.

Advantages

1. More reproducible.
2. Separations are very efficient because of the much smaller particle size of the stationary phase.

HPLC (Fig. 19.8)

High performance liquid chromatography (HPLC) is a separation technique that involves injection of a small volume of liquid sample into a tube packed with tiny particles (3 to 5 µm in diameter called the stationary phase) where individual components of the sample are moved down the packed tube (column) with a liquid (mobile phase) forced through the column by high pressure delivered by a pump. These components are separated from one another by the column packing that involves various chemical and/or physical interactions between their molecules and the packing particles. These separated components are detected at the exit of this tube

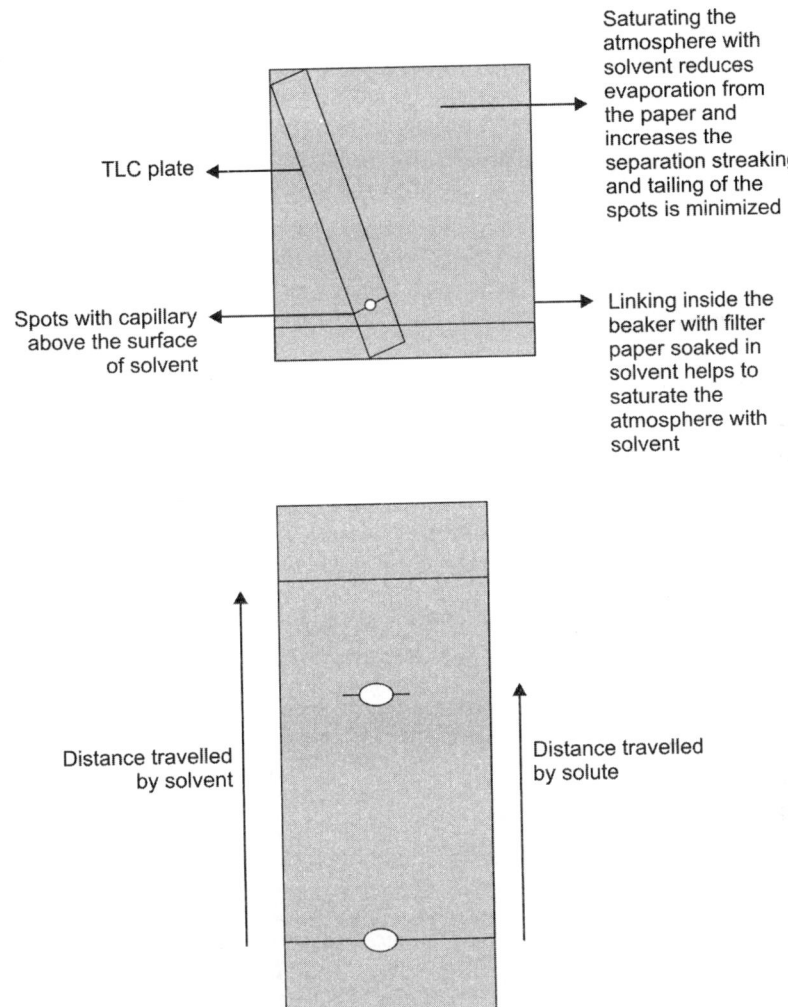

Fig. 19.7: Thin layer chromatography

(column) by a flow-through device (detector) that measures their amount. An output from this detector is called a "liquid chromatogram".

HPTLC

HPTLC (High performance thin layer chromatography) is an advanced and automated form of TLC that provides superior separation power and suitable for qualitative and quantitative analytical tasks. It is a flexible, versatile and economical process in which the various stages are carried out independently. It promotes for sample preparation requirements are often minimal, simultaneous processing of sample and standard, no prior treatment for solvents like filtration and degassing, higher separation efficiencies, shorter analysis time, less consumption of mobile phase, visual detection possible, efficient data acquisition and processing, low cost per analysis and low maintenance cost of the instrument. It is a valuable tool for reliable identification as it provides chromatographic fingerprints that can be visualized and stored as electronic image.

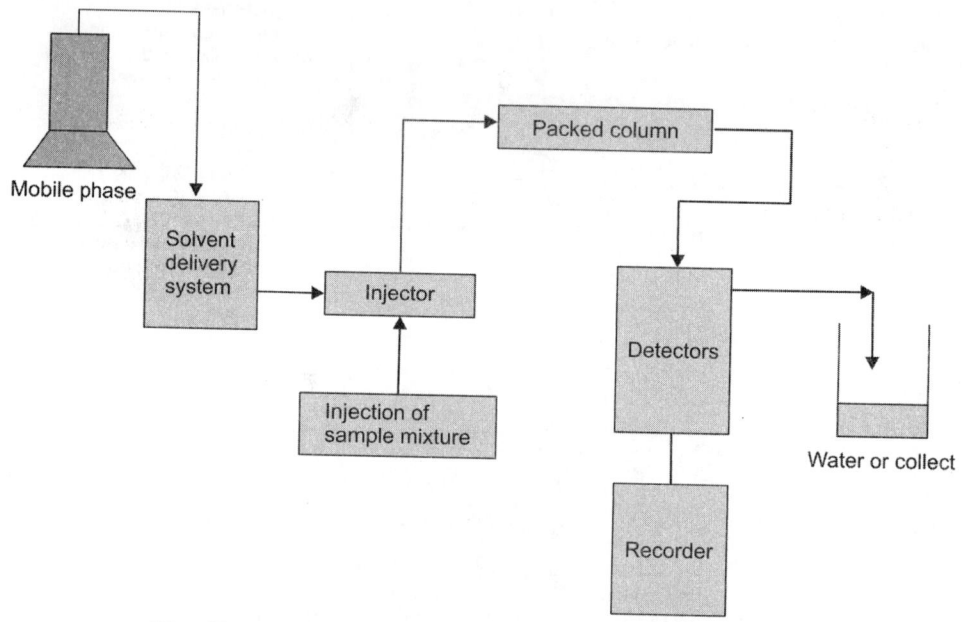

Fig. 19.8: High performance liquid chromatography (HPLC)

Table 19.2: Application of chromatography in evaluation of herbal drugs

S. no.	Herbal drug	Chromatography	Solvent system	Detecting reagent
1.	Ginseng	TLC	Chloroform: methanol: ethyl acetate: water (15:22:40:1)	UV at 366 nm
2.	Rhubarb	TLC	Acetone: water: formic acid (18:1:1)	UV at 366 nm
3.	Cinchona alkaloids	TLC	Chloroform: diethylamine (90:10)	UV at 366 nm
4.	Rhubarb	TLC	Acetone: water: formic acid (18:1:1)	UV at 366 nm
5.	Atropine	TLC	Methanol: acetone: diethylamine (25:24:1)	Dragendorffs reagent
6.	Acacia	TLC	Ethyl acetate: methanol: water (50:28:20:2)	Vanillin: Hydrochloric reagent
7.	Apamarga	TLC	n-Hexane: ethyl acetate: glacial acetic acid (10:5:0.1)	Sulfuric acid reagent

(Contd.)

Table 19.2: Application of chromatography in evaluation of herbal drugs *(Contd.)*

S. no.	Herbal drug	Chromatography	Solvent system	Detecting reagent
8.	Vasaka	HPLC	Methanol: water (2:3)	UV at 298 nm
9.	Bael	TLC	Toluene: ether (1:1)	Potassium hydroxide reagent
10.	Kalmegh	TLC (7:1)	Chloroform: methanol	20% sulfuric acid in methanol and heat 120°C
		HPLC	Chloroform: methanol (9:1)	UV at 254 nm
11.	Guggul	HPLC	Acetonitrile: water (65:35)	UV at 242 nm
12.	Coriander	TLC	Toluene: ethylacetate (9.3:0.7)	Vanillin sulfuric acid reagent
13.	Curcuma	TLC	Chloroform: ethanol: glacial acetic acid	Under UV 366 nm light
14.	Amla	TLC	n-propanol: n-butanol: 4N ammonia (7:1:2)	UV 254 nm
15.	Liquorice	TLC	Toluene: ethyl acetate: glacial acetic acid (12.5:7.5:0.5)	UV 254 nm
16.	Tulsi	TLC	Toluene: ethyl acetate (9.9:0.1)	Vanillin sulfuric acid reagent
17.	Black pepper	TLC	Toluene: ethyl acetate (7:3)	UV 254 nm
18.	Kantakari	TLC	Toluene: ethyl acetate: diethylamine (7:2:1)	Modified Dragendroffs reagent

20

Herbal Drug Interactions

Herb: An herb refers to non-woody seed-producing plants that die to the ground at the end of the growing season. In the culinary arts, it refers to vegetable products used to add flavor or aroma to food. But in the field of medicine, it is most accurately defined as crude drugs of vegetable origin utilized for the treatment of disease states, often of a chronic nature, or to attain or to maintain a condition of improved health.

Herbal Quality

The United States Pharmacopeia (USP) and *The National Formulary* (NF) monographs established legal standards of identity and, subject to the limitations of the methods of the period, quality of the vegetable drugs. The matter of proper identification and appropriate quality, lack of adulteration, sophistication, or substitution is an extremely important one in the field of herbal medicine. The matter of standardization of herbs or herbal extracts, the concentration of active constituents in different lots of supposedly identical plant material is highly variable. Also of great importance to the quality of an herb is the environmental conditions, e.g. fertility of the soil, length of growing season, temperature, amount of moisture, and time of harvest are some of the significant factors. Processing also plays a role. Some constituents are heat labile, and the plant material containing them needs to be dried at low temperatures. Other active principles are destroyed by enzymatic processes that continue for long periods of time, if the herb is dried too slowly. If the chemical identity of the constituent is known, it or a marker compound indicative of the activity of the herb can usually be isolated and quantified by appropriate physical or chemical methods. If it is unknown, if it is a complex mixture of constituents, or if no marker compound is available, biological assays, such as that employed for digitalis must be utilized, at least initially. Once the potency of the herb is known, it can be mixed with appropriate quantities of material of greater or lesser potency to produce a product with defined activity.

General Guidelines in the Use of Herbal Medicines (Table 20.1)

Unfortunately, in the United States, the FDA does not regulate herbal medicines as drugs but rather as dietary supplements; consequently, health or therapeutic claims cannot be placed on the package label. The FDA neither establishes nor regularly enforces any standards of quality for herbal products. This means that one must rely upon the reputation of the producer for any quality assurance. Products are often misbranded, and often the quantities of the ingredients are not listed. In mixtures containing large numbers of herbal constituents, quantities sufficient to render a therapeutic effect may be lacking. Safety considerations include warnings and precautions relative to the use of a particular herb, drug–drug interactions between

Table 20.1: Safety precautions of herbs with justification

Safety precautions of herbs	Reason
Herbal use is not recommended for pregnant women	In the pregnant woman, most drugs cross the placental barrier to some extent, and these expose the developing fetus to potential teratogenic effects of the drug. **First trimester:** Teratogenic susceptibility, anatomical malformations
Lactating mothers	The potential exists for the secretion of the drug in the mother's milk, resulting in adverse effects in the nursing infant.
Infants or children under the age of six	The body and organ functions of infants and young children are in a continuous state of development. Changes in the relative body composition (lipid content, protein binding, and body-water compartments) will produce a different drug distribution in their bodies than in adults also produce a slower drug metabolism
Elderly patient	Aging process results in a significant increase in the proportion of body fat to muscle mass and in decreases in renal function, total body water, lean body mass, organ perfusion, and hepatic microsomal enzyme activity. Such changes may lead to altered ADME of drugs that, in turn, could result in an accumulation of a drug in the body all the way to toxic levels.

prescription medications and the herbal medication, and the fact that certain groups of individuals often experience a higher incidence of adverse drug effects that could have dire consequences.

Mechanisms of Botanical–Drug Interactions

Interactions between pharmacologically active botanicals and drugs involve the same pharmacokinetic and pharmacodynamic mechanisms as drug–drug interactions.

Pharmacokinetic interactions: It involves alteration in absorption, distribution, metabolism, or excretion of the affected drug or botanical.

Pharmacodynamic interactions: Alter the relationship between the drug concentration and the pharmacological response for a drug or botanical.

Most pharmacokinetic and pharmacodynamic botanical–drug interaction studies and clinical cases in the literature evaluated the challenge of not knowing the identify and constitution of the botanical or botanical product, the difficulty of measuring concentration of a specific botanical or its active ingredient(s).

The pharmacist and doctors need to emphasis on the risks and benefits of herbal medicines, just as they do with conventional medicine. The fact that herbal medicines also have adverse effects and may give rise to potential drug-herb interactions does not imply that their use should be discouraged. Herbal medicines are found to be efficacious, sometimes being a suitable alternative to conventional drugs. Most herbal drugs have good safety profiles, therefore, they are often taken over a long period of time in combinations, but can provide an vacancy for enzyme induction/inhibition. The fundamental issue to consider them as medicines after having a look on their adverse effects and potential interactions (Table 20.2).

Table 20.2: Herb with their interactions

Herb	Chemical constituents	Uses	Herb drug interaction
Aloe vera	Polysaccharides like polymannans, and other constituents include glycoproteins and various carboxypeptidases, sterols, saponins, tannins, organic acids, vitamins, minerals and anthraquinone glycosides	Anti-inflammatory antitumor, immunomodulatory and antibacterial mild analgesic, antioxidant and antidiabetic effects.	Aloe vera juice reduces blood-glucose levels in patients with diabetes taking glibenclamide. Aloe vera does not interact with food and herbal medicine
Arjuna	**Triterpenoid saponins:** Arjunic arjunolic acid, and arjun glycosides **Flavonoids:** Quercetin asarjunone arjunolone, and luteolin **Polyphenols:** Gallic acid, ellagic acid	Heart tonic, it is used in diabetes mellitus, diarrhea, dysentery and obesity.	The interaction between arjuna and antithyroid drugs may deplete thyroid hormones based on experimental evidence. Arjuna when given with conventional CVS drugs appears to have some effects on cardiovascular function
Asafoetida	Gum resin contains ferulic acid esters and asaresinotannols, farnesiferols A, B and C, natural coumarin derivatives	Used to aid digestion, it is used in asthma and bronchitis	Asafoetida may interact with anticoagulants, and with conventional antihypertensives may be expected to produce additive hypotensive effects
Asparagus	**Saponins:** Asparagosides, steroidal glycosides, asparagusic acid. **Flavonoids:** Rutin, kaempferol and quercetin. Amino acids and polysaccharides	Diuretic, laxative, cardiac tonic and sedative	In larger quantities, it reduces the effectiveness anticoagulants like warfarin. It may be avoided with coumarins and indanediones because it contains vitamin K_1 content
Tea or coffee	Trimethylxanthine like caffeine, theobromine and theophylline	Stimulant and diuretic effects	It may antagonize the effects of antihypertensive drugs. Caffeine-containing herbs may produce a degree of additive diuresis with other diuretics. It is not recommended to be used with phenylpropanolamine, bitter orange and ephedra
Garlic	Sulfur-containing compounds, alliin, allicin	Antihypertensive, antithrombotic, fibrinolytic, antimicrobial, anticancer,	It may cause bleeding in those taking warfarin or fluindione. It is not

(Contd.)

Table 20.2: Herb with their interactions (Contd.)

Herb	Chemical constituents	Uses	Herb drug interaction
		expectorant, antidiabetic and lipid-lowering properties	recommended with alcohol, benzodiazepines, caffeine, chlorzoxazone, dextromethorphan, docetaxel, gentamicin, paracetamol and rifampicin
Ginger	Volatile oils, like zingiberene and bisabolene. The other, like zingerone, zingiberol, zingiberenol, curcumene, camphene and linalool are minor components	Carminative, anti-emetic, antiinflammatory, anti-spasmodic and antiplatelet	Antiplatelet effects for ginger that were synergistic with those of nifedipine
Senna	Anthraquinone glycosides are major components of senna. In the leaf, the anthraquinones include sennosides A, B, C and D, and palmidin A, rhein anthrone and aloe-emodin glycosides	Laxative	Senna has been predicted to interact with a number of drugs that lower potassium and digoxin. Senna may slightly reduce quinidine levels
Rhubarb	Anthraquinone glycosides, chrysophanol, emodin, rhein, aloe-emodin, physcion and sennosides A to E. Various tannins, stilbene glycosides, resins, starch and trace amounts of volatile oil	Treat diarrhea and as a flavoring in food	It shows interactions with corticosteroids and potassium-depleting diuretics
Pepper	Alkaloids and alkylamides, the most important being piperine, with piperanine, piperettine, piperlongumine, pipernonaline, lignans and minor constituents, such as the piperoleins	Used as a stimulant and carminative, and is reputed to have anti-asthmatic, antimicrobial, hepatoprotective and hypocholesterolemic effects	Piperine markedly increased the AUC of a single dose of nevirapine and of theophylline oxidant. High dose piperine also increased the AUC of rifampicin
Liquorice	Glycyrrhizin (glycyrrhizic or glycyrrhizinic acid), numerous phenolics and flavonoids of the chalcone and isoflavone type, and umbelliferone, glabrocoumarones A and B, herniarin and glycyrin	Expectorant, antispasmodic and anti-inflammatory, and to treat peptic and duodenal ulcers	Liquorice appears to diminish the effects of antihypertensives and may have additive effects on potassium depletion, if given in large quantities with laxatives and corticosteroids. liquorice may enhance the effects of warfarin

21

Phytonutrients: The Natural Drugs of Future

NUTRACEUTICALS

Dr. Stephen De Felice first coins the term nutraceutics in 1989 and he defined nutraceuticals as "food or parts of food that provide medical or health benefits including the prevention and treatment of diseases". The term functional food is also used to refer nutraceuticals. The US Congress in 1990 defined a medical food as a "food which is formulated to be consumed or administered orally under the supervision of a physician and which is intended for specific dietary management of a disease or condition for which distinctive nutritional requirements based on a recognized scientific principle established by medical evaluation". Since the introduction of nutraceuticals is very simple and risk free.

The old proverb "an apple a day will keep the doctor away" is now replaced by "a nutraceutical a day may keep the doctor away". Consumers are turning massively to food supplements to improve well-being where pharmaceuticals fail. Nutraceuticals are products and their derivatives that occur in nature and are constituents of plants and animal, including humans. These constituents confer a health benefit above and beyond basic nutrition or basic fortification. Nutraceuticals are the active ingredients in functional food or nutritional supplements that deliver a health benefit. Some examples are n-3 long-chain fatty acids in milk to reduce cardiovascular risks, probiotics in yogurt to improve growth of beneficial intestinal flora, phytosterols in margarine to reduce cholesterol uptake, and folic acid in flour to prevent spina bifida and reduce homocysteine, a risk factor for cardiovascular disease. Combinations of essential nutrients and nutraceuticals may strengthen the health promoting potential by synergy and could be expected to contribute to risk reduction of chronic diseases, ageing, etc.

Economic and Legal Factors

In 1994, the United States Congress, influenced by growing "consumerism" as well as strong manufacturer lobbying efforts, passed the Dietary Supplement and Health Education Act (DSHEA). Dietary supplements are governed under Current Good Manufacturing Practice in Manufacturing, Packaging or Holding Human Food (CGMP) regulations. Labeling of dietary supplements is under the purview of the FDA. In 1999, the FDA announced labeling recommendations for dietary supplements marketed in the USA.

Clinical Aspects of the Use of Botanicals

Many United States consumers have embraced the use of botanicals and other supplements as a "natural" approach to their health care. Unfortunately, misconceptions regarding safety and efficacy of the agents are common, and the fact that a substance can be called "natural" of course does not guarantee its safety. In fact, these products can be adulterated, misbranded, or contaminated either intentionally or unintentionally in variety of ways. Furthermore, the doses recommended for active botanical substances may be much higher than those considered clinically safe. For example, the doses recommended for several Ma-huang preparation contain three to five times the medically recommended daily dose of the active ingredient, ephedrine–dose that impose significant risk for patients with cardiovascular disease.

Adverse effects have been documented for a variety of botanical medications. Unfortunately, chemical analysis is rarely performed on the products involved. This leads to uncertainty about whether the primary herb or an adulterant caused the adverse effect. In some cases, the chemical constituents of the herb can clearly lead to toxicity.

Nutraceuticals are non-specific biological therapies used to promote wellness, prevent malignant processes and control symptoms. These can be grouped into the following three broad categories:

1. Substances with established nutritional functions, such as vitamins, minerals, amino acids and fatty acids—nutrients.

Table 21.1: Classes and components of phytonutrients

S. no.	Class/components	Sources	Potential benefits
1.	Fatty acids	Milk and meat	Improve body composition, reduce cancers
2.	Polyphenols		
	1. Flavonone	Citrus fruits	Neutralize free radicals, reduce risk of cancer
	2. Flavones	Fruits, vegetables, soyabean	
	3. Catechins/tannin	Tea, babul pods	
	4. Anthocyanidine	Fruits	
	5. Pro-anthocyanidine	Cocoa, chocolate, tea, rapeseed	Reduce cardiovascular disorders
3.	Saponins	Soybeans, chick pea	Lower cholesterol, anticancer
4.	Probiotics/prebiotics/synbiotics		
	Lactobacillus	Yogurt	Improve GI health
	Fructo-oligosaccharides	Whole grains, onions	
5.	Phytoestrogen		
	i. Daidzein, zenistein	Soybean, flax, maize	Reduce menopause symptoms, maintain bone health
	ii. Lignans	Flax, rye, vegetables	Reduce cancer and heart diseases
6.	Caroteinoids		
	β-caroteine	Oat, maize fodder, carrots, vegetables and fruits	Neutralize free radicals
	Luteine	Vegetables	Healthy vision
	Zeoxanthine	Eggs, citrus, corn	
	Lycopene	Tomatoes	Reduce prostate cancer
7.	Dietary fiber		
	Insoluble fiber	Wheat bran	Reduce breast, colon cancer
	β-glucan	Oats	Reduce cardiovascular disorders
	Whole grain	Cereal grains	

2. Herbs or botanical products as concentrates and extract—herbals.
3. Reagents derived from other sources, e.g. pyruvate, chondrotin sulfate, steroid, hormones, precursors) serving specific functions, such as sports nutrition—dietary supplements.

The detailed classification is summarized in Table 21.1.

Product Classes

Vitamins

Vitamins are essential organic compounds that are not synthesized in the human or animal organism. They must are consumed with the diet either as such or as a precursor, a so-called provitamin, which can be converted to the vitamin, e.g. β-carotene is a provitamin that is converted biochemically to vitamin A.

13 compounds or groups of compounds have been classified as vitamins (for humans) (Table 21.2):

Table 21.2: Types of vitamins

Water-soluble	Fat-soluble
Vitamin B_1 (thiamin)	Vitamin A (retinols)
Vitamin B_2 (riboflavin)	Vitamin D (calciferols)
Vitamin B_6 (pyridoxal group)	Vitamin E (tocopherols)
Vitamin C (L-ascorbic acid)	Vitamin K (phylloquinone)
Vitamin B_{12}	
Pantothenic acid	
Biotin	
Folic acid	
Niacin C	

$R^1 = R^2 = R^3 = CH_3$: α-tocopherol
$R^2 = H, R^1 = R^3 = CH_3$: β-tocopherol
$R^1 = H, R^2 = R^3 = CH_3$: γ-tocopherol
$R^1 = R^2 = H, R^3 = CH_3$: δ-tocopherol

Vitamin E: Vitamin E is a group of compounds based on 6-chromanol. Differences between α-, β-, γ-, δ-tocopherol are given in the number of methyl groups on the chromane ring.

Vitamin E is thought to function primarily as a chain-breaking antioxidant that prevents the propagation of free radical reactions in this manner protecting membrane lipids and blood lipids (e.g. LDL cholesterol) against oxidative damage. Vitamin E is believed to help prevent diseases associated with oxidative stress, such as cardiovascular disease, cancer, chronic inflammation, and neurologic disorders.

Vitamin K_1: Vitamin K is the term for 2-methyl-1, 4-naphthoquinone. Vitamin K is lipophilic compounds, heat resistant, stable in air, but sensitive to alkali and light. Vitamin K_1 is localized in chloroplasts of green leafy vegetable (84) and is also found in plant oils,

Vitamin K_1

Lutein

e.g. from soybeans, or olives. Vitamin K has a significant role to play in human health that is beyond its well-established function in blood clotting. Vitamin K may also positively affect Ca balance, a key mineral in bone metabolism.

Folic acid: Folic acid, N-[4-[[(2-amino-1,4-dihydro-4-oxo-6-pteridinyl) methyl] amino] benzoyl]-L-glutamic acid, is *de novo* synthesized in microorganisms and plants. These compounds are essential coenzymes for the C1-unit transfer at various oxidation levels.

Carotenoids: Dietary carotenoids are thought to provide health benefits by decreasing the risk of chronic diseases, particularly cancer, cardiovascular disease, and age-related eye diseases. The carotenoids are β-carotene, lycopene, lutein, and zeaxanthin.

Lutein: Lutein is one of the important and widespread natural carotenoids. Lutein can be extracted from natural sources, e.g. from tagetes, or marigold flower petals using various organic solvents.

Zeaxanthin: Zeaxanthin (3R, 30R)-dihydroxy-β, β-carotene) is widespread in nature, is found, e.g. as the yellow coloring in egg yolk and corn. Zeaxanthin reduces the risk of age-related macular degeneration.

Lutein and zeaxanthin are two nutritional carotenoids that are found in a wide variety of fruits and vegetables. Their antioxidant properties, their specific occurrence within the macula at high concentration has led to expectations that the intake of these carotenoids could contribute to reducing the risk for age-related macular degeneration (AMD).

Lycopene: Lycopene (ψ, ψ-carotene) is the red, acyclic carotenoid highly abundant in the tomato. Besides lycopene, tomatoes also contain the carotenoid precursors phytoene and phytofluene, as well as β-carotene and some other minor carotenoids. Other dietary sources are watermelon (23–72 mg/g wet weight), pink guava (~54 mg/g wet weight), pink grapefruit (~33 mg/g wet weight), and papaya (20–53 mg/g wet weight). The high antioxidant properties of lycopene are suggested to be linked with its effect on prevention of cancer and chronic diseases, such as cardiovascular disease. Lycopene might provide protection against oxidative DNA damage suggested to be an early event in carcinogenesis.

Polyunsaturated fatty acids: Polyunsaturated fatty acids (PUFA) are of interest because of their beneficial physiological activities.

20:4ω6; 20:4n6; 20Δ 5,8,11,14
arachidonic acid, AA

Zeaxanthin

Lycopene (*all-E*)

ARA: Arachidonic acid (AA), (all-Z)-5,8,11,14-eicosatetraenoic acid, in an essential fatty acid and a precursor in the biosynthesis of prostaglandin, thromboxanes, and leukotriens. AA occurs in liver, brain, glandular organs, and was isolated from liver lipids and beef.

DHA/EPA: Docosahexaenoic acid (DHA) is an omega-3 PUFA. Fish oils are rich on

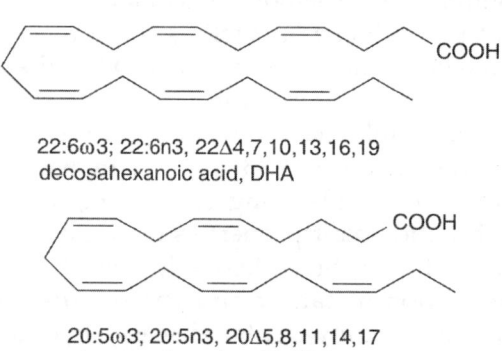

22:6ω3; 22:6n3, 22Δ4,7,10,13,16,19
decosahexanoic acid, DHA

20:5ω3; 20:5n3, 20Δ5,8,11,14,17
eicosapentaenoic acid, EPA

PUFA, especially eicosopentanoic acid (EPA) docosahexanoic acid (DHA). The content of EPA varies from 5 to 26% and of DHA from 6–26% of total fatty acid. PUFA and their ethyl esters are soluble in CO_2, and therefore, it is possible to concentrate and separate them using this nonflammable and nontoxic eluent.

CLA: Conjugated linoleic acid (CLA) was identified as a potential mutagen inhibitor. CLA is a term describing several isomers of linoleic acid (LL).

Health effects of PUFA: There are two main classes of PUFA, the omega-6 and the omega-3 that are formed from the two essential fatty acids linoleic and α-linolenic acids, respectively. These fatty acids have a structural role in cell membranes, where they regulate fluidity and affect the function of membrane-related proteins. In addition, PUFA are the precursors of eicosanoids, which have a variety of important biological activities and play a role in a number of diseases. The most relevant PUFA in cell membranes are arachidonic acid (AA) and docosahexaenoic acid (DHA), which are important structural and functional components of membranes especially in the central nervous system. Both DHA and AA make up one-third of all lipids in the brain's gray

18:2ω6; 18:2n6; 18Δ9,12
linolenic acid, LA

matter. These fatty acids must be supplied in sufficient amounts during fetal and infant brain growth. A deficit of omega-3 PUFAs during the perinatal brain growth or the retinal development can lead to disorders of the central nervous system and to impairment of vision, which may be irreversible.

Polyphenols: Polyphenols have been found to have beneficial health effects.

EGCG: (–)-Epigallocatechin gallate is one of the complex mixtures of polyphenols found in green tea (*Camelia sinensis*). Other catechins found in *Camelia sinensis*, are epicatechin (EC), and epicatechin gallate (ECG), and epigallocatechin (EGC). EGCG exerts a broad range of activities that include antioxidant, anti-inflammatory, antiangio-

X = H, Y = OH, epicathechin
X = H, Y = $C_7H_5O_5$, epicatechin gallate
X = OH, Y = OH, epigallocatechin
X = OH, Y = $C_7H_5O_5$, epigallocatechin gallate

genic, antiartherogenic, antithrombotic, and anti-infectious properties. These activities are agreed upon to play an important role in fending off disease.

Flavonoids and isoflavonoids are natural antioxidants and are suggested as agents responsible in the diet for the prevention of coronary diseases, breast cancer, and prostate cancer. Chemically, flavonoids and isoflavonoids are derivatives of 4H-chromene. Most important are the 4-oxo-chromens, such as flavones and 3-hydroxyflavones. Another important flavone is the plant dye quercetin, 3, 5, 7, 30, 40-penthydroxy-flavone, one of the most important and widely distributed of the flavonoid family. The following show structures of flavone, 4H-chromene, chromone, 3-hydroxyflavone, and quercetin.

Genistein: Genistein has been associated with reduced incidence of breast and prostate cancers, cardiovascular disease, and osteoporosis.

Phytosterols: Phytosterols are derived from isoprenoid biogenesis and are ubiquitous in higher plants. Usually, they are C27–29 substances with a 3-hydroxyl-steran core with C8–10 alkyl and alkenyl side chains at C-17. Various phytosterols, such as brassicasterol, stigmasterol, and beta-sitosterol. Phytosterols occur mostly in intracellular organelles, where they appear to play important roles in the stabilization of membranes. They have been found in nearly all plant tissues and organs, including leaves, stems, roots, blossoms, fruits, and seeds. The common dietary phytosterols are most widely established and known for their effects on serum cholesterol. These phytosterols have been shown to competitively inhibit the normally occurring adsorption of endogenous and dietary cholesterol from the intestines. Thus they can lead to lowering of serum cholesterol levels.

Others

Creatine: Creatine is a substance that occurs in the human body. The total amount of creatine in a normal healthy person is ~120 g (70 kg) person (256–258). Phosphocreatine, the phosphorylated creatine and creatine, are important for cellular energy storage, transport,

Creatine
(N-aminoiminomethyl–N-methylglycine)

and buffering. In the human organism, creatine is formed from the amino acids argenin, glycin, and methionin. Creatine pyruvate and its salts have several physiological property for treatment of obesity and overweight, and can be used to prevent free radicals and to enhance long-term performance.

Lipoic acid

(R)-α-Lipoic acid: Lipoic acid is a growth factor (274). (R)-(α)-Lipoic acid is the biologically active form and racemic lipoic acid is used as an antidote for liver diseases and poisoning. L-Lipoic acid serves as a coenzyme in the oxidative decarboxylation of ketoacids and can be found in every cell of vegetable and animal organisms.

Glucosamin: Glucosamin from exogeneous sources, e.g. food, is incorporated into the metabolic pathway of glycosaminglycan

Glucoseamin
(2-amino–2-deoxyglucose)

synthesis. Glucosamin increased the production of proteoglycans and sulfate uptake by articular cartilage.

Coenzyme Q10: Ubiquinone is a generic term for a family of quinines (2, 3-dimethoxy-

Coenzyme Q10

5-methyl-6-polyprenyl-benzoquinone) in which the number of prenyl groups varies from 1 to 10.

Conclusion

Nutraceuticals play an important role in therapeutic development but their future will be assured by level of purity, safety and efficacy. Nutraceuticals will continue to appeal because they are convenient for today's lifestyle.

Health care authorities consider prevention and treatment of diseases with nutraceuticals as a powerful measure for promoting optimal health, longevity and quality of life. It is well documented in literature that lack of nutraceuticals on our every day diet leads to various diseases. The present age is facing stress, pollution, hyperactivity and tension, where nutraceuticals play beneficial role in prevention and cure of the diseases.

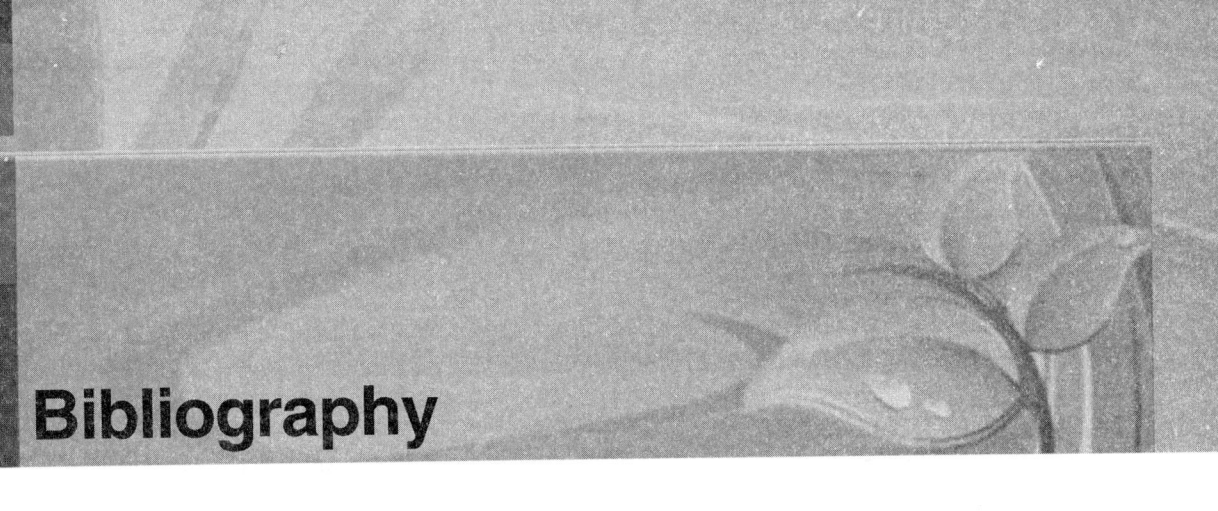

Bibliography

- Amrit Pal Singh, A Treatise on Phytochemistry, Emedia Science Ltd in the UK, 2002.
- Ansari SH. Essentials of Pharmacognosy, Birla Publcation, 2nd, 2007, 08.
- Barbour, MG, JH Burk, WD Pitts. Terrestrial plant ecology. The Benjamin/Cummings Publishing Co., Menlo Park, CA, 1987.
- Biren Shah. Textbook of Pharmacognosy and Phytochemistry, Elesivier Publications.
- Coultate, TP. Food. The chemistry of its components, 2nd Ed, London, 1995.
- Coyne, PI, MJ Trlica, CE Owensby. Carbon and nitrogen dynamics in range plants in DJ. Bedunah and RE Sosebee (eds.). Wildland plants: physiological ecology and developmental morphology. Society for Range Management. Denver, CO; PP 59–169; 1995.
- Daubenmire, RF. Plants and Environment. John Wiley and Sons, New York, 1974. NY. 422p. dems-pc-consulting.info/Ayurvedic_Medicine.pdf.
- Esposito, DeKorte. Aromatherapy: Art or Science? Highlights of Aromatherapy in Medicine Today, InetCE 221-999-04-095-H01, *www.inetce.com/articles/pdf/221-999-04-095-H01.pdf*.
- Evans, WC. Trease and Evans: Pharmacognosy, Elsevier, 15th, 2007.
- Fennema, Owen R. Food chemistry, 3rd Ed, Marcel Dekker, Inc. New York, 1996.
- Frank S. D'Amelio. Botanicals: A Phytocosmetic Desk Reference, CRC Press LLC, 1999.
- Fusetani N. Marine toxins: an overview Prog Mol Subcell Biol. 46, 2009.
- Handa, SS, Kapoor,VK. TB of Pharmacognosy, Vallabh Prakashan, 2nd, 2007.
- Harborn, JB. Phytochemical Methods: A guide to modern techniques of plant analysis, Springer, 3rd, 1998.
- Henry Kamer, Scientific and Appilied Pharmacognosy. John Wiley and Sons, New York, 1920.
- http://preuniversity.grkraj.org/html/3_PLANT_ANATOMY.htm.
- http://www.erowid.org/library/books_online/golden_guide/g151–160.shtml.
- http://www.fda.gov/RegulatoryInformation/Legislation/FederalFoodDrugandCosmeticActFDCAct.
- http://www.iloveindia.com/medicine-systems/homeopathy/homeopathy-history.html.
- http://www.iloveindia.com/medicine-systems/naturopathy/concept.html.
- http://www.iloveindia.com/medicine-systems/naturopathy/concept.html.
- http://www.pharmagateway.net/ArticlePage.aspx?DOI = 10.1208/ps050325.
- http://www.pharmatutor.org/pharmacognosy/scope-of-pharmacognosy.html.
- http://www.scribd.com/doc/167866521/Corrected-General-Study-on-Formation-of- secondary-Metabolites.

- http://www.scribd.com/doc/21742180/Histrocial development of pharmacognosy [cited 2010 july 29].
- http://www.scribd.com/doc/50884163/01Plant-Anatomy.
- http://www.techno-preneur.net/technology/project-profiles/chemical/ayurvedic.html.
- http://www.webzeest.com/article/1957/plant-anatomy.
- Indian Herbal Pharmacopoeia, IDMA, I, 2002.
- Janet Emerson. Top Aromatherapy Essential Oils, Balms And Lotions, Louchuck.
- Jensen, RE. Climate of North Dakota. National Weather Service, North Dakota State University, Fargo, ND. 48p, 1972.
- Kalia, AN. TB of Industrial Pharmacognosy, CBS Publishers & Distributors, 1st; 1–285; 2010 Rangari, VD. Pharmacognosy and Phytochemistry-Vol. I, Career Publication, 2nd; 2009.
- Kanam Salma. General study of formatin of secondary metabolites, Pharmacognosy, available on 12/09/2007.
- Kawakita, Tetsuya; Sano, Chiaki; Shioya, Shigeru; Takehara, Masahiro;Yamaguchi, Shizuko (2005). "Monosodium Glutamate". Ullmann's Encyclopedia of Industrial Chemistry.
- Khandelwal KR. Practical Pharmacognosy, Nirali Prakashan, 2008.
- Khandelwal. Practical Pharmacognosy, Nirali Prakashan, 22nd, 2013.
- Kokate, CK. Textbook of Pharmacognosy. Nirali Prakashan, Pune, 42th, 2008.
- Kokate, CK. Practical Pharmacognosy, Nirali Prakashan, 4th, 2008.
- Leopold, AC; PE Kriedemann. Plant growth and development. McGraw-Hill Book Co., New York, NY. 545p, 1975.
- Llewellyn L. Manske, Range Plant Growth and Development are Affected by Environmental Factors, Dickinson Research Extension Center, Grassland section, 2001 Annual Report (http://www.ag.ndsu.edu/archive/dickinso/research/2000/range00b.htm)
- Meyer, Lillian Hoagland. Food chemistry, The AVI publishing company, Inc.Westport, Connecticut, 1982.
- Mohammed Ali. Textbook of Pharmacognosy, CBS Publishers & Distributors, 2nd, 1–518; 2007.
- Mukherjee, PK. Quality Contorl of herbal drugs: An Approch to evaluation of botanicals, Business Horizons, 1st , 2012.
- Nandkarni, AK. Indian Materia Medica Vol I, Papular Prakashan, I, 1st, 2007.
- Nandkarni, AK. Indian Materia Medica Vol II, Papular Prakashan, I, 1st, 2007.
- Nutritional Cosmetics: Beauty from Within, William Andrew, Oxford, Elsevier, 2009, 1–47.
- Odum, EP. Fundamentals of ecology. WB. Saunders Company. Philadelphia, PA. 574p, 1971.
- Paola Pittia Flavors in food, University of Teramo, Italy, 2007.
- Parliament, TH. Thermal generation of aromas, VI series, Americanchemical society. USA, 1989.
- Paul M Dewick, Medicinal Natural Products, A Biosynthetic Approach, second edition, John Wiley and Sons Ltd, 2002.
- Petrovska BB. Historical Review of Medicinal Plants' Usage, Pharmacognosy review, 6(11), 1–5;2012.
- Qadry JS. Pharmacognosy, SB. Shah Prakashan, 12th, 2005.
- Rajeev Kumar Jha, Xu Zi-rong. Biomedical Compounds from Marine Organisms, Marine Drugs. 2004; 2(3).
- Rangari, VD. Pharmacognosy and Phytochemistry-Vol. II, Career Publication, 2nd, 2009.

- SBP board of consultants and engineers, Aromatic chemical perfumes and flavourtechnology, Small business publications, New Delhi.
- Sebastian Pole, Lic Ohm, A History of Ayurveda and the growth of the *Materia Medica*, Churchil Livingstone, Elesivier, 6.
- Shah, BN; Seth, AK. TB of Pharmacognosy and Phytochemistry, Elsevier Health Science, 1st, 2010.
- Tailang, D. Phytochemistry Theory and Practice, Birla Publication, 1st, 1–255, 2008.
- Terry Robson BA. An Introduction to Complementary Medicine, Allen and Unwine, 2003.
- The Ayurvedic Pharmacopoeia of India, Part 1, Volume 1, Government of India, Ministry of Health and Family Welfare, Department of AYUSH.
- The Ayurvedic Pharmacopoeia of India, Part 1, Volume II, Government of India, Ministry of Health and Family Welfare, Department of AYUSH.
- The Ayurvedic Pharmacopoeia of India, Part 1, Volume III, Government of India, Ministry of Health and Family Welfare, Department of AYUSH.
- Vinod D. Rangari, Pharmacognosy and Phytochemistry, Career Publications, I, II.
- Wallis, TE. TB of Pharmacognosy, CBS Publishers & Distributors, 5th, 2005.
- Weier, TE; CR Stocking; MG Barbour. Botany: an introduction to plant biology. John Wiley and Sons, New York, NY, 1974.
- www.dpi.nsw.gov.au/__data/assets/pdf_file/.../soil-pak-sis-Part-E.pdf.
- www.fantastic-flavour.com.

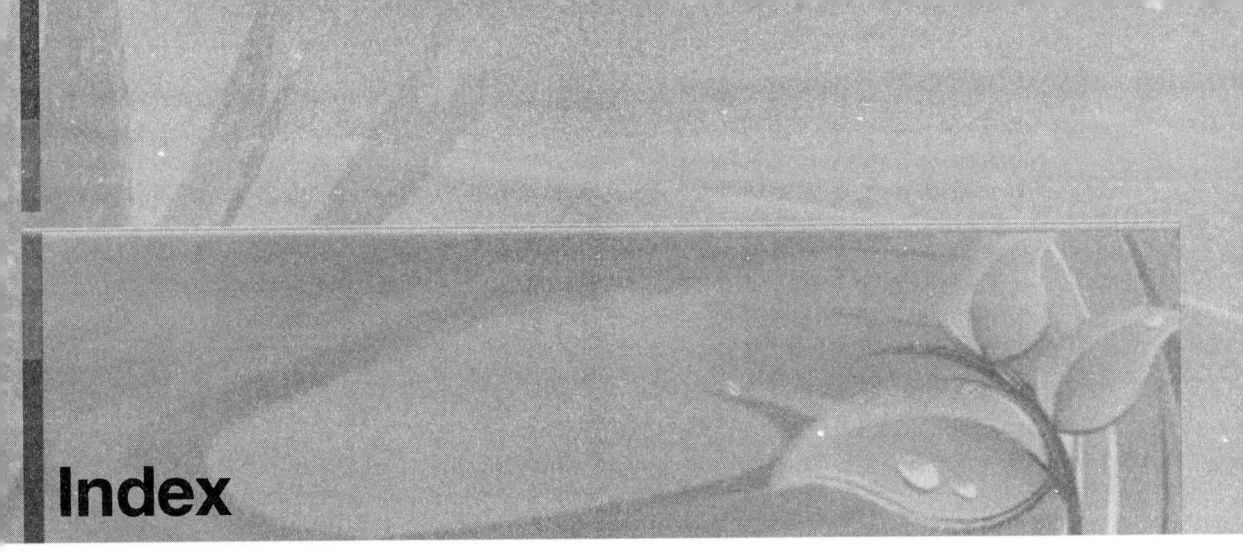

Index

A

Abscisic acid 62, 73
Acacia; *Acacia senegal* 98
Achyranthes aspera 339
Adhatoda vasica 333
Adhatodine 80
Adsorption chromatography 345
Aegle marmelos 330
Agar; *Gelidium amansii* 97
Algal toxins 210
Alkaloids 158
Allicin 88
Allium sativum 341
Aloe 114, 356
Aloin 84
Amino alkaloids 184
Amla 189
Amylopectin 93
Amylose 93
Anatomy of dicot leaves 255
Anatomy of monocot stem 253
Anethol 147
Anthraquinone glycosides 110
Apamarga 339
Aristha 284
Arjuna 128, 187, 356
Arjungenin 129
Arjunolic acid 128
Aromatherapy 225
Artemisinin 46, 48
Asafoetida 356

Asava 285
Ashoka bark 188, 328
Ashwagandha 329
Asparagus 356
Asparagus racemosus 120
Atropine 36, 41, 80
Auxin 62, 69
Avaleha 286
Ayurvedic pharmacy 279
Azadirachta indica 336

B

Bacopa monnieri 126, 333
Bacoside A and B 127
Bael fruit 330
Bael; *Aegle marmelos* 94
Bahera 190
Bees wax 203
Belladonna 178
Bentonite 215
Berberine 80
Bhasmas 288
Bitter almond 131
Black pepper 342
Brahmi 126, 333
Brucine 81

C

Caffeine 81
Calamine 215
Callus culture 295, 299

Camphor 86, 237
Capsaicin 86, 237
Caraway 147
Carbohydrates 91
Cardamom fruits and seeds 142
Cardiac glycosides 107
Carnauba wax 203
Cartenoids 361
Carveol 148
Cascara 117
Cascarosides A 118
Cassia acutifolia 111
Cassia angustifolia 111
Castor oil 195
Catechu 192
Catharanthus roseus 172
Choline 122
Chromatography 344
Chrysophanol 116
Churnas 287
Cinchona 150, 183
Cinnamomum
   camphora 237
   zeylanicum 150
Citraka 331
Citral 44, 46
Clove 152, 237
Cocaine 81
Cocoa butter 200
Cod liver oil 198
Codeine 33, 82
Copernicia cerifera 203
Coriander 149, 332
Coriandrum sativum 149, 332
Cosmeceuticals 260
Crucifereae 309
Cultivation 61
Cyanogenetic glycosides 130
Cytokinnins 62, 73

D

Datura 179
Datura metel 340
Deoxyribonuclease 220

Dhatura 340
Digitalis 108
Digitalis glycosides 108
Digitalis purpurea 108
Digitoxin 49, 52, 83
Dill 143
Dioscorea 119
Disogenin 51, 55

E

Elettaria cardamomum 142
Ellagic acid 87
Enzymes 218
Ephedra 185
Ephedrine 35, 38
Ergometrine 36
Ergot 163
Ergotamine 165
Ergotoxin 165
Ethylene 62, 73
Eucalyptol 238
Eugenia caryophyllata 147, 237
Eugenol 87
Exogenous factors 62

F

Fennel 145
Flavaniod glycosides 133
Flavoring agents 233
Foeniculum vulgare 145
Folic acid 361
Fruits 318

G

Garlic 341, 356
Geranium 229
Geranium maculatum 229
Ghatugum; *Anogeissus latifolia* 96
Gibberellins 62, 73
Ginger 154, 357
Gingerol 86, 155
Ginseng 120
Ginsenosides 121

Glucosamin 364
Glycolysis 31, 33
Glycosides 104
Glycyrrhiza 124
Glycyrrhiza glabra 124
Glycyrrhizin 85
Glycyrrhizin 126
Gokhru 122
Gramineae 308
Gymnemic acid 85

H

Hair 263
Hairy root culture 292, 303
Herbal drug interaction 354
Hesperidin 134
History of PTC 290
Honey (*Apis mellifera, Apis dorsata*) 95
HPLC 350
HPTLC 351
Hydrolyzable tannin 186
Hyocyamine 82
Hyoscyamus 181

I

Indole alkaloids 158
Ion exchange chromatography 346
Ipecacuanha 175
Isapgol; *Plantago ovata* 101
Isoquinoline alkaloids 173
Isothiocyanate glycosides 135

J

Jasmine 230
Jasminum officinale 230

K

Kaolin 215
Kieselguhr 216

L

Labiatae 309
Lard 202

Leguminosae 311
Lepas 287
Liliaceae 313
Linseed oil 196
Linum usitatissimum 196
Lipids, fats and waxes 193
Liquorice 357
Lutein 361
Lyopene 361

M

Marine drug 206
Marine toxins 210
Marker 79
Menthol 43, 45, 87, 238
Methi 122, 335
Morphine 32, 33, 82
Myrobalan 191
Mystristica fragrans 141

N

Neem 336
   oil 199
Non-hydrolyzable or condensed tannin 186
Nutmeg 141
Nux vomica 167

O

Ocimum sanctum 337
Olea europaea 197
Olive oil 197
Opium 173, 174
Oryza sativa 102

P

Palmitic acid 198
Panax ginseng 120
Panax quinquefolius 120
Pancreatin 221
Papaverine 82
Paper chromatography 349
Pedalium murex 123
Pepper 357

Peppermint 232
Pepsin 221
Peucedanum graveolens 143
Pharmacognosy
Physostigma 169
Phytonutrients 358
Phytopharmaceuticals 79
Phytosterols 363
Phytostigma venenosum 169
Piper nigrum 342
Piperine 83, 239
Plant anatomy 243
Plant bitters 240, 241
Plant tissue culture 289
Podophyllin 86
Poisonous plant 269
Polygala senega 129
Primary metabolites 26
Protein 222
Protoplast culture 293, 304
Prunasin 132
Prunus amygdalis var amara 131
Prunus serotina 132
Pseudohallucinogens 274
Pseudotannins 186

Q

Quality control and standardization 314
Quinine 42, 43, 83
Quinoline alkaloids 182

R

Radioactive tracer techniques 53
Rauwolfia 170
Rauwolfia serpentine 170
Renin 221
Reserpine 38, 39, 171
Rhamnus purshiana 112
Rhein 84
Rheum emodi 115, 116
Rhizomes and roots 319
Rhubarb 115, 357
Ricinolein 196

Ricinus communis 195
Rosa damascena 230
Rose 230
Rubiaceae 300, 312
Rutin 47, 50, 85, 133

S

Sandal wood 231
Saponin glycosides 118
Saraca indica 328
Sarsasapogenin 51, 54
Scillitoxin 110
Secondary metabolites 26, 27
Seeds 318
Senega 129, 130
Senna 111, 357
Sennosides 49, 53, 84
Serpentine 171
Shagaols 155
Shatavari 120
Shatavarin 120
Shikmic acid pathway 30
Shilajit 213
Size exclusion chromatography 347
Skin 261
Solanaceae 306
Solanum tuberosum 102
Squill 109
Starch 92, 93, 102
Stems 319
Stevioside 88
Stomata 315
Streptokinase 222
Strychnine 41, 42, 81
Strychnos nuxvomica 167
Study of different families 306
Sus scrofa 202
Suspension culture 295, 300
Sweetning agent 239

T

Tailas 286
Talc 214

Tannic acid 88
Tannins 185
Taxol 44, 47, 89
Tea 356
Terminilia arjuna 128
Terpeniods 135
Theobroma cacao 200
Thin layer chromatography 350
Tragacanth; *Astragulus gummifer* 100
Tribulus terrestris 123
Trichomes 317
Trigonella foenum graecum 122
Trigonelline 122
Triticum astivum 102
Tropane alkaliods 177
Tulsi 337
Turmeric 157

U

Umbelliferae 310
Urginea
    indica 109
    maritima 109
Urosolic acid 89

V

Vanillin 239
Vasaka 333
Vasicine 80
Vinca 172
Vincristine 172
Vitamin E 360
Vitamin K_1 360
Vitamins 360
Volatile oils 137

W

Withaferine 87
Withania somnifera 329
Wlid cherry bark 132
Woods 318
Wool fat 201

Z

Zea mays 102
Zingiber officinalis 150
Zingiberene 155, 239